This authoritative new publication is the first to review comprehensively the important relationship between maternal alcohol abuse during pregnancy and the resulting damage to the child *in utero*, and the results of this damage during the development of affected children. It includes important contributions by leading and internationally acclaimed clinicians and researchers. The first part of the book discusses clinical issues of alcohol teratogenicity, the clinical picture of fetal alcohol syndrome, and the epidemiology of maternal alcohol abuse and the developmental outcome of the children. The second part addresses pathogenesis and neuropathology, whilst the third reviews developmental issues in the growing child. The final part evaluates approaches to rehabilitation and intervention, and reviews social and public health issues. This comprehensive account will be invaluable for gynecologists, obstetricians, midwives, neonatologists and pediatricians, and for child and adolescent psychiatrists and psychologists.

ALCOHOL, PREGNANCY AND THE DEVELOPING CHILD

ALCOHOL, PREGNANCY AND THE DEVELOPING CHILD

Edited by

HANS-LUDWIG SPOHR

Professor of Paediatrics, Women's and Children's Hospital of the German Red Cross, Berlin, Germany

and

HANS-CHRISTOPH STEINHAUSEN

Professor, Department of Child and Adolescent Psychiatry, University of Zurich, Switzerland

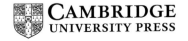

CAMBRIDGE
UNIVERSITY PRESS

Published by the Press Syndicate of the University of Cambridge
The Pitt Building, Trumpington Street, Cambridge CB2 1RP
40 West 20th Street, New York, NY 10011-4211, USA
10 Stamford Road, Oakleigh, Melbourne 3166, Australia

First published 1996

Printed in Great Britain at the University Press, Cambridge

A catalogue record for this book is available from the British Library

Library of Congress cataloguing in publication data

Alcohol, pregnancy, and the developing child/edited by Hans-Ludwig
Spohr and Hans-Christoph Steinhausen.
p.   cm.
Includes bibliographical references and index.
ISBN 0 521 56426 3 (hc)
1. Fetal alcohol syndrome – Etiology.   2. Alcohol – Pathogenesis.
3. Alcoholism in pregnancy – Complications.   I. Spohr, Hans-Ludwig.
II. Steinhausen, Hans-Christoph.
[DNLM: 1. Fetal Alcohol Syndrome.   2. Alcoholism – in pregnancy.
3. Prenatal Exposure Delayed Effects.   WQ 211 A355 1996]
RG628.3.F45A43   1996
618.3'2 – dc20
DNLM/DLC
for Library of Congress   96–4950   CIP

ISBN 0 521 56426 3 hardback

Contents

Contributors

Ernest L. Abel, PhD

C. S. Mott Center for Human Growth and Development, Department of Obstetrics-Gynecology, Wayne State University, 275 Hancock Avenue, Detroit, MI 48201, USA

Ilona Autti-Rämö, MD

Children's Castle Hospital, SF-00250 Helsinki 25, Finland

Linda C. Band, PhD

Alcohol and Brain Research Laboratory, Texas A&M University Health Science Center, College Station, TX 77843-1114, USA

Helen M. Barr, MA, MS

Fetal Alcohol and Drug Unit, Department of Psychiatry and Behavioral Sciences GG-20, University of Washington, 180 Nickerson, Suite 309, Seattle, WA 98109, USA

Fred L. Bookstein, PhD

Centre for Human Growth & Development, University of Michigan, Ann Arbor, MI 48109, USA

Marja-Liisa Granström, MD

Department of Child Neurology, University of Helsinki, Children's Castle Hospital, SF-00250 Helsinki 25, Finland

John H. Hannigan, PhD

C. S. Mott Center for Human Growth and Development, Department of Obstetrics-Gynecology, Wayne State University, 275 Hancock Avenue, Detroit, MI 48201, USA

Monique Kaminski, MD
INSERM U.149, 16, ave Paul Vaillant Couturier, F-94807 Villejuif Cedex, France

Béatrice Larroque, MD
INSERM U.149, 16, ave Paul Vaillant Couturier, F-94807 Villejuif Cedex, France

Frank Majewski, MD
Institute of Human Genetics, Moorenstrasse 5, D-40225 Düsseldorf, Germany

Barbara A. Morse, PhD
Division of Psychiatry and Fetal Alcohol Education Program, Boston University School of Medicine, 7 Kent Street, Brookline, MA 02146, USA

Anne-Marie Nybo Andersen, MD
Danish Epidemiology Science Centre, Statens Seruminstitut, 5, Artillerivej, DK-2300 Copenhagen S, Denmark

Mary J. O'Connor, PhD
Neuropsychiatric Institute, University of California at Los Angeles, 760 Westwood Plaza, Los Angeles, CA 90024, USA

Jørn Olsen, PhD
Danish Epidemiology Science Centre, Statens Seruminstitut, 5, Artillerivej, DK-2300 Copenhagen S, Denmark

Robert J. Sokol, MD
Wayne State University, School of Medicine, 275 Hancock Avenue, Detroit, MI 48201, USA

Hans-Ludwig Spohr, MD
Women's and Children's Hospital, DRK-Kliniken Westend, Pulsstrasse 4, D-14059 Berlin, Germany

Hans-Christoph Steinhausen, MD, PhD
Department of Child and Adolescent Psychiatry, University of Zürich, Freiestrasse 15, Postfach, CH-8028 Zürich, Switzerland

Gisela Stoltenburg-Didinger, MD
Institute of Neuropathology, Free University Berlin, Klinikum Steglitz, Hindenburgdamm 30, D-12203 Berlin, Germany

Ann P. Streissguth, PhD
Fetal Alcohol and Drug Unit, Department of Psychiatry and Behavioral Sciences GG-20, University of Washington, 180 Nickerson, Suite 309, Seattle, WA 98109, USA

Lyn Weiner, MPH
Division of Psychiatry and Fetal Alcohol Education Program, Boston University School of Medicine, 7 Kent Street, Brookline, MA 02146, USA

James R. West MD
Alcohol and Brain Research Laboratory, Texas A&M University Health Science Center, College Station, TX 77843-1114, USA

Janice E. Whitty, MD
Wayne State University, School of Medicine, Hutzel Hospital, 4707 St Antoine, Detroit, MI 48201, USA

Foreword

In many countries, alcohol and drug abuse during pregnancy is one of the main threats to child health. Despite this fact, maternal substance abuse has not yet attracted the attention from health and social workers which corresponds to its serious consequences. The reports published in this monograph may act as an alarm and thus increase awareness of the risk of alcohol drinking during pregnancy.

In several chapters in this monograph, various studies on growth and development after fetal exposure to alcohol are reported. The high incidence of mild to moderate mental retardation with marked cognitive defects and severe child psychiatric symptoms is evident. It may also be mentioned that in a study from Sweden, the results of Griffiths' test in 4-year-old boys who had been subjected to fetal alcohol exposure were found to be lower than normal on all scales, whereas the performance of corresponding girls did not differ significantly from that of girls in the control material. In the same study, it was also found that the number of psychopathological symptoms according to DSM III-R criteria were much higher in boys with fetal alcohol syndrome (FAS) than in control families, whereas the girls did not differ from the controls. These findings provide additional evidence that females are more resistant to fetal exposure to alcohol than males.

Symptoms seen in children with maternal alcoholism may be the result not only of FAS but also of the psychosocial stress to which children in such families are subjected, with a high risk of being victims of child abuse and neglect. Paternal alcohol abuse may have serious consequences for the family as well. Due to the chaotic situation which alcohol abuse creates in the home, the risk for pre- and perinatal complications is higher than normal. Preschool children in such families have, irrespective of social class, far more psychosomatic symptoms than expected, as found by Nylander in 1961.

In maternal alcohol addiction, the adverse effects of abuse of other substances that may have an influence on the outcome of pregnancy and on postnatal growth and development also have to be considered. The life situation of pregnant alcoholic women, who have a high prevalence of various diseases or nutritional deficiencies, may constitute additional risk factors for the fetus. Most alcoholic women are heavy cigarette smokers, which increases the risk for low birth weight and small-for-gestational-age (SGA) infants. Some of the criteria for FAS, such as prenatal growth retardation, may thus at least partly be due to tobacco smoking during pregnancy, a risk factor which is dose-dependent. Another factor which has to be taken into account is excessive coffee drinking among alcoholic women, because exposure to caffeine reduces birth weight (Peacock *et al.*, 1991).

Alcoholic mothers may also abuse other substances in addition to nicotine and caffeine, such as heroin, cocaine, amphetamine, marijuana and tranquillizers. For instance, in the offspring of amphetamine-addicted mothers, the risk for perinatal death, birth defects, low birth weight, SGA births and other neonatal complications is almost as high as when the mothers are alcoholics (Eriksson & Zetterström, 1994). Thus, in the offspring of pregnant alcoholics with mixed abuse, it may be impossible to establish the effect of each of the substances to which the fetus has been exposed. It may also be possible that an additional abuse potentiates the adverse effect of alcohol. Thus, in children of amphetamine-addicted mothers, the most obvious predictors of poor adjustment at 4 years of age were found to be additional alcohol abuse and a high dose of the drug (Billing *et al.*, 1988). Mixed abuse, including that of nicotine, should always be taken into account in studies of FAS.

In this monograph, several chapters give data on the dose of alcohol which is critical to the fetus, while in others the pathogenetic mechanism behind FAS is elucidated. Undoubtedly such studies are of extreme value for understanding the background to FAS, and also for the prevention of this condition. In the 1970s and early 1980s most reported cases of FAS presented with typical features. On the other hand Olegård *et al.* (1979), when reporting a number of such typical cases, also concluded that FAS may perhaps be the most common cause of mild to moderate mental retardation in the three largest Swedish cities. In later studies, the features of FAS have been less typical in some of the identified cases. Thus, in a longitudinal prospective study performed at a maternity centre in a suburb of Stockholm, 21 (3%) of the pregnant women in the cohort were found to be addicted to alcohol (Aronson *et al.*, 1985). In the offspring, the perinatal mortality rate was significantly increased as were the rates of low birth weight and SGA infants, but none of the children had microcephaly, craniofacial dysmorphism or congenital malformations of the types that are seen in FAS (Nordberg *et al.*, 1994). One can only speculate upon the reason why the special features of FAS were lacking in this material. In this context, it may be mentioned that Pullarkat & Azar (1992) (8) have suggested that alcohol induces birth defects by inhibiting the conversion of retinol into retinal and thus the synthesis of retinoic acid, which is crucial to the development of the fetus. In subclinical vitamin A deficiency, which may occur in alcoholic women with poor nutrition and low intake of green vegetables, the risk of fetal retinoic acid deficiency is obvious.

From the different chapters in this monograph it is obvious that the knowledge of FAS has increased very rapidly during the last decade. However, many problems remain to be solved. For efficient prevention of FAS, it is necessary to improve the methods of identifying maternal alcohol addiction. Until now, pregnant women have not been particularly reluctant to give accurate information about cigarette smoking. Drugs that are injected may be fairly easy to identify due to the presence of needle pricks. On the other hand, the means by which alcohol addiction can be identified are rather unreliable. In interviews at maternity health stations, only about 30% of women with such abuse give accurate information (Nylander & Zetterström, 1983). Nor can clinical biochemical tests be used, because pregnancy interferes with the results.

In all families with alcohol abuse the situation is very complex, and the presence of different confounders has to be discussed. Nor is the background to the confusing variability of symptoms and signs seen in children with FAS well understood. It may be partly explained by factors other than simply the amount of alcohol that has been consumed during the course of pregnancy. For efficient prevention of FAS and other consequences of familial alcohol addiction, much more has to be known about the psychology behind addiction, and about the means of helping parents to abstain from an abuse which causes extremely serious consequences for their children.

Newborn infants who have been exposed to alcohol during fetal life may be much more vulnerable to adverse environmental factors than other babies, which means that they should be taken care of under the best possible psychosocial conditions. On the other hand, if these infants remain in the custody of their alcohol-addicted mother, they run a great risk of being subjected to severe psychosocial stress. To prevent such a situation, the children have to be surrounded by an efficient social network. Special attention has to be given to the presence of signs of bonding failure, feeding problems, failure to thrive, and other symptoms of abuse and neglect. In all families with maternal alcohol addiction, the possibility that the father also is an alcoholic should always be kept in mind, because such a situation may constitute an additional threat to the children.

Karolinska Hospital
Stockholm, Sweden
November 1995

Rolf Zetterström, MD

References

Aronson, M., Kyllerman, M., Sabel, K. G., Sandin, B. & Olegård, R. (1985) Children of alcoholic mothers: development, perceptual and behavioural characteristics as compared to matched controls. *Acta Paediatrica Scandinavica*, **74**, 27–35.

Billing, L., Eriksson, M., Steneroth, G. & Zetterström, R. (1988). Predictive indicators for adjustment in 4-year-old children whose mothers used amphetamine during pregnancy. *Child Abuse and Neglect*, **12**, 503–7.

Eriksson, M. & Zetterström, R. (1994). Amphetamine addiction during pregnancy: 10-year follow-up. *Acta Paediatrica, Supplement*, **404**, 27–31.

Nordberg, L., Rydelius, P.-A. & Zetterström, R. (1994). Parental alcoholism and early child development. *Acta Paediatrica Supplement*, **404**, 14–18.

Nylander, I. (1960). Children of alcoholic fathers. *Acta Paediatrica*, **49** (Supplement 121), 1–134.

Nylander, I. & Zetterström, R. (1983). Home environment of children in a new Stockholm suburb: a prospective longitudinal study. *Acta Paediatrica Scandinavica Supplement*, **310**, 1–40.

Olegård, R., Sabel, K. G., Aronson, M., Sandin, B., Johansson, P. R., Carlsson, C., *et al.* (1979). Effect on the child of alcohol abuse during pregnancy. *Acta Psychiatrica Scandinavica Supplement*, **275**, 112–21.

Peacock, J. L., Bland, J. M. & Anderson, H. R. (1991). Effects on birth weight of alcohol and caffeine consumption in smoking women. *Journal of Epidemiology and Communiy Health*, **45**, 159–163.

Pullarkat, R. K. & Azar, B. (1992). Retinoic acid, embryonic development and alcohol-induced birth defects. *Embryonic Development*, **16**, 317–23.

Preface

In the western industrialized countries chronic alcoholism is currently one of the leading diseases afflicting the population and is, in addition to this, a serious socioeconomic burden. Chronic alcohol abuse is on the rise and affects increasingly younger sectors of the population. An estimated 20% of alcohol-dependent women are of child-bearing age. Alcohol consumption during pregnancy has serious effects on the developing child.

The objective of the present book is to reveal the relation between chronic maternal alcohol abuse during pregnancy and the damage to the child *in utero*. Furthermore, the long-term consequences for the affected children are outlined, and measures of rehabilitation and successful prevention of fetal alcohol syndrome (FAS) as an important social and public health issue are discussed. The monograph, which is collaboratively written by researchers of international acclaim, aims to present the latest knowledge about long-term prenatal effects of maternal alcohol abuse to a broad readership.

The first section, which is concerned with clinical issues, introduces the general problem of alcohol teratogenicity in humans, presents a detailed description of the clinical symptoms of FAS and discusses the epidemiology of maternal alcohol abuse and its consequences for the child.

Pathogenesis and neuropathology are the topics of the second section. The etiology of alcohol damage to the fetus is still unknown. The major theories and clinical findings are discussed in the first chapter. Animal research has not only provided a model of FAS to support clinical findings of physical and neurobehavioral deficits in children suffering from this syndrome, but has also helped researchers to decipher the *in utero* mechanisms of alcohol damage. The current knowledge in this exciting research area is reviewed in another chapter.

Further contributions on the neuropathology of experimental fetal alcohol syndrome and neuropathological findings in human FAS not only summarize scientific findings in this important research area but also reflect the fundamental importance of teratogenic alcohol effects on the developing brain.

The large third section of the book is devoted to clinical issues. The chapters in this section are mainly based on large-scale clinical studies. Some of these studies cover long periods of development in childhood and adolescence, so that there is sufficient evidence on the late effects of intrauterine exposure to alcohol. The dimensions of development cover both physical and psychological domains, so that a full picture of all potential effects is provided by these contributions.

The topic of the fourth and last section is intervention. Rehabilitation and prevention measures are described that aim to alleviate the detrimental effects of disabling features due to intrauterine exposure to alcohol. Furthermore, the main aspects of social and public health policies are discussed.

The editors of the present monograph are extremely grateful to all the authors who provided chapters for this book on an important issue of health in developing children. Furthermore, they would like to thank both Mr Peter Silver of Cambridge University Press for his excellent collaboration and stimulation to produce this book as well as Ms Carol Rauss at the University of Zurich for her editorial assistance.

November 1995

Hans-Ludwig Spohr
Hans-Christoph Steinhausen

Part I

Clinical issues

1

Alcohol teratogenicity in humans: critical period, thresholds, specificity and vulnerability

JANICE E. WHITTY AND ROBERT J. SOKOL

Introduction

In 1980, the Fetal Alcohol Study Group of the Research Society on Alcoholism proposed formal criteria for the diagnosis of fetal alcohol syndrome (FAS) (Rosett, 1980). These criteria are listed in Table 1.1.

Although FAS occurs only in children born to alcoholic women, relatively few alcoholic women (about 4%) give birth to children with FAS (Abel, 1995). The reasons for this differential susceptibility are unclear. Some of the contributory factors may include variations in time of exposure during critical periods of development when the fetus is most susceptible to the teratogenic effects of alcohol; differences in the amount and pattern of alcohol ingestion; and specific maternal, fetal or genetic vulnerability factors which make a particular fetus more or less susceptible to the effects of alcohol exposure *in utero*. This chapter surveys these factors and considers their implications not only for the occurrence of FAS, but also for its prevention.

Critical periods

The embryo/fetus is susceptible to alcohol's toxicity throughout its development, but structural anomalies arise primarily when exposure occurs during 'critical periods' of development. These periods are well known. The first trimester, especially the period between the second and eighth week of gestation, is a time when bodily organs and appendages are forming (Wilson, 1973). This period of 'organogenesis' is highly susceptible to perturbation by teratogens. Exposures prior to or after this period may have other effects on the conceptus, but these may not be readily observable malformations.

Since development of different organs occurs at different times during this period of organogenesis, unless exposure to alcohol always occurs at the

3

Table 1.1. *Minimum criteria for diagnosing fetal alcohol syndrome, as recommended by the Fetal Alcohol Study Group of the Research Society on Alcoholism*

Area	Manifestations
Growth	Prenatal or postnatal growth retardation or both: weight, length or head circumference, or any combination of these, less than the 10th percentile for gestational age
Central nervous system function	Signs of neurological abnormality, developmental delay or intellectual impairment
Craniofacial appearance	Characteristic abnormalities (at least two of these): *microcephaly*, head circumference less than the 3rd percentile; *microphthalmia* or short palperbral fissures or both; poorly developed philtrum, thin upper lip and flattening of maxillary area

From Sokol (1981).

same moment during development there will be considerable variation in both the kinds and severity of malformations that arise in conjunction with prenatal alcohol exposure. In addition, very high exposures to a teratogen can cause malformations prior to or following the time of greatest susceptibility (Wilson, 1973).

Intrauterine growth retardation from alcohol occurs primarily when exposure occurs during the third trimester, whereas functional damage can occur at any time during development once organs have formed. In other words, maternal alcoholism can result in damage to the developing fetus which does not necessarily manifest itself in the form of structural defects or FAS, because drinking has not occurred regularly throughout pregnancy. Whereas FAS will not occur unless drinking has occurred during all three trimesters of pregnancy, individual anomalies may occur as a result of drinking (usually at relatively high levels: see below) during more discrete periods. Thus, one reason why FAS occurs at such a relatively low incidence among alcoholic women (Abel, 1995) is that many of these women somehow manage to restrict their drinking to a particular period of pregnancy.

However, the fact that FAS does not occur in every pregnancy characterized by alcoholism is important only from a research perspective. Identifying the time in gestation when the fetus is most susceptible to anatomical derangements secondary to alcohol exposure may be useful from an epidemiological standpoint, but for purposes of preventive perinatal medicine it is negligible. No physician would advise a patient to avoid alcohol intake only during organogenesis. If advice is given to abstain, it is given for the duration of pregnancy. If there is a potential danger associated with drinking during pregnancy, reducing consumption at any time during pregnancy would be potentially beneficial. Since there is no 'safe' time to drink, there is no advantage from a prevention standpoint in advising a patient that drinking later in pregnancy, for example, is less dangerous than drinking during early pregnancy.

Amount and pattern of drinking

Cautioning women that there is no 'safe' time to drink, however, is not the same as saying there is no 'safe' amount to drink. Thresholds exist for all teratogens, below which they do not produce adverse effects (Wilson, 1973). In the absence of reliable information as to what these thresholds are, most physicians may counsel their patients to be on the 'safe side' and not drink at all. However, other physicians interpreting the same data have concluded there is a 'safe' level for drinking and that aggressively counselling total abstention may cause undue anxiety to those women who may have engaged in 'social' drinking prior to learning of their pregnancy – anxiety which may itself result in abnormal fetal development (e.g., Rosett & Weiner, 1982; Lipson & Webster, 1989).

One of the reasons for this controversy is that FAS has only been reliably linked to 'heavy' drinking during gestation. Nevertheless, numerous warnings about the adverse effects of drinking on the fetus have been made in professional journals and in the media concerning 'moderate' or 'social' drinking in relation to FAS.

In part, this confusion stems from terms such as 'heavy', 'moderate' and 'social' drinking, which may have different meanings for those who issue these warnings and those who receive them (Abel & Kruger, 1996). Instead of relying on such vague terms, identifying the number of 'drinks' that places a fetus at risk for FAS or alcohol-related birth defects (ARBD), i.e., 'thresholds', would be of considerable benefit if only from the standpoint of communication. Pregnant women, and those who counsel them, would be able to respond to guidelines that contain relatively specific information concerning amounts of alcohol that may be 'safe' or 'dangerous' rather than more vaguely worded advice. Equally important, counsellors may be able to reduce the incidence of these disorders by providing women with sound, experimentally based information with respect to drinking behavior that poses a risk for the fetus. From a credibility standpoint, women may also be more amenable to accepting advice concerning their drinking behavior when they are made to feel they are being treated as rational people who are able to modify their behavior, i.e., cut down their drinking, rather than as incompetents who must abstain totally because they are incapable of making judgments and regulating their drinking behavior (Abel & Hannigan, 1995*a*).

Determining the point at which drinking begins to be dangerous for the developing fetus is in itself problematic, however, because drinking behavior varies greatly. Conclusions about levels harmful to a fetus cannot be based on experimental paradigms in which women are given graded amounts of alcohol, as is possible when comparable studies are conducted in animals (Abel, 1984). Instead, researchers must rely on what their subjects tell them they have consumed, and these self-reports must then be related to outcomes. Since the self-reported information is subject to distortion due to denial, underreporting or inadvertent inaccuracy, relationships are often tenuous and dependent on how the self-report data are examined, so that conclusions are always tentative.

To complicate matters further, the extent of underreporting of substance abuse in general may vary considerably according to the gestational period for which information is gathered, and in some cases consumption may be at least 3 times higher than what is reported to researchers (e.g., Day *et al.*, 1993; Dicker & Leighton, 1994).

Underreporting may also vary according to socioeconomic class, race, cultural acceptance or criticism of certain drinking practices, and general lifestyle factors, all of which may affect what individuals self-report about their drinking behavior. For example, both abstention rates and rates of heavier drinking tend to be higher among pregnant African-Americans and Native Americans compared with Caucasians (Day *et al.*, 1993; Faden *et al.*, 1994). As a result, people in cultures where drinking is not commonplace, and excessive drinking is socially censured, may be motivated to underreport to a much greater extent than those in cultures where drinking is accepted and overindulgence subject to less social condemnation.

Underreporting means that thresholds based on estimated dose–response relationships should be considered 'guidelines' rather than hard and fast cutoff points between 'safe' and 'dangerous' levels of consumption. A reasonable conclusion, however, is that the threshold will usually be higher, rather than lower, than that extrapolated from the data.

Yet another consideration has to do with the way data are analyzed. For example, Ernhart *et al.* (1985) evaluated the threshold question with respect to physical anomalies using three different indicators of alcohol consumption. When the data were examined in terms of average absolute intake per day, the authors estimated the threshold for anomalies at about 1 drink per day. When the analysis was restricted to drinking very early in pregnancy, which they termed the 'estimated embryonic AA/day', the threshold was an average of 4 drinks per day in the embryonic period. A third index, based on reinterviewing subjects 5 years later, resulted in a threshold estimate of about an average of 1 drink per day. On the basis of these data the authors estimated the threshold for FAS-related physical anomalies at an average of 3 drinks per day.

To complicate the issue even further, it is also evident that the threshold for some anomalies may be higher or lower than for others. Exposure producing functional anomalies in behavior may also be much lower than levels producing structural changes. Jacobson *et al.* (1993), for example, found that children whose mothers drank at least an average of 1 drink per day during pregnancy were 4 times more likely to score in the bottom 10 percentiles on the Bayley scales of infant development. However, the authors report that most of the women in this study averaged over 6 drinks per drinking day, and some averaged as many as 14 drinks per drinking day. Unlike Ernhart *et al.* (1985), Jacobson *et al.* (1993) did not find that retrospective maternal recall of drinking in pregnancy provides a lower threshold than measures taken earlier.

Thresholds may also be affected by concurrent use of other drugs which act synergistically with alcohol to affect fetal development. Women who abuse alcohol, frequently abuse tobacco and drugs, have poor health and may be malnourished. Any of these factors could result in birth defects on their own. Clarifying the issue of whether alcohol abuse specifically causes a particular constellation of defects is difficult to achieve in human research; determining a threshold for these effects is even more difficult.

These considerations are also relevant for estimating the number of women at risk for having FAS children, and from a public policy standpoint. Recent studies indicate that only 0.2–0.3% of pregnant women consume 60 or more drinks per month, or about 2 or more drinks per day (Faden *et al.*, 1994). Although these percentages are small in relative terms, the number of births that occur each year in the United States is about 3.5 million. If 2 drinks per day were the threshold for damaging effects to the fetus, this would place about 7000 newborns at risk for ARBDs. The higher the threshold, the fewer the children at potential risk.

On the basis of Abel's recent analysis of the epidemiological literature specifically dealing with FAS (see Abel & Hannigan, this volume), the number of children born with FAS each year in the United States is between 2000 and 24000. This implies that the threshold for FAS is undoubtedly greater than 2 drinks per day, since there are fewer, not more, women involved as drinking amounts increase.

Another potential variable that must be considered in addition to the amount of alcohol ingested, is the pattern of ingestion. In most cases, thresholds are based on dose–response studies that collect data in terms of average amount of alcohol consumed per day. However, several studies in humans and animals have found that binge drinking is more deleterious than continuous drinking, even though the same amount of alcohol may be consumed over a given period (e.g., Streissguth *et al.*, 1989; West *et al.*, 1990). These studies indicate that it is the maximum peak blood alcohol concentration that is obtained, rather than total daily or weekly ingestion, that determines whether exposure is deleterious. One of the reasons some women are less likely than others to give birth to children with FAS is therefore possibly related to regular consumption of alcohol compared with sporadic binges.

Although each child is special and deserves the opportunity of a healthy birth, there are a great many other potential causes of birth defects, and only limited resources with which to deal with them. The higher or lower the threshold at which a factor results in birth defects, the lesser or greater the impact on the health of the nation and, therefore, the lesser or greater the concern from a public policy standpoint.

On an individual basis, regardless of how many women are at risk, it is still important to identify those individual and social factors that enable some women and prevent others from reducing their drinking during pregnancy, as well as those individual factors that make mothers and fetuses more or less susceptible to alcohol's teratogenic effects.

Individual and social factors related to continued drinking during pregnancy

There are several well-known characteristics associated with drinking among women. Caucasian women are more likely to drink prior to and during early pregnancy than African-American women (Streissguth *et al.*, 1991), but heavy drinking during pregnancy tends to be more common among African-Americans and Native Americans (Day *et al.*, 1993; Faden *et al.*, 1994). Marital status is also related to drinking behavior, with unmarried women more likely to drink than married women (Serdula *et al.*, 1991). Specifically with respect to pregnancy, drinking in early pregnancy tends to occur more commonly among less educated women (Streissguth *et al.*, 1991). Older pregnant women are more likely to drink than younger pregnant women (Faden *et al.*, 1994; National Institute on Drug Abuse, 1994), and women who are heavy smokers are often heavy drinkers as well (Serdula *et al.*, 1991; Faden *et al.*, 1994). Heavy drinkers are more likely to associate with men who are also heavy drinkers (Abel, 1983) or to use illicit drugs (Day *et al.*, 1993), and are less likely to seek and obtain prenatal care (e.g., Day *et al.*, 1993; Faden *et al.*, 1994). All these factors can interact with alcohol to affect fetal development (Abel & Hannigan, 1995*b*).

In addition, there are numerous other predictive factors related to drinking behavior which become stronger with higher levels of alcohol consumption, such as nontraditional employment, unemployment, divorce/separation, depression, anxiety, low self-esteem, eating disorders and abusive spousal relationships (Gomberg & Nirenberg, 1993; Galanter, 1996; Wilsnack, 1995*a, b*). These interpersonal and sociocultural factors are relevant for identifying women potentially at risk for abusive drinking, and are probably related to maternal risk factors in addition to drinking that contribute to ARBDs, but this latter relationship has yet to be explored.

Genetic susceptibilities

Reports of human twins with different severities of ARBDs (Christoffel & Salafsky, 1975) implies a genetic difference in fetal susceptibility to alcohol. Whereas women may differ genetically in terms of the kinds of enzymes they may have for metabolizing alcohol, this would not explain the differential susceptibility of twins to maternal alcohol consumption, although differences in maternal metabolic activity may explain why some offspring of women who drink heavily during pregnancy are severely affected while others are not.

With respect to the latter possibility, we compared 25 cases of FAS with 50 non-FAS control infants in a 'synthetic' case–control study to examine possible factors related to FAS (Sokol *et al.*, 1986). We found that in addition to drinking more, the mothers of the FAS cases were characterized by increased age, increased frequency of black race, higher gravidity and higher parity. In the presence of four factors – number of drinking days, MAST positivity (see below), parity and race – the chance of having an FAS-affected offspring rose to 85.2%.

Studies in animals, using inbred strains, have likewise indicated that genetic differences can affect vulnerability to the effects of alcohol exposure during pregnancy (Chernoff, 1980).

Table 1.2. *T-ACE questions*

T	How many drinks does it take to make you feel high (Tolerance)?
A	Have people Annoyed you by criticizing your drinking?
C	Have you felt you ought to Cut down on your drinking?
E	Have you ever had a drink first thing in the morning to steady your nerves or get rid of a hangover ('Eye opener')?

Clinical identification

A reliable screen for alcohol abuse would be useful for identifying those women whose fetuses are at risk for FAS and ARBDs. Currently available laboratory tests have not been shown to be of value for the detection of alcohol consumption unless administered within a few hours of drinking. Alternatively, structured interviews in the clinic have been developed for the detection of risk drinking.

The Michigan Alcoholism Screening Test (MAST) is a validated questionnaire which is arguably the 'gold standard' for screening for alcoholism (Selzer, 1971). The MAST contains 25 questions, with a score of greater than or equal to 5 considered positive for alcohol abuse. However, the complexity of the MAST makes it relatively time consuming to administer and, therefore, limits its clinical utility.

Simpler, briefer questionnaires have been developed that are easier to administer in a clinical situation. One is the widely used CAGE, a four-part questionnaire that takes only minutes to complete (Ewing, 1984). When the MAST and CAGE were compared, 50–60% of a group of about 1500 women enrolled in a prenatal clinic who were found to be MAST positive were also detected by the CAGE (Bottoms *et al.*, 1988). More recently, we have developed a variation of the CAGE, which we called T-ACE (Sokol *et al.*, 1989). The T-ACE items are shown in Table 1.2.

When we tested the T-ACE we found that when none of the answers was positive, an individual had a very low likelihood of being a risk drinker. Patients who answered positively on the tolerance question alone, had an eightfold increased risk to about 12%. A positive answer to all four items meant about a 63% probability of being a risk drinker.

We have compared the T-ACE with other instruments, including the MAST, and found we were able to identify 7 out of 10 risk drinkers during pregnancy (Sokol *et al.*, 1989).

Identification of risk drinkers holds promise for preventive efforts and improved pregnancy outcome. Reliable identification of alcohol abusers is also of value for study purposes since it would allow investigators to focus on women most at risk for FAS and ARBD very early on in their pregnancies.

Summary and conclusions

Defining alcohol teratogenicity in the human with the precision desirable for offering patients rational advice and for clinical risk assessment and management has been difficult. First the drinking of alcoholic beverages is a complex human behavior, difficult to ascertain accurately or to represent quantitatively. Second, the pattern of ARBDs in individuals is not invariant. Different collections of anomalies are a result of variations in times of exposure during gestation, number and patterning of drinks consumed, additional risk factors such as poverty, diet and smoking, and individual genotypic susceptibilities.

In the light of all these difficulties in defining a valid 'threshold', it is tempting to advise patients that the only safe course to follow with respect to drinking during pregnancy is that of total abstention. But this advice reflects as much the clinician's frustration as it does a concern for protecting every pregnancy from the potentially harmful effects of alcohol. Under these circumstances, it is very likely that the 'science' of medicine may have to recognize the 'art' that enables an experienced physician to counsel one patient differently from another, depending on that physician's awareness of the patient's risk factors for ARBDs and her past and current drinking behavior.

Acknowledgments

The authors would like to acknowledge Dr Ernest Abel of Wayne State University School of Medicine Department of Obstetrics and Gynecology for his valuable contributions to this chapter.

References

Abel, E.L. (1984). *Fetal Alcohol Syndrome/Fetal Alcohol Effects*. New York: Raven Press.

Abel, E.L. (1995). An update on incidence of FAS: FAS is not an equal opportunity birth defect. *Neurotoxicology and Teratology*, **17**, 437–43.

Abel, E.L. & Hannigan, J.H. (1995a). 'J-shaped' relationship between drinking during pregnancy and birth weight: reanalysis of prospective epidemiological data. *Alcohol and Alcoholism*, **30**, 345–55.

Abel, E.L. & Hannigan, J.H. (1995*b*). Maternal risk factors in fetal alcohol syndrome: provocative and permissive influences. *Neurotoxicology and Teratology*, **17**, 445–62.

Abel, E.L. & Kruger, M.L. (1996). Hon v. Stroh Brewery Co.: what do we mean by 'moderate' and 'heavy' drinking? *Alcoholism: Clinical and Experimental Research*, in press.

Bottoms, S.F., Sokol, R.J. & Martier, S. (1988). Use of the 'CAGE' to screen for risk-drinking in pregnancy. In *Proceedings of the Annual Meeting of Society of Perinatal Obstetricians*, p. 331.

Chernoff, G.F. (1980). The fetal alcohol syndrome in mice: maternal variables. *Teratology*, **22**, 71–5.

Christoffel, K.K. & Salafsky, I. (1975). Fetal alcohol syndrome in dizygotic twins. *Journal of Pediatrics*, **87**, 963–7.

Day, N.L., Cottreau, C.M. & Richardson, G.A. (1993). The epidemiology of alcohol, marijuana, and cocaine use among women of childbearing age and pregnant women. *Clinical and Obstetric Gynecology*, **36**, 232–45.

Dicker, M. & Leighton, E.A. (1994). Trends in the US prevalence of drug-using parturient women and drug-affected newborns, 1979 through 1990. *American Journal of Public Health*, **84**, 1433–8.

Ernhart, C.B., Wolf, A.W., Li, P.L., Sokol, R.J., Keard, M.J. & Filipovich, H.F. (1985). Alcohol-related birth defects: syndromal anomalies, intrauterine growth retardation and neonatal behavioral assessment. *Alcoholism: Clinical and Experimental Research*, **9**, 447–53.

Ewing, J.A. (1984). Detecting alcoholism: the CAGE questionnaire. *JAMA*, **252**, 1905–7.

Faden, V.B., Graubard, B.I. & Dufour, M. (1994). Drinking by expectant mothers: what does it mean for their babies? Working paper, Division of Biometry and Epidemiology, National Institute on Alcohol Abuse and Alcoholism.

Faden, V.B. & Hanna, E.Z. (1994). Alcohol and pregnancy: to drink or not to drink? Paper presented at the Conference on Psychosocial and Behavioral Factors in Women's Health, American Psychological Association, Washington, DC, May, 1994.

Galanter, M. (ed.) (1996). *Recent Developments in Alcoholism*, vol. XII, *Alcoholism and Women: The Effect of Gender*. New York: Plenum Press. (in press).

Gomberg, E.S.L. & Nirenberg, T.D. (eds.) (1993). *Women and Substance Abuse*. Norwood, NJ: Ablex Press.

Jacobson, J.L., Jacobson, S.W., Sokol, R.J., Martier, S.S., Ager, J.W. & Kaplan-Estrin, M.G. (1993). Teratogenic effects of alcohol on infant development. *Alcoholism: Clinical and Experimental Research*, **17**, 174–83.

Lipson, A.H. & Webster, W.S. (1989). A contemporary note regarding the ACP policy statement on alcohol consumption in relation to pregnancy. *Australian Pediatric Journal*, **25**, 302–4.

National Institute on Drug Abuse (1994). NIDA survey examines extent of women's drug use during pregnancy. NIDA media advisory. Rockville, MD, September 6, 1994.

Rosett, H.L. (1980). A clinical perspective of the fetal alcohol syndrome. (editorial). Alcoholism: *Clinical and Experimental Research*, **4**, 119–22.

Rosett, H.L. & Weiner, L. (1982). Prevention of fetal alcohol effects. *Pediatrics*, **69**, 813–16.

Selzer, M.L. (1971). The Michigan alcoholism screening instrument: the quest for a new diagnostic instrument. *American Journal of Psychiatry*, **127**, 89–94.

Serdula, M., Williamson, D.F., Kendrick, J.S., Anda, R.F. & Byers, T. (1991). Trends in alcohol consumption by pregnant women, 1985 through 1988. *JAMA*, **265**, 876–9.

Sokol, R.J. (1980). Alcohol and spontaneous abortion. *Lancet*, **ii**, 1709.

Sokol, R.J. (1981). Alcohol and abnormal outcomes of pregnancy. *Canadian Medical Association Journal*, **125**, 143–8.

Sokol, R.J., Ager, J., Martier, S., Debanne, S., Ernhart, C., Kuzma, J. & Miller, S.I. (1986). Significant determinants of susceptibility to alcohol teratogenicity. *Annals of the New York Academy of Sciences*, **477**, 87–102.

Sokol, R.J., Martier, S.S. & Ager, J.W. (1989). The T-ACE questions: practical prenatal detection of risk drinking. *American Journal of Obstetrics and Gynecology*, **160**, 863–70.

Streissguth, A.P., Brookstein, F.L., Sampson, P.D. & Barr, H.M. (1989). Neurobehavioral effects of prenatal alcohol. III. PLS analyses of neuropsychologic tests. *Neurotoxicology and Teratology*, **11**, 493–507.

Streissguth, A.P., Grant, T.M., Barr, H.M., *et al.* (1991). Cocaine and the use of alcohol and other drugs during pregnancy. *American Journal of Obstetrics and Gynecology*, **164**, 1239.

West, J.R., Goodlett, C.R., Bonthius, D.J., *et al.* (1990). Cell population depletions associated with fetal alcohol brain damage: mechanisms of BAC-dependent cell loss. *Alcoholism: Clinical and Experimental Research*, **14**, 813–18.

Wilsnack, S.C. (1995*a*). Alcohol use and alcohol problems in women. In *Psychology of Women's Health: Progress and Challenges in Research and Application*, ed. A. L. Stanton & S. J. Gallant. Washington, DC: American Psychological Association (in press).

Wilsnack, S.C. (1995*b*). Patterns and trends in women's drinking: recent findings and some implications for prevention. In *Prevention Research on Women and Alcohol*, ed. E. Taylor, J. Howard, P. Mail & M. Hilton. Washington, DC: US Government Printing Office (in press).

Wilson, J.G. (1973). *Environment and Birth Defects*. New York: Academic Press.

2

Clinical symptoms in patients with fetal alcohol syndrome

FRANK MAJEWSKI

Introduction

Maternal alcohol illness and excessive alcohol abuse during pregnancy can cause severe physical and psychological damage in children. The teratogenic damage can vary from minimal cerebral disturbances to severe mental and morphological damage. The combination of growth retardation, dysmorphias/malformations and mental retardation is referred to as fetal alcohol syndrome (FAS), or as alcohol embryopathy (AE) in the German literature. The term fetal alcohol effects (FAE) describes mild behavioral and mental disturbances.

Fetal alcohol syndrome (FAS)

The main symptoms of FAS are intrauterine growth retardation (IUGR), microcephaly, mental retardation, muscular hypotonia, hyperactivity, a characteristic face, and a variety of internal malformations. The diagnosis of FAS is likely if all or most of these characteristics as well as a history of severe maternal alcohol abuse during pregnancy are present and if other syndromes with IUGR and microcephaly – in particular the much rarer de Lange syndrome and Dubowitz syndrome – are excluded.

Lemoine et al. (1968) in France and independently Jones et al. (1973) in the United States were the first to report on alcohol embryotoxicity in humans. Lemoine et al. (1968) reported on the characteristics of 127 children of alcoholic parents. They noted a recognizable craniofacial anomaly, i.e., microcephaly, a short and upturned nose, small lips, and retrogenia. The facial anomalies were 'typical during the first two years . . . and changed with age.' Most of their patients exhibited marked pre- and postnatal growth retardation, underweight, mental retardation (IQ around 70), and various malformations such as heart defects, microphthalmia, cleft palate, hip dislocation, and visceral anomalies. Because this paper appeared in a local French medical journal, there was international interest only in the papers of Jones *et al.*, which were published in the *Lancet* in 1973 and 1974. In their first report they described 11 children of alcoholic mothers. All exhibited growth retardation, underweight, and microcephaly. All showed motor and mental developmental delay. Characteristic dysmorphic facial features included ptosis of upper lids, epicanthic folds, short upturned nose, small vermilion border of upper lip and retrogenia. Furthermore, some children suffered from congenital heart defect, anomalous palmar creases, and limited supination. In their 1974 paper Jones *et al.* examined 26 offspring of 23 chronic alcoholic mothers. The perinatal mortality was 17%. Thirty-two percent of the surviving children showed symptoms of FAS. After these publications, numerous case reports appeared that confirmed the clinical picture of FAS. This specific embryofetal disturbance was observed worldwide, and a large series of cases was published.

International review

Clarren and Smith (1978) in the *United States* observed 65 cases of FAS. Streissguth *et al.* in 1978 and later in numerous papers reported on the psychological development of children with FAS. In 1985 Streissguth *et al.* reported on a 10 year follow-up of 8 cases first described in 1973/4. All children remained microcephalic and mentally handicapped; only 4 children with milder disturbances showed some improvement in intelligence. There was no catch-up in growth but some in weight in females after normal puberty. Abel & Sokol (1991) calculated the frequency of FAS in the 'Western World' at 0.33 per 1000, but the French data were not included.

In *France* Dupuis *et al.* (1978) studied the heart malformations of 50 children with FAS. Dehaene *et al.* (1981) prospectively observed 45 new cases of FAS within 3 years. Dehaene *et al.* (1991) observed a frequency of all types of FAS of 4.8 per 1000 (1/208) and of severe FAS of 1 in 820 in the maternity hospital of Roubaix. Kaminski *et al.* (1981) in a prospective epidemiological study observed no correlation between maternal alcohol consumption and major malformations in the offspring. But they found increased frequencies of prematurity and stillbirths, as well as decreased birth weights, when the mothers drank more than 40 ml wine or the equivalent of other alcoholic beverages per day.

In *Sweden* Kyllerman *et al.* (1979) examined 52 children of alcoholic women. Two thirds were mentally handicapped and 6 children presented with symptoms of FAS. Olegård *et al.* (1979) studied the symptoms and the frequency of FAS. Larsson (1987) led a group of nurses, social workers and physicians who tried to identify and help pregnant women with alcohol problems in the hospital of Huddinge/Stockholm. After this intervention study the frequency of FAS in this region decreased to zero, although the team had 50 pregnant 'alcohol or drug abusers' in treatment per year (Larsson, 1987). Aronson *et al.* (1985) carried out a psychometric study of 21 children of alcoholic mothers. Ten children presented with symptoms of FAS and with significantly lower IQ and perceptual delay than the morphologically unaffected children.

Autti-Rämö & Granström (1991) in *Finland* examined 53 children at $1\frac{1}{2}$ years of age who had various durations of prenatal exposure to alcohol. The mothers either drank moderately (28–150 g per week) or heavily (more than 150 g per week) during the first trimester (group I), or heavily during the first and second trimester (group II), or heavily during the entire pregnancy (group III). There were no developmental differences between group I children and non-exposed controls. The children of groups II and III showed significantly lower scores in language and total mental assessment. The number of developmentally delayed children increased with increasing duration of prenatal alcohol exposure. In group II there was one child with FAS, whereas in group III 5 of the 19 children (38%) were diagnosed with FAS. In *Spain* an international meeting on FAS was organized in 1984 (Grisolia, 1985). Cahuana & Gairi (1985) reported on a total of 63 Spanish cases. Tanaka *et al.* (1981, 1982) examined 26 *Japanese* cases and studied some pathogenic mechanisms in a rat model. In particular they observed low zinc levels and hypoglycemia in rats with FAS.

There have been few reports from the *United Kingdom*. Beattie *et al.* (1983) reported on a series of 40 affected children whose mothers were all alcohol addicted. Plant (1985) carried out a prospective study on 1012 newborns. Ninety-two percent of the mothers drank alcohol during pregnancy, but mostly in moderate amounts. Despite a sophisticated study program, Plant failed to observe a single case of FAS. Sulaiman *et al.* (1988) examined 952 consecutive primigravidas in Scotland and correlated the maternal alcohol intake with the perinatal outcome. There was no negative influence on the newborn if the mothers consumed less than 14 g alcohol per day during pregnancy. Among the newborns of mothers who consumed 14–17 g daily, there was an insignificant decrease in birth weight and head circumference. This decrease in birth weight and head circumference, in addition to the decrease in length and Apgar scores, was significant among the newborns of mothers who drank more than 17 g per day (without an upper limit).

Florey *et al.* (1992) edited the EUROMAC study, a concerted action in nine European centers. They observed an adverse effect on growth in infants whose mothers drank more than 120 g alcohol per week. In contrast there was a trend of increasing attention span with increasing maternal alcohol consumption. Children at age 18 months were not impaired either mentally or physically if the mothers drank up to 140 g per week.

In *Germany* the first large series (68 cases) was reported by Majewski *et al.* (1976). Since then more than 600 cases have been observed in three centers in Germany. The Berlin study group concentrated on electroencephalographic abnormalities (Spohr *et al.*, 1979), pediatric, neurological, psychological and psychiatric findings (Nestler *et al.*, 1981; Spohr & Steinhausen, 1984), and long-term follow-up (Spohr *et al.*, 1993; Steinhausen *et al.*, 1994). Löser first examined the type and frequency of congenital heart defects (Löser *et al.*, 1977; Löser, 1987). Later he included somatic and psychiatric anomalies as well as long-term follow-up findings (Löser, 1995). Majewski (1981, 1993) focused on dysmorphic features, growth data, and pathogenesis.

Diagnosis

In numerous case reports and in all larger series cited so far a similar and recognizable pattern of mental and growth retardation, facial dysmorphias, and malformations in children of alcohol-addicted mothers was observed, which is summarized by the term FAS or AE. The main characteristics of FAS are:

1. marked prenatal growth retardation;
2. postnatal growth retardation and underweight;
3. microcephaly;
4. motor and mental retardation, hyperactivity, muscular hypotonia;
5. typical face with rounded forehead, short upturned nose, epicanthal folds, marked nasolabial furrows, flat philtrum, small vermilion border of lips, and retrogenia;
6. malformations, especially of the heart and the genitals.

No single symptom is specific for FAS. The diagnosis is likely only if various characteristics are present and combined with a history of maternal alcohol abuse prior to and during pregnancy. The ascertainment of cases and the clinical description vary from author to author. Some studies reported only on severely affected children, while in others only milder forms were examined. In the latter, internal malformations are rare or lacking. Therefore, a direct comparison of the frequencies of clinical symptoms in the different studies is not meaningful. The following summarizes the clinical symptoms of 230 children who manifested three degrees of severity of FAS (see below). These children were examined by the author over a period of 20 years. Because most authors arrived at the same results, only major differences between studies will be discussed.

Classification

The degree of prenatal damage caused by maternal alcoholism is highly variable. Although there is a continuum from severe to mild damage, a classification into three degrees of severity is relevant to the prognosis (Majewski *et al.*, 1976). In the left-hand column of Table 2.1, 25 symptoms were scored on a scale from 1 to 4. Only extremely severe brain damage was graded with a score of 8. It should be emphasized that this scoring system allows a classification into the degrees I to III but not the initial diagnosis of FAS (e.g., a child with Dubowitz or de Lange syndrome can easily reach a score equivalent to FAS III). Furthermore, this classification is possible only during the first years of life because later the facial anomalies change (see below). This classification has been followed by most German authors. Dehaene *et al.* (1977) also used a classification into three degrees, but their criteria involved clinical judgments only.

FAS III

The severe type of FAS is characterized by marked pre- and postnatal growth retardation, microcephaly, and mental retardation. The face is so typical that the diagnosis of maternal alcoholism during pregnancy can be deduced: the forehead is rounded, there may be blepharophimosis, the nose is short and upturned, the philtrum is flat, the vermilion border of the lips (mainly the upper) is very narrow, the mandible is hypoplastic. Children with FAS III frequently suffer from internal malformations (Table 2.1). Mental impairment is always severe and most children are hypotonic and hyperactive (Fig. 2.1 *a–d*).

FAS II

Patients with the moderate type of FAS are growth retarded as well as microcephalic. Their mental retardation is not as severe as in FAS III. The face is dysmorphic (Fig. 2.2 *a, b*) but, without proven maternal alcoholism the diagnosis can only be suspected. However, hyperactivity and muscular hypotonia may be of diagnostic help. Internal malformations are not as frequent as in FAS III (Table 2.1).

Table 2.1. *Frequencies of symptoms in 230 children with FAS*

Points	Symptoms	FAS III a/b	%	FAS II a/b	%	FAS I a/b	%	Total a/b	%
4	IUGR	54/57	95	56/69	81	58/75	77	168/201	84
-	Postnatal growth retardation	53/55	96	67/77	87	57/79	72	177/211	84
4	Microcephaly	52/59	88	63/83	76	58/82	71	173/224	77
2/4/8	Statomotor/mental retardation	34/40	98	56/61	92	49/71	69	144/172	84
4	Hyperactivity	47/58	81	65/82	79	46/80	58	158/220	72
2	Muscular hypotonia	41/57	72	46/80	58	34/76	45	121/213	57
2	Epicanthic folds	32/62	52	44/82	54	30/81	37	103/225	46
2	Ptosis	27/59	46	18/81	22	11/81	14	56/221	25
2	Blepharophimosis	20/57	35	33/79	42	9/76	12	62/212	29
-	Antimongoloid palpebral fissures	29/61	48	19/74	26	14/67	21	62/212	29
-	Strabismus	13/51	25	13/73	18	8/72	11	34/196	17
-	Dysplastic ears	23/56	41	21/65	32	11/73	15	56/194	29
3	Short upturned nose	42/61	69	41/73	56	32/83	39	117/219	53
1	Nasolabial furrows	53/60	88	51/80	64	43/79	54	142/219	65
1	Small lips	48/61	79	57/83	69	39/81	48	144/225	64
4	Cleft palate	11/63	17	4/81	5	0/83	0	15/227	7
2	High arched palate	25/61	41	15/76	20	12/81	15	52/218	24
-	Hypoplasia of maxilla	1/56	2	2/76	3	2/80	3	5/212	2
2	Hypoplasia of mandible	57/64	89	65/82	79	27/83	33	149/229	65
3	Anomalous palmar creases	51/59	86	59/83	71	38/80	48	148/222	67
2	Brachyclinodactyly V	30/62	48	32/82	39	19/81	23	81/225	36
2	Camptodactyly	15/59	25	9/83	11	4/83	5	28/225	12
1	Hypoplasia of terminal phalanges	15/58	26	6/83	8	5/77	7	26/218	12
2	Limited supination	11/52	21	5/83	6	5/82	6	21/217	10
2	Hip dislocation	6/48	13	7/75	9	7/80	9	20/203	10
-	Flat feet	14/42	33	29/47	62	18/60	30	61/149	41
-	Pectus excavatum	10/49	20	14/78	18	19/79	24	43/206	21
-	Pectus carinatum	6/52	12	5/72	7	4/77	5	15/201	7
4	Congenital heart defect	36/57	63	15/80	19	8/82	10	59/219	27
-	Hemangiomas	14/58	24	11/72	15	6/75	8	31/204	15
2/4	Genital anomalies	36/59	61	31/82	38	22/82	27	89/223	40
1	Sacral dimple	35/36	63	43/81	53	25/76	33	103/214	48
2	Hernias	11/51	22	5/63	8	6/78	8	22/192	11
4	Genitourinary malformations	7/45	16	5/53	9	0/78	0	12/174	7

a, symptoms observed; b, symptoms looked for.
FAS I ($n = 83$), 10–29 points; FAS II ($n = 83$), 30–39 points; FAS III ($n = 64$), $\geqslant 40$ points.

FAS I

The mild form of FAS is characterized by pre- and postnatal growth retardation, underweight, and microcephaly. Mental development is normal or only slightly subnormal. The face of most children is normal (Fig. 2.2c), and there are few or no internal malformations (Table 2.1). Diagnosis is possible only by verification of severe maternal alcoholism.

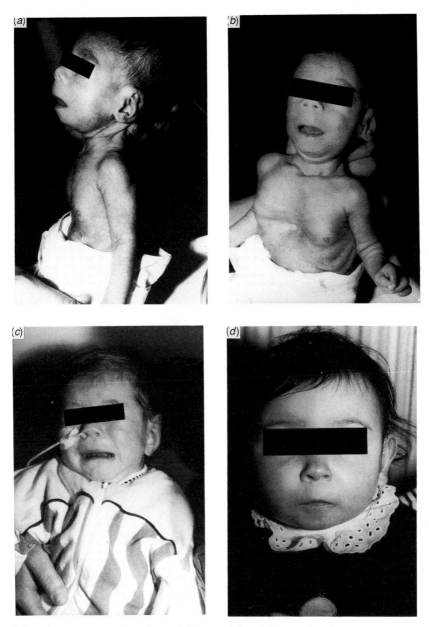

Fig. 2.1.   Appearance of various children with FAS III. (*a*), (*b*) Face and profile of a newborn with FAS III. (*c*) Face of a baby with FAS III. (*d*) Appearance of a young child with FAS III.

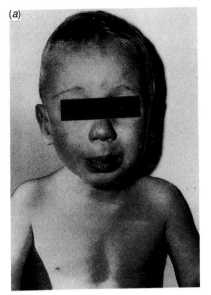

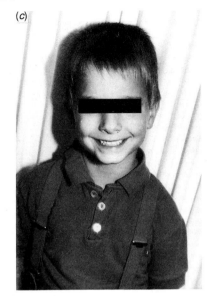

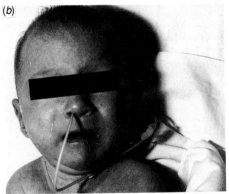

Fig. 2.2.   Appearance of various children with FAS II (*a, b*) and FAS I (*c*). (*a*) Boy with FAS II. (*b*) Appearance of a girl with FAS II who needed tube feeding for more than 6 months. (*c*) Face of a boy with FAS I.

If the diagnosis by facial anomalies is questionable, the examiner should look at the crying baby: the skin of the rounded forehead is wrinkled, the nasolabial furrows are increased, and the lateral parts of the lower lips are turned down (Fig. 2.2). Furthermore, hyperexcitability and restless spontaneous movements may help in the diagnosis of questionable cases.

Fetal alcohol effects (FAE)

The term FAE includes all the alcohol-induced cerebral disturbances without the typical morphological abnormalities of FAS (Abel, 1984; Streissguth,

1987). These effects are observed as developmental delay (especially of speech), attention deficits, hyperactivity, learning disabilities, and emotional and social adaptive disturbances. Because the development of the brain can be disturbed during the entire pregnancy, the symptoms of this 'embryotoxic encephalopathy' (Löser, 1991) are various. Therefore, the definition of FAE is somewhat weak and seems to be nonspecific. In addition, the effects on the offspring of mild or moderate alcohol consumption during pregnancy are mostly mild, and they are often hard to verify.

Streissguth *et al.* (1981, 1990) prospectively examined 500 children. Two hundred and fifty of the mothers had consumed alcohol moderately to heavily during pregnancy, and 250 had consumed little or none. Newborns of mothers who drank more than 1 ounce (29.6 g) of alcohol daily during pregnancy showed delayed reactions to the stimuli of a light, a rattle, and a bell. At the ages of 8 months and 4 years these children had some behavioral disturbances, especially attentional deficits. At a mean age of 7.5 years all the 482 children re-examined were healthy, but there was a decrease in IQ of 7 points in 30 children whose mothers had consumed more than 1 ounce of alcohol per day. Mentally subnormal children were observed only among the offspring of mothers who had consumed more than 2 ounces (59 g) of absolute alcohol per day during pregnancy. Olson *et al.* (1992) reported on the follow-up of 458 children at age 11 years by questionnaires mailed to their class teachers. A wide variety of classroom-related problems, including attention, activity, information-processing, and academic difficulties were salient for prenatal exposure. Maternal binge drinking (5 or more 'drinks per occasion') and drinking during very early pregnancy were particularly salient for the poorer school performance of these children. In contrast, Autti-Rämö & Granström (1991) observed no influence of first trimester 'moderate to heavy drinking' on 21 children at the age of 1.5 years compared with non-exposed controls.

Clinical symptoms

In Table 2.1 the frequencies of 34 common symptoms of 230 children with different degrees of FAS are listed. In the following the various dysmorphic features of FAS will be described.

Frequent malformations and anomalies

Eighty-four percent of our patients manifested intrauterine and postnatal growth retardation, 77% were microcephalic, and 84% were mentally retarded. Twenty-seven percent of all patients suffered from congenital heart defects, mostly septal defects. In addition, we observed more complex heart defects, such as transposition of great vessels, pentalogy of Fallot, and aplasia of one lung artery. A nearly identical percentage (29%) of congenital heart defects was observed by Löser *et al.* (1992) in their sample of 216 cases of FAS. These authors observed septal defects in 47 out of 63 patients with heart defects. The frequency of congenital heart defects in our patient group was related to the degree of FAS: 63% in patients with FAS III, 19% in those with FAS II, and 10% in patients with FAS I (see Table 2.1). Forty percent of all patients exhibited mostly minor anomalies of external genitalia (i.e., hypospadias, cryptorchidism, hypoplasia of labia minora) and at least 7% suffered from malformations of the genitourinary tract (diverticula of bladder, hypoplastic kidney, polycystic kidney, megaureter, hydronephrosis). Genital anomalies also correlated with the degree of FAS; they were present in 61% of children with FAS III, in 38% of children with FAS II, and in 27% of children with FAS I. Spina bifida was present in 2% of our cohort. Most of these frequencies are in concordance with other larger series, such as those of Clarren & Smith (1978), Spohr (1990), and Löser *et al.* (1992).

Craniofacial dysmorphology

The face in patients with FAS III is characterized by a rounded forehead, antimongoloid slant to the palpebral fissures (48%), blepharophimosis (35%), a short upturned nose (69%), deep nasolabial furrows (88%), and hypoplastic mandible (89%). All symptoms may be present in milder forms also, but at lower frequency. We observed hypoplasia of the maxilla in only 2–3% of our cases, whereas other authors, including Spohr *et al.* (1993), observed this symptom in 19%. Mid-face hypoplasia was mentioned by Streissguth *et al.* (1991), but not quantified. This difference is probably caused by the higher proportion of milder cases in the cohort of Spohr *et al.* (1993). The impression of small palpebral fissures is caused by ptosis and epicanthic folds, whereas blepharophimosis is defined by horizontally shortened palpebral fissures. We have measured the length of the palpebral fissures (Majewski, 1981) and observed blepharophimosis in only 29% of our cases of all degrees of severity. In our patients of FAS III we observed blepharophimosis in 35% (Table 2.1). Blepharophimosis was noted by Clarren & Smith (1978) in more than 80% of their cases and by Spohr *et al.* (1993) in 41% at the initial examination of their 71 cases, and in 29% at the follow-up examination.

Facial appearance changes with age. In older patients the nose is no longer short and upturned, the lips are no longer thin, and the chin often becomes rather prominent (Fig. 2.3*a,c*). The same changes in facial appearance were noted by Streissguth *et al.* (1985, 1991), Lemoine & Lemoine (1992), Löser (1995) and Spohr *et al.* (1993). Because retrogenia changes to progenia, the

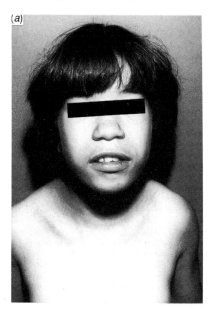
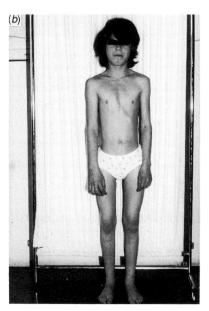
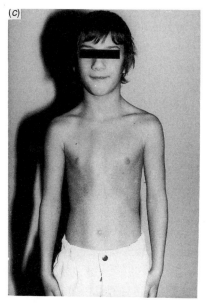

Fig. 2.3. Appearance of older children. (*a*) Girl with FAS III at age 13 years. (*b*) Girl with FAS III at age 10 2/12 years. (*c*) Girl with FAS II at age 9 years.

impression of hypoplastic maxilla may be more frequent in older cases. The only unchanged features in all cohorts are small palpebral fissures and microcephaly. In older patients, photographs taken in babyhood often serve as a necessary diagnostic tool. The face in severely affected children is so characteristic that the diagnosis can be made from photographs alone. Six of seven expert clinicians were able to identify accurately most of 21 7-year-old children who had been prenatally exposed to high levels of alcohol (Clarren *et al.*, 1987).

With time, further symptoms turned out to be typical of FAS (not listed in Table 2.1), such as flat philtrum (95% in the cohort of Löser *et al.*, 1992), small teeth (31% in the series of Spohr, 1990), and thick and brittle hair.

Infrequent malformations and anomalies

We observed tortuosity of retinal vessels in about 10%, and milder anomalies, including myopia and strabismus, infrequently. Significant hypoplasia of the optic nerve disc was found in only 1 patient. Strömland (1987) was the first to report ocular involvement in FAS, i.e., myopia, strabismus, hypoplasia of optic nerve disc, and increased tortuosity of retinal vessels in nearly 90% of her 30 patients. But this figure may be elevated due to ascertainment bias in an ophthalmological clinic.

Other less frequently observed symptoms were cleft palate (7%), clinodactyly V (36%), camptodactyly (12%), hypoplasia of terminal phalanges (12%), limited supination (10%), in some cases due to radioulnar synostosis, pectus excavatum (21%) or carinatum (8%), sacral dimple (48%), hernias (11%) and (mostly small) hemangiomas (15%).

Clinical features by severity

Frequencies of symptoms according to the different degrees of FAS are given in Table 2.1. Though the classification of FAS was initially based on dysmorphic criteria, it appeared that nearly all clinical features were more frequent in FAS III than in FAS II, and were rare in FAS I. Except for cleft palate, genitourinary malformations, and spina bifida, all features were also observed in cases of FAS I, but were less frequent and mostly of milder degree than in cases of FAS II or III. In cases of FAS II the frequencies of nearly all symptoms lie between those of FAS III and I. For a more detailed clinical description and a literature review see Majewski (1987*a*).

Anatomical and functional CNS findings

Our case 181 with FAS III (Fig. 2.1) died from congenital heart defect (atrial septal defect, ventricular septal defect) at age 8 months. Neuropathological examination (unpublished) revealed marked hydrocephalus internus e vacuo and agenesis of corpus callosum. A similar spectrum of malformations was observed by Clarren *et al. (*1978, case 1). There are only 16 published brain dissections (Jones *et al.*, 1973; Clarren *et al.*, 1978; Majewski *et al.*, 1978; Volk, 1987; Peiffer *et al.*, 1979; Wiesniewski *et al.*, 1983). The malformations observed ranged from microdysplasias and heterotopias (10/16 cases) to severe brain malformations (5/16). These malformations included hydrocephalus internus (3 cases: Clarren *et al.*, 1978; Peiffer *et al.*, 1979), hypoplasia of cerebellum (4 cases: Clarren *et al.*, 1978; Peiffer *et al.*, 1979; Wiesniewski *et al.*, 1983), and agenesis of corpus callosum (3 cases: Clarren *et al.*, 1978; Peiffer *et al.*, 1979; Wiesniewski *et al.*, 1983). The severest malformations were observed in our case 18 (Peiffer *et al.*, 1979): agenesis of corpus callosum, hypoplasia of cerebellum, hydrocephalus internus et externus, and a porencephalic cyst. In a few cases holoprosencephaly has been reported as a possible pathogenic consequence of heavy maternal alcohol abuse (Bönnemann & Meinecke, 1990; Ronen & Andrews, 1991). For a more detailed description of malformations of the CNS in cases with FAS see Stoltenberg-Didinger (this volume).

Four children suffered from neural tube defects. The frequency of spina bifida in our series was 2%; compared with the general population this is a 20-fold increase. Friedman (1982) also suggested an increased frequency of neural tube defects in children with FAS.

Ten percent of our patients suffered from convulsions, and 72% demonstrated hyperexcitability, hyperactivity, and ataxia. In most children these symptoms decreased after the age of 2–3 years. Muscular hypotonia was observed in 57% of our patients. The degree of mental retardation was related to the physical abnormalities in the children. The mean IQ of patients with FAS III was 66, whereas it was 79 in patients with FAS II, and 91 in patients with FAS I (Majewski, 1981). A similar correlation between the degree of morphological abnormalities and mental retardation was observed by Streissguth *et al.* (1978) in 20 cases. In a follow-up study of 8 children the initial mean IQ of these children was 56; 10 years later at follow-up it was 61 (Streissguth *et al.*, 1985).

After an interval of several years Löser & Ilse (1991) re-examined 22 patients aged 14–20 years with FAS of different degrees. Four patients were able to attend a regular school, 2 attended a school for children with learning disabilities, 2 a special school for children with physical handicaps, 9 a school for the mentally handicapped, and 1 patient was unable to be educated. Unfortunately, no figures for the degree of FAS in 15 of the patients are given, but all 7 patients with FAS III attended a school for the mentally handicapped.

Streissguth *et al.* (1991) re-examined adolescents and adults with FAS (mean age 18 years, range 12–40 years). The average IQ of these patients was 66 (range 30–90). Arithmetic deficits were most characteristic. Maladaptive behaviors such as poor judgment, destructiveness, and difficulty of perceiving social cues were common. None of the adults was able to live independently.

Most children with FAS are impaired in their cognitive, emotional, and behavioral development. In early childhood they are hyperexcitable and hyperactive. They show delay of speech and language, attention deficits and/or specific learning disorders such as dyslexia, dyscalculia, and poor achievement in motor skills and in logic and planning abilities. They tend to act impulsively and lack personal distance and/or recognition of danger. For a more detailed evaluation of psychological disturbances see Steinhausen (this volume).

Auxological data

The mean birth weight of 124 children with FAS born at term was 2354.6 g. This weight corresponds to the 50th percentile of children born at $34\frac{1}{2}$ weeks of gestation. Mean head circumference (31.97 cm) and length (46.05 cm) were similarly retarded by 5 to $5\frac{1}{2}$ weeks. In most newborns with FAS there was a proportionate retardation of all three parameters and no relative microcephaly (i.e., occipitofrontal circumference related to length).

There was a decrease in the mean values of weight, length, and head circumference from FAS I to FAS II to FAS III (Table 2.2). In Fig. 2.4, measurements are given in standard deviation scores (SDS). At birth there was a deviation of all parameters by more than 3 SDS. During the first 6 months of life there was a decrease in weight and even more in head circumference to about -4 SDS. From the second month of life onwards there was some catch-up growth for height, from the sixth month of life for weight, and from the twelfth month of life for head circumference. In all age groups (except newborns) head circumference was the most retarded parameter. At the age of 6.5 years height increased over the 3rd percentile; at the age of 8 years head circumference followed and weight came nearly up to the -2 SD line.

Table 2.2. *Auxological data on 124 children with FAS I, II and II born at term*

	Mean weight (g)		Mean length (cm)		Mean OFC (cm)	
	M	F	M	F	M	F
FAS I ($n=42$)	2.545	2.676	48.3	48.1	32.9	33.1
FAS II ($n=49$)	2.371	2.329	46.0	46.0	32.0	31.5
FAS III ($n=33$)	2.125	1.955	44.4	43.8	31.5	31.0

OFC, occipitofrontal circumference; M, male; F, female.

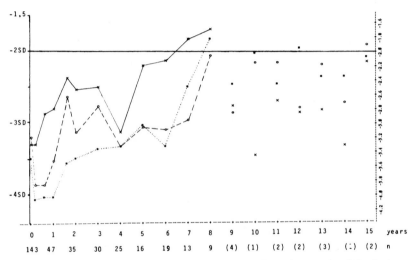

Fig. 2.4.   Growth data of 175 children with FAS, given in standard deviation scores (SDS). Crosses, height; circles, weight; asterisks, occipitofrontal circumference.

A comparison of the mean values in SDS of all age groups (Table 2.3) shows that children with FAS III are more retarded in all three parameters than children with FAS II or FAS I. Retardation was most pronounced for head circumference in children with FAS III, reaching a value of more than −4 SDS.

The last examination of our oldest female patient with FAS III was at an age of nearly 18 years. Her final height was 145 cm. She had a normal puberty, normal female proportions, was slightly overweight, but was still microcephalic and mentally retarded. The same catch-up growth for weight was observed by Streissguth *et al.* (1985) and Spohr *et al.* (1993) in their female patients. The predicted final height of our oldest male patient with FAS III is 160 cm. Streissguth *et al.* (1991) reported on 31 adolescent or adult

Table 2.3. *Anthropometric measurements of all newborns with FAS I–III in standard deviation sources (SDS)*

	Weight	Height	OFC
FAS I	−2.54	−2.01	−2.71
FAS II	−3.23	−2.88	−3.57
FAS III	−3.89	−3.58	−4.14

patients with FAS. The mean growth retardation corresponded to −2.1 SD (range −6 to 0 SD), retardation of head circumference to −1.9 SD (range −5 SD to +2 SD), and retardation of weight to −1.4 SD (−4 to 0 SD). Weight deficiency, which is typical for young children with FAS, was less marked in these adolescents and adults. Twenty-five percent of the patients with FAS did not suffer from underweight. The mean weight–height proportion was 48% (range 3–90%). The time of onset of puberty in all patients was within normal limits.

In Fig. 2.5 the development of carpal bone age, weight, height, and head circumference of a female with FAS III is depicted. Carpal bone age was nearly normal. As in the cases of adolescent American females after the age of 12 years, weight gain was faster than height gain; the same was observed

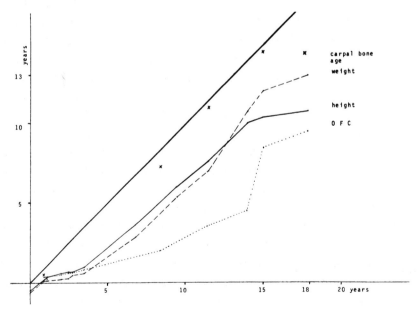

Fig. 2.5.   Growth data of an individual patient with FAS III. OFC, occipitofrontal circumference.

Table 2.4. *The association of head circumference (OFC) with weight in SDS by degree of severity of FAS*

	OFC		
	FAS I	FAS II	FAS III
Weight > −2 SDS	−1.86	−1.96	−
Weight < −2 SDS	−3.14	−3.87	−4.11

by Streissguth *et al.* (1991) in their adult female patients. Typically, the most impaired parameter is head circumference.

Correlation of weight with head circumference

With the exception of severe congenital heart defects, microcephaly and mental retardation are the main problems for most children with FAS. The enlargement of head circumference and corresponding brain weight is an important goal of medical care in children with FAS. Brain growth velocity is at its maximum between the 32nd gestational week and the sixth month after the normal date of birth. After the age of 19 months brain growth velocity decreases to less than 10%. In a group of 27 otherwise healthy small-for-dates children Brandt (1981) observed a catch-up growth of head circumference that approaches normal values after early and high-calorie postnatal feeding. However, this observation has not been confirmed by other authors and is controversial. To study whether there was an influence of weight on head circumference patients with FAS I, II and III were divided into two main weight groups corresponding to > −2 SDS or < −2 SDS (Table 2.4). The corresponding head circumferences are given as SDS values. In general, children with FAS I had less pronounced microcephaly than those with FAS II or III. Heavier children above −2 SDS with FAS I and FAS II had markedly larger head circumferences than children below −2 SDS. This may reflect some correlation of weight and brain growth. However, these differences are nearly the same at birth, and catch-up growth of head circumference in heavier children is not observed to be greater than in the underweight children. Thus, our patients with greater weight do not have better brain growth. Nevertheless, one should attempt to increase head circumference by early and high-calorie feeding, especially in the first 6 months of life. Increased head circumference parallels increased brain growth

Table 2.5. *Degree of severity of FAS (I–III) in families with several affected children*

Family	Sibling 1	Sibling 2	Sibling 3
Li	I	II	
Ha.	I	II	III
Sp.	I	II	III
CI	I	II	
Ko.	I	I	
Fe.	I	II	
Ba.	I	II	
Be.	III	III	
Rö.	I	I	
Cr.	I	II	
Da.	I	II	
Eb.	II	III	
Fa.	I	II	
Ma.	I	I	III
Mü	FAE[a]	FAE[a]	I
Sch.	FAE	FAE	II
Br.	II	I	

[a] Dizygotic twins.

(Brandt, 1981) and probably parallels improved mental development due to an increase in myelinization and the growth of dendrites and synapses.

Degree of FAS in twins and siblings

The twin study by Streissguth & Dehaene (1993), which describes 16 twins with a history of 'maternal alcoholism or alcohol abuse' during the target pregnancy, demonstrated that the teratogenic effects of maternal alcoholism may be influenced by genetic factors. All five pairs of monozygotic twins were equally affected: in two pairs both twins had FAS, in one pair both had FAE, and in two pairs neither twin was affected. By contrast, only 7 of 11 dizygotic twin pairs were concordant: in two pairs one twin had FAS and one had FAE, and in two further pairs one twin had FAE and the other was not affected. Among the twins concordant for diagnosis, there was one pair with FAS, whereas only one child had a cleft lip and palate. We observed a possibly dizygotic pair of male twins who were similarly affected by FAE; the younger sister had FAS I (sibship Mü. in Table 2.5).

   We observed 38 affected siblings (Table 2.5). Mostly (with one exception in sibship Br.) the younger sib was more severely impaired than the older one

(Fig. 2.6). In the families Mü. and Sch. the first two children (dizygotic twins in family Mü.) had FAE, whereas the third child in the two families suffered from FAS I and FAS II, respectively. In another study we observed no influence of the (extremely high) daily amounts of alcohol intake during pregnancy on severity of FAS, whereas we detected a significant influence of the increasing stage of maternal alcohol abuse on the degree of FAS (Majewski, 1981). The latter correlation is supported by our observation in the affected siblings. From our studies it is evident that high daily alcohol intake and an advanced stage of maternal alcohol illness are prerequisites for FAS.

Differential diagnosis

In each child with intrauterine and postnatal growth retardation, microcephaly, and a dysmorphic face the tentative diagnosis of FAS is the most probable because FAS is rather frequent, and all other types of intrauterine growth retardation (IUGR) are rare or very rare (except trisomy 18).

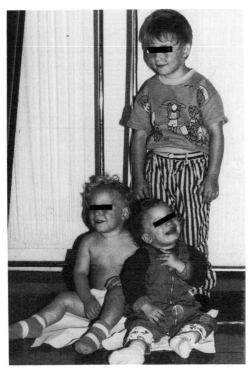

Fig. 2.6. Three siblings, the younger ones with FAS I (left) and II (right).

In *trisomy 18* (frequency 1 : 2000 newborns) there is no hyperexcitability, no flat philtrum and no blepharophimosis. In contrast to FAS the mouth in patients with trisomy 18 is small, there may be ptosis of upper lips, the sternum is short and the ribs are small. Heart defects and genitourinary malformations are more frequent in trisomy 18 than in FAS. The typically clenched hands with the index finger overlying the third, and the little finger overlying the fourth, is only occasionally seen in newborns with FAS. Very typical of trisomy 18 are dorsiflexed short big toes and rocker-bottom feet.

Various *structural chromosomal aberrations* present with marked IUGR; the craniofacial dysmorphias in most of these aberrations are clearly different from those in FAS. Only about 60 cases of *Dubowitz syndrome* have been reported. This rare syndrome has autosomal recessive inheritance. The degree of IUGR, microcephaly and hyperactivity are nearly the same as in FAS. The lips in Dubowitz syndrome are rather full, the teeth relatively large. Typically there is telecanthus and eczema on the chin and cheeks; heart defects are incommon in Dubowitz syndrome, as is syndactyly of toes 2 and 3 in FAS.

Children with *Brachmann–de Lange syndrome* are in some respects quite similar to children with FAS: small lips, receding chin, shortened nose, IUGR and microcephaly. In Brachmann–de Lange syndrome the eyebrows are arched and usually grow together by synophrys. A median prominence of the upper lip is typical only for Brachmann–de Lange syndrome. Most children with this syndrome show muscular hypertonia. Oligodactyly and brachymetacarpy I in Brachmann–de Lange syndrome are inconstant, but clearly distinguish the two diseases. Prognosis is poor in many children with Brachmann–de Lange syndrome; intellectual performance is usually severely limited (mean IQ in survivors is below 35). Brachmann–de Lange syndrome is a disorder that appears sporadically.

Children with *Rubinstein–Taybi syndrome* usually present with IUGR, microcephaly and profound mental retardation. They are easily recognized by broad thumbs and big toes, and by a beaked and sharp nose. But the facial dysmorphias in this syndrome change and become typical only with increasing age. Almost all cases of Rubinstein–Taybi syndrome occur sporadically (except for a very few instances of apparently dominant inheritance). A small interstitial deletion at 16p13.3 was observed in some patients with this syndrome (Hennekam *et al.*, 1993).

Patients with *Silver–Russell syndrome* are clearly distinguishable by the relative macrocephaly, triangular face, café-au-lait spots, asymmetry of limbs (inconstant), and normal intelligence in the majority of cases. The etiology of Silver–Russell syndrome is unknown; almost all cases are sporadic.

There are some 20 further delineated types of IUGR, which are all extremely rare. For instance, the well-known recessively inherited *Seckel syndrome* has so far been reported (and correctly diagnosed) in only about 20 cases. Mean birth weight of patients with this syndrome is far below 2000g and microcephaly and hypoplasia of mandible are more pronounced than in newborns with FAS.

In newborns with FAS III the diagnosis is strongly suggested by marked IUGR, microcephaly, hyperactivity, rounded forehead, shortened nose, nasolabial furrows, small lips, and retrogenia. In newborns with FAS II and I the diagnosis can be made only after verification of severe maternal alcohol abuse and the exclusion of other types of IUGR.

In only 3 cases have we made a false diagnosis. In 2 of these we currently have no clear idea from which syndrome with IUGR the patient suffers. In the third case we detected a ring chromosome 22. Although we have subsequently verified that two of the mothers are abstinent, we have been unable to verify abstinence in the mother of the child with the ring chromosome.

References

Abel, E.L. (1984). Prenatal effects of alcohol. *Drug and Alcohol Dependence*, **14**, 1–10.

Abel, E.L. & Sokol, R.J. (1991). A revised conservative estimate of the incidence of FAS and its economic impact. *Alcoholism: Clinical and Experimental Research*, **15**, 514–24.

Aronson, M., Kyllerman, M., Sabel, K.-G., Sandin, B. & Olegard, R. (1985). Children of alcoholic mothers. *Acta Paediatrica Scandinavica*, **74**, 27–35.

Autti-Rämö, I. & Granström, M.L. (1991). The effect of intrauterine alcohol exposition in various durations on early cognitive development. *Neuropediatrics*, **22**, 203–10.

Beattie, J.O., Day, R.E., Cockburn, F. & Gary, R.A. (1983). Alcohol and the fetus in the West of Scotland. *British Medical Journal*, **287**, 17–20.

Bönnemann, C. & Meinecke, P. (1990). Holoprosencephaly as a possible embryonic alcohol effect: another observation. *American Journal of Medical Genetics*, **37**, 431–2.

Brandt, J. (1981). Kopfumfang und Gehirnentwicklung. *Klinische Wochenschrift*, **59**, 995–1007.

Cahuana, A. & Gairi, J.M. (1985). Sindrome alcoholico fetal en Espana. In *Sindrome alcoholico fetal*, Jornadas Internationales, pp. 163–76. Madrid: Fundacion Valgrande.

Clarren, S.K., Alvord, E.C., Sumi, S.M., Streissguth, A.P. & Smith, D.W. (1978). Brain malformations related to prenatal exposure to ethanol. *Journal of Pediatrics*, **92**, 64–7.

Clarren, S.K., Sampson, P.D., Larsen, J., Donnell, D.J., Barr, H.M., Bookstein, F.L., Martin, D.C. & Streissguth, A.P. (1987). Facial aspects of fetal alcohol exposure: assessment by photographs and morphometric analysis. *American Journal of Medical Genetics*, **26**, 651–66.

Clarren, S.K. & Smith, D.W. (1978). The fetal alcohol syndrome: experience with 65 patients and a review of the world literature. *New England Journal of Medicine*, **298**, 1063–7.

Dehaene, P., Crépin, G., Delahousse, G., Querleu, D., Walbaum, R., Titran, M. & Samaille-Vilette, C. (1981). Aspects epiémiologiques du syndrome d'alcoolisme foetal: 45 observations en 3 ans. *Nouvelle Presse Médical (Paris)*, **10**, 2639–43.

Dehaene, P., Samaille-Vilette, C., Boulanger-Fasquelle, P., Subtil, D., Delahousse, G. & Crépin, G. (1991). Diagnostique et prévalence du syndrome d'alcoolisme foetal en maternitée. *Nouvelle Presse Médical (Paris)*, **20**, 1002.

Dupuis, C., Dehaene, P., Deroubaiy-Tella, P., Blanc-Garin, A.P., Rey, C. & Carpentier-Courault, C. (1978). Les cardiopathies des enfants nées des mères alcooliques. *Archives des Maladies du Coeur et des Vaisseaux (Paris)*, **71**, 565–72.

Florey, C. du V., Taylor, D., Bolumar, F., Kaminski, M. & Olsen, J. (eds.) (1992). EUROMAC: a European concerted action: maternal alcohol consumption and its relation to the outcome of pregnancy and child development at 18 months. *International Journal of Epidemiology*, **21**, Suppl. 1.

Friedman, J.M. (1982). Can maternal alcohol ingestion cause neural tube defects? *Journal of Pediatrics*, **101**, 232–4.

Grisolia, D.S. (ed.) (1985). *Sindroma alcoholico fetal*, Jornadas Internationales, Serie Cientifica. Madrid: Fundacion Valgrande.

Hanson, J.W., Streissguth, A.P. & Smith, D.W. (1978). The effects of moderate alcohol consumption during pregnancy on fetal growth and morphogenesis. *Journal of Pediatrics*, **92**, 457–60.

Hennekam, R.C.M., Tilanus, M., Hamel, B.C.J., Voshart-van Heeren, H., Mariman, E.C.M., van Beersum, S.E.C., van den Boogaard, M.-J.H. & Breuning, M.H. (1993). Deletion at chromosome 16q13.3 as a cause of Rubinstein–Taybi syndrome: clinical aspects. *American Journal of Human Genetics*, **52**, 255–62.

Jones, K.L., Smith, D.W., Ulleland, C. & Streissguth, A.P. (1973). Pattern of malformations in offspring of chronic alcoholic mothers. *Lancet*, **i**, 1267–71.

Jones, K.L., Smith, D.W., Streissguth, A.P. & Myrianthopoulos, N.C. (1974). Outcome in offspring of chronic alcoholic women. *Lancet*, **i**, 1076–8.

Kaminski, M., Franc, M., Lebouvier, M., du Mazaubrun, C. & Rumeau-Rouquette, C. (1981). Moderate alcohol use and pregnancy outcome. *Neurobehavioral Toxicology and Teratology*, **3**, 173–81.

Kyllerman, M., Aronsson, A., Karlberg, E., Olegärd, R., Sabel, K.-G., Sandin, B., Johansson, P.R., Carlsson, C. & Iversen, K. (1979). Epidemiologic and neuropediatric aspects of the fetal alcohol syndrome. *Neuropädiatrie*, Suppl. **10**, 435–36.

Larsson, G. (1987). Program for early identification and treatment of pregnant abusers. In *Die Alkoholembryopathie*, ed. F. Majewski, pp. 189–96. Frankfurt: Umwelt und Medizin.

Larsson, G., Bohlinger, A.B. & Tunell, R. (1985). Prospective study of children exposed to variable amounts of alcohol *in utero*. *Archives of Diseases in Childhood*, **60**, 316–21.

Lemoine, P., Harousseau, H., Borteyru, J.P. & Menuet, J.C. (1968). Les enfants des parents alcooliques: anomalies observées à propos de 127 cas. *Quest Médical*, **21**, 476–92.

Lemoine, P. & Lemoine, P. (1992). Avenir des enfants des méres alcooliques (étude de 105 cas retrouvés à l'âge adulte) et quelques constations d'intérêt prophylactique. *Annales de Pédiatrie*, **39**, 226–35.

Löser, H. (1987). Herzfehler und toxische Herzmuskelschäden bei Alkoholembryopathie. In *Die Alkoholembryopathie*, ed. F. Majewski, pp. 124–33. Frankfurt: Umwelt und Medizin.

Löser, H. (1991). Alkoholeffekte und Schwachformen der Alkoholembryopathie. *Deutsches Ärzteblatt*, **88**, 1921–9.

Löser, H. (1995). *Alkoholembryopathie und Alkoholeffekte*. Stuttgart: Fischer.

Löser, H., Grävinghoff, K. & Rustemeyer, P. (1989). Schwachformen der Alkoholembryopathie nach exzessivem Alkoholgenuss. *Monatsschrift für Kinderheilkunde*, **137**, 764–9.

Löser, H. & Ilse, R. (1991). Körperliche und geistige Langzeitentwicklung bei Kindern mit Alkoholembryopathie. *Sozialpädiatrie in Praxis und Klinik*, **13**, 8–14.

Löser, H. & Majewski, F. (1977). Type and frequency of cardiac defects in embryofetal alcohol syndrome: report on 16 cases. *British Heart Journal*, **39**, 1374–9.

Löser, H., Pfefferkorn, J.R. & Themann, H. (1992). Alkohol in der Schwangerschaft und kindliche Herzschäden. *Klinische Pëdiatrie*, **204**, 335–9.

Majewski, F. (1981). Alcohol embryopathy: some facts and speculations about pathogenesis. *Neurobehavioral Toxicology and Teratology*, **3**, 129–44.

Majewski, F. (1987*a*). Teratogene Schäden durch Alkohol. In *Psychiatrie der Gegenwart*, ed. K.P. Kisker *et al.*, pp. 243–72. Berlin: Springer.

Majewski, F. (1987*b*). Die Alkoholembryopathie: eine häufige und vermeidbare Störung. In *Die Alkoholembryopathie*, ed. F. Majewski, pp. 109–23. Frankfurt: Umwelt und Medizin.

Majewski, F. (1993). Alcohol embryopathy: experience in 200 patients. *Developmental Brain Dysfunction*, **6**, 248–65.

Majewski, F., Bierich, J.R., Löser, H., Michaelis, R., Leiber, B. & Bettecken, F. (1976). Zur Klinik und Pathogenese der Alkoholembryopathie (Bericht über 68 Patienten). *Münchener Medizinische Wochenschrift*, **118**, 1635–42.

Majewski, F., Fischbach, H., Peiffer, J. & Bierich, J.R. (1978). Zur Frage der Interruptio bei alkoholkranken Frauen. *Deutsche Medizinische Wochenschrift*, **103**, 895–8.

Nestler, V., Spohr, H.-L. & Steinhausen, H.-C. (1981). *Die Alkoholembryopathie*. Stuttgart: Enke.

Olegärd, R., Sabel, K.G., Aronsson, M., Sandin, B., Johannsson, P.R., Carlsson, C., Kyllerman, M., Iversen, K. & Hrbek, A. (1979). Effects on the child of alcohol abuse during pregnancy: retrospective and prospective studies. *Acta Paediatrica Scandinavica, Supplement*, **275**, 112–21.

Olson, H.C., Sampson, P.D., Barr, H., Streissguth, A.P. & Bookstein, F.L. (1992). Prenatal exposure to alcohol and school problems in late childhood: a longitudinal prospective study. *Developmental Psychopathology*, **4**, 341–59.

Peiffer, J., Majewski, F., Fischbach, H., Bierich, J.R. & Volk, B. (1979). Alcohol embryopathy: neuropathology of 3 children and 3 fetuses. *Journal of the Neurological Sciences*, **41**, 125–37.

Plant, M. (1985). *Women, Drinking, and Pregnancy*: London: Tavistock.

Ronen, G.M. & Andrews, W.L. (1991). Holoprosencephaly as a possible embryonic alcohol effect. *American Journal of Medical Genetics*, **40**, 151–4.

Spohr, H.-L. (1985). Die Alkoholembryopathie: Aspekte zur Entwicklung pränatal alkoholgeschädigter Kinder. *Öffentliches Gesundheitswesen*, **47**, 430–4.

Spohr, H.-L. (1987). Neurologische und psychiatrische Befunde bei pränataler Alkoholexposition. In *Die Alkoholembryopathie*, ed. F. Majewski, pp. 134–42. Frankfurt: Umwelt und Medizin.

Spohr, H.-L. (1990). Das fetale Alkoholsyndrom – die Alkoholembryopathie – ein klinischer Überblick. In *Alkohol in der Schwangerschaft und die Folge fü das Kind*, ed. M. Steiner. Frankfurt: Fischer.

Spohr, H.-L., Majewski, F. & Nolte, R. (1979). EEG-examination of children with fetal alcohol syndrome. Paper presented at the seventh conference of the European Teratologic Society, Herzlia, Israel.

Spohr, H.-L. & Steinhausen, H.-C. (1984). Der Verlauf der Alkoholembryopathie. *Monatsschrift für Kinderheilkunde*, **132**, 844–9.

Spohr, H.-L., Willms, J. & Steinhausen, H.-C. (1993). Prenatal exposure and long-term developmental consequences. *Lancet*, **i**, 907–10.

Steinhausen, H.C., Willms, J. & Spohr, H.-L. (1994). Correlates of psychopathology and intelligence in children with fetal alcohol syndrome. *Journal of Child Psychology and Psychiatry and Allied Disciplines*, **35**, 323–31.

Streissguth, A.P. (1987). Fetal alcohol syndrome and fetal alcohol effects: teratogenetic cause of mental retardation and developmental disabilities. In *Die Alkoholembryopathie*, ed. F. Majewski, pp. 143–65. Frankfurt: Umwelt und Medizin.

Streissguth, A.P., Aase, J.M., Clarren, S.K., Randels, S.P., LaDue, R.A. & Smith, D.F. (1991). Fetal alcohol syndrome in adolescents and adults. *JAMA*, **265**, 1961–7.

Streissguth, A.P., Barr, H.M. & Sampson, P.D. (1990). Moderate prenatal alcohol exposure: effects on child IQ and learning problems at age $7\frac{1}{2}$ years. *Alcoholism: Clinical and Experimental Research*, **14**, 662–9.

Streissguth, A.P., Bookstein, F.L., Sampson, P.D. & Barr, H.M. (1989). Neurobehavioural effects of prenatal alcohol. III. Partial least squares analysis of neuropsychologic tests. *Neurotoxicology and Teratology*, **11**, 493–507.

Streissguth, A.P., Clarren, S.K. & Jones, K.L. (1985). Natural history of the fetal alcohol syndrome: a 10-year follow-up of 11 patients. *Lancet*, **ii**, 85–91.

Streissguth, A.P. & Dehaene, P. (1993). Fetal alcohol syndrome in twins of alcoholic mothers: concordance of diagnosis and IQ. *American Journal of Medical Genetics*, **47**, 857–61.

Streissguth, A.P., Herman, C.S. & Smith, D.W. (1978). Intelligence, behaviour and dysmorphogenesis in the fetal alcohol syndrome: a report on 20 patients. *Journal of Paediatrics*, **92**, 363–7.

Streissguth, A.P., Martin, J.C., Martin, D.C. & Barr, H.M. (1981). The Seattle longitudinal prospective study on alcohol and pregnancy. *Neurobehavioral Toxicology and Teratology*, **3**, 323–33.

Strömland, K. (1987). Ocular involvement in the fetal alcohol syndrome. *Survey of Ophthalmology*, **31**, 277–84.

Sulaiman, N.D., Flore, E.V., Taylor, D.J. & Ogston, S.A. (1988). Alcohol consumption in Dundee primigravidas and its effects on outcome of pregnancy. *British Medical Journal*, **296**, 1500–3.

Tanaka, H., Arima, M. & Suzuki, N. (1981). The fetal alcohol syndrome in Japan. *Brain and Development*, **3**, 305–11.

Tanaka, H., Nakazawa, K., Suzuki, N. & Arima, M. (1982). Prevention possibility for brain dysfunction in rat with the fetal alcohol syndrome: low-zinc-status and hypoglycemia. *Brain and Development*, **4**, 429–38.

Véghelyi, P.V., Osztovics, M., Kardos, G., Leisztner, L., Szaszovensky, E., Igali, S. & Imrei, J. (1978). The fetal alcohol syndrome: symptoms and pathogenesis. *Acta Paediatrica Hungarica*, **19**, 171–89.

Volk, B. (1987). Klinisch-neuropathologische Befunde und experimentelle Untersuchungen zur Alkoholembryopathie. In *Die Alkoholembryopathie*, ed. F. Majewski, pp. 89–101. Frankfurt: Umwelt und Medizin.

Wiesniewski, K., Dambska, M., Shev, J.H. & Quazi, Q. (1983). A clinical neuropathological study of the fetal alcohol syndrome. *Neuropediatrics*, **14**, 197–201.

3

Alcohol use during pregnancy and its effects on developmental outcome

MONIQUE KAMINSKI AND BEATRICE LARROQUE

Introduction

The consequences for the child of very heavy drinking during pregnancy are now well established, and are described in Chapters 2, 11 and 12 of this book. The present chapter concentrates on the potential effects of moderate alcohol consumption during pregnancy. These effects are expected to be of the same nature as those observed in fetal alcohol syndrome (FAS) but more moderate. They include intrauterine growth retardation, specific craniofacial features, and signs of central nervous system dysfunctioning. These effects are much less dramatic than FAS but may affect many more children.

The first part of the chapter describes the population at risk, the level of alcohol use by women of reproductive age, and the characteristics of the heavier drinkers. The second part reviews the association of alcohol consumption with subfecundity and adverse pregnancy outcome. The third part discusses the links between alcohol consumption during pregnancy and the condition of the child at birth and during the neonatal period. The potential consequences of moderate alcohol exposure *in utero* for later child development are discussed in Chapters 8–10. Although child development is the major public health issue related to prenatal alcohol exposure, the physical and neurobehavioral characteristics of the newborn can help identify at-risk children and enable suitable care to be initiated. Furthermore, knowing how these characteristics are affected by prenatal alcohol exposure helps to improve our knowledge about the mechanisms involved in the effects of alcohol on the fetus.

The issue of alcohol consumption during pregnancy has been the subject of a large number of studies. The selection of papers cited here gives priority to recent studies in which a quantitative assessment of alcohol consumption was attempted. We selected studies that included data on alcohol consumption

41

during pregnancy, and not only prior to pregnancy, and that were not centered on women who were alcoholics or very heavy drinkers. Most of the studies reviewed are prospective, i.e., data on alcohol consumption were collected *before* delivery, thus minimizing the risk of direct bias when measuring the association between alcohol consumption and the condition of the child. However, a small number of retrospective studies have been included that were especially informative on specific points.

The analysis of the effects of moderate alcohol consumption in pregnancy raises many methodological questions that have serious consequences for the interpretation of the results of epidemiological studies. These methodological considerations will be discussed whenever relevant.

In most studies alcohol consumption is recorded in number of drinks (glasses) per type of alcoholic beverage per day or week. It is often assumed that the average absolute alcohol content of a standard glass of beer, wine, or spirit is approximately the same, i.e., about 10 g (Goddard, 1991). We have adopted this approximate measure in this chapter.

Alcohol use by women

Alcohol use by women of reproductive age

In general, in European and North American countries women drink less alcohol than men. Even the most recent data (Plant, 1990) report that they are more often abstainers, that, when they do drink alcohol, they drink less in quantity, and that they are less often affected by diseases linked to heavy alcohol consumption. The types of alcoholic beverages consumed by women and by men differ, and there are variations by age and by country (Goddard, 1991; Guignon, 1994).

In some countries, surveys on random samples of the general population provide estimates of alcohol consumption and characteristics of the heavier drinkers. In England and Wales in 1990 (Smyth & Browne, 1992), 9% of women aged 18–24 years and 7% of women aged 25–44 years were abstainers, whereas 17% of the younger group and 13% of the older group consumed at least 15 drinks per week. After controlling for age, the percentage of these heavier drinkers was higher among married than among unmarried women, especially for married women without dependent children. This percentage also increased with higher socioeconomic status and higher household income.

In France, in 1991–2 (Guignon, 1994), contrary to the observation made in England and Wales, daily alcohol consumption of women increased with age: the percentage of women who consumed at least three drinks per day increased from 1.5% at 20–24 years to 6% at 35–44 years of age. The level of alcohol consumption was higher among women with less qualified occupations and for those at the two extremes of the household income distribution. There was no difference regarding marital status. Data from the United States in 1988 and 1990 (Williams & Debakey, 1992; Midanik & Clark, 1994) showed that regular heavier consumption (at least 14 drinks per week) did not vary with age between 18 and 44 years, whereas binge drinking was more frequent among the younger women. As in France, heavier regular drinking was more frequent when family income was either very low or very high.

Alcohol consumption during pregnancy

There are no recent national data available on the level of alcohol consumption by pregnant women. However, there is now good evidence from many countries that many women stop drinking or decrease their alcohol consumption when they are pregnant; these changes in behavior often occur during the first trimester of the pregnancy and are associated with a decrease in tobacco and coffee consumption (Rosett *et al.*, 1983; Halmesmaki *et al.*, 1987; Johnson *et al.*, 1987; Plant, 1987; Smith *et al.*, 1987; Kaminski *et al.*, 1989; Waterson & Murray-Lyon, 1989*b*, 1990). These changes in behavior are often associated with either nausea or loss of taste for alcohol during pregnancy (Little & Hook, 1979; Plant, 1987; Heller *et al.*, 1988; Waterson & Murray-Lyon, 1989*b*; Lelong *et al.*, 1995). But when pregnant women are asked why they decreased alcohol consumption during pregnancy, concern for the health of the child is often mentioned (Waterson & Murray-Lyon, 1989*b*; Lelong *et al.*, 1995).

Most pregnant women know that alcohol use during pregnancy may not be safe for the child, although the level of consumption described as reasonable during pregnancy may vary from 0 to 4 or more drinks per day (Lelong *et al.*, 1995; Kaminski *et al.*, 1995). Awareness of the risks linked to 'heavy' drinking during pregnancy is also high in the general population, at least in the United States (Little *et al.*, 1981; Fox *et al.*, 1987).

In contrast with this optimistic image of knowledge about and behavior towards alcohol during pregnancy, it should be noted that the women who are the heavier drinkers before pregnancy are those who modify their behavior least while pregnant (Smith *et al.*, 1987; Waterson & Murray-Lyon, 1989*b*; Lelong *et al.*, 1995). They are also those who describe least often a loss of taste for alcohol, and they are less aware of the potential dangers of alcohol during pregnancy. These women are also the least affected by interventions aimed at a reduction of alcohol consumption by pregnant women (Streissguth *et al.*, 1983*b*; Olsen *et al.*, 1989). Moreover, in contrast to smoking, pregnant women mention having received very little advice regarding alcohol consumption, either from doctors and midwives or from their family (Waterson & Murray-Lyon, 1989*b*; Lelong *et al.*, 1995).

In most countries, heavier alcohol use is often associated with tobacco use and coffee consumption (Smith *et al.*, 1987; Heller *et al.*, 1988; Walpole *et al.*, 1989; Lelong *et al.*, 1995). In the United States, the use of illegal drugs is also more common among the heavier alcohol consumers (Johnson *et al.*, 1987; Smith *et al.*, 1987; Day *et al.*, 1989). In addition, as for smoking, the alcohol consumption of the pregnant women is highly correlated with that of the father of the child (Smith *et al.*, 1987; Waterson *et al.*, 1990; Lelong *et al.*, 1995).

In contrast to these common patterns of behavior in different countries, the social and demographic characteristics of the heavier alcohol users during pregnancy vary according to country, as they do in the general population. In a European study that included seven countries (EUROMAC, 1992) the heavier drinkers during pregnancy were older than the abstainers or lighter drinkers in all countries except Denmark, and they were of a lower social status in all countries apart from Germany. In contrast, in the United States and Australia the heavier drinkers seem to have a higher social level (Johnson *et al.*, 1987; Walpole *et al.*, 1989).

The above description of characteristics associated with alcohol use during pregnancy points to the need for appropriate control of confounders in the analysis of the relations between alcohol consumption and pregnancy outcome. Unfortunately, major confounding factors were not always controlled for in the literature reviewed below, and confounding due to absence of control or insufficient control for covariates may partly explain apparently contradictory results.

Alcohol use and pregnancy outcome

Infertility and subfecundity

Only a small number of studies have investigated the role of women's moderate alcohol consumption in infertility or subfecundity. In two studies, infertility was found to be more frequent among moderate alcohol consumers. In the first study the increased risk was limited to primary (as opposed to secondary) infertility (Olsen *et al.*, 1983*b*). In the second study, the increase in risk involved infertility associated with ovulatory factors or endometriosis (as opposed to other causes) (Grodstein *et al.*, 1994). A third study (Joesoef *et al.*, 1993) did not find any relation between primary infertility and alcohol consumption; however the threshold of 'heavy' consumption was low, (5 drinks per week, compared with at least 10 in the other two studies). Among fertile women, there was no association between alcohol consumption and time to conception, an indicator of subfecundity (Olsen *et al.*, 1983*b*; Joesoef *et al.*, 1993).

Spontaneous abortion and fetal wastage

Two early, well-controlled studies showed an increased risk of spontaneous abortion with relatively low levels of alcohol consumption during pregnancy: an increased risk of second trimester abortion for the consumption of 1–2 drinks per day (Harlap & Shiono, 1980) and even an increased risk of first or second trimester abortion for the consumption of about 4 drinks per week (Kline *et al.*, 1980). Three studies have recently confirmed these results, although for slightly higher levels of consumption (Russell & Skinner, 1988; Armstrong *et al.*, 1992; Windham *et al.*, 1992). Although one study failed to demonstrate an association between alcohol consumption and unexplained recurrent spontaneous abortions (Parazzini *et al.*, 1990), the overall evidence is in favor of an effect of alcohol during pregnancy on spontaneous abortion. In addition, Anokute (1986) found a dose–effect relationship between alcohol consumption and total fetal wastage (spontaneous abortions and stillbirths), but confounders other than tobacco were not considered. Walpole *et al.* (1989) did not find a similar relation, but the number of cases of fetal wastage in their study was low. To the best of our knowledge, no study has investigated the potential risk of ectopic pregnancy in relation to alcohol consumption.

Stillbirths were also found to be more common among women who drank heavily during pregnancy (Kaminski *et al.*, 1976), and the main cause of death associated with alcohol was abruptio placentae (Goujard *et al.*, 1978). These results were found in a large-scale study carried out in the 1960s. This study included a high number of moderate drinkers, and at that time the stillbirth rate was still high. These results have not been replicated in more recent, smaller-scale studies with lower stillbirth rates (Kaminski *et al.*, 1981; Davis *et al.*, 1982; Marbury *et al.*, 1983; Plant, 1987). However, a higher risk of abruptio placentae was also found by Marbury *et al.* (1983).

Condition of the child at birth

Apgar scores and respiratory distress syndrome

Conflicting results have been observed for Apgar scores and respiratory distress syndrome. Streissguth *et al.* (1981), Marbury *et al.* (1983), Lumley *et al.* (1985), Plant (1987), Russell & Skinner (1988), and Sulaiman *et al.* (1988) found depressed Apgar scores at 1 minute or 5 minutes in association with maternal alcohol consumption, whereas other studies did not find such an association (Ouellette *et al.*, 1977; Davis *et al.*, 1982; Coles *et al.*, 1985). No relation was found by Marbury *et al.* (1983) between alcohol consumption and respiratory distress syndrome. Ioffe & Chernick (1987) observed a higher rate of respiratory distress syndrome with heavier maternal alcohol consumption among term infants, whereas the rate of respiratory distress syndrome for preterm babies was lower with heavier maternal alcohol consumption. The authors explained this last result by the role of alcohol in accelerating fetal lung maturation.

Length of gestation and preterm delivery

A significant relation between alcohol consumption during (and in one instance before) pregnancy and length of gestation has been described in several studies; the results showed either a shorter mean length of gestation (Tennes & Blackard, 1980; Hingson *et al.*, 1982; Rosett *et al.*, 1983; Lumley *et al.*, 1985; Little *et al.*, 1986; Sulaiman *et al.*, 1988) or a higher preterm delivery rate (Ouellette *et al.*, 1977; Berkowitz, 1981; Kaminski *et al.*, 1981; Little *et al.*, 1986; Shiono *et al.*, 1986; McDonald *et al.*, 1992*a*) among heavier alcohol consumers. However, other studies failed to find such a relation (Kaminski *et al.*, 1976; Davis *et al.*, 1982; Marbury *et al.*, 1983; Mills *et al.*, 1984; Kaminski *et al.*, 1989; Verkerk *et al.*, 1993). Also, in several of the studies that did find a significant relation between alcohol consumption and length of gestation, the association was not very strong (Tennes & Blackard, 1980; Lumley *et al.*, 1985; Shiono *et al.*, 1986). In one of the studies (Ouellette *et al.*, 1977), the level of consumption was very high. In several instances, potential confounders were not or insufficiently controlled for, especially regarding social characteristics, which are major risk factors for preterm delivery and which are often associated with heavier drinking, as described above.

Intrauterine growth characteristics

Birth weight

Birth weight is the outcome variable that has been considered most often in relation to prenatal alcohol exposure. In the majority of studies that have analyzed average birth weight by level of maternal alcohol consumption, a significant decrease in birth weight with increasing alcohol consumption has been found (Kaminski *et al.*, 1976, 1981; Little, 1977; Streissguth *et al.*, 1981; Kuzma & Sokol, 1982; Olsen *et al.*, 1983*a*, 1991; Rosett *et al.*, 1983; Mills *et al.*, 1984; Lumley *et al.*, 1985; Little *et al.*, 1986; Smith *et al.*, 1986; Plant, 1987; EUROMAC, 1992; Larroque *et al.*, 1993). However, no significant association was found in other studies (Tennes & Blackard, 1980; Kaminski *et al.*, 1981; Davis *et al.*, 1982; Hingson *et al.*, 1982; Marbury *et al.*, 1983; Ernhart *et al.*, 1985; Russell & Skinner, 1988; Sulaiman *et al.*, 1988; Day *et al.*, 1989). In most studies that looked at variations of the rate of low birth weight or low weight for gestational age, as related to the level of maternal alcohol consumption, a significantly higher rate of low birth weight among babies of heavier drinkers was found (Kaminski *et al.*, 1976; Ouellette *et al.*, 1977; Rosett *et al.*, 1983; Wright *et al.*, 1983; Mills *et al.*, 1984; Lumley *et al.*, 1985; Little *et al.*, 1986; Day *et al.*, 1989; Olsen *et al.*, 1991; McDonald *et al.*, 1992*a*). Such an association was not found in only a small number of studies (Tennes & Blackard, 1980; Kaminski *et al.*, 1981; Marbury *et al.*, 1983). Results were consistent in most studies that analysed birth weight both in a quantitative way and as a qualitative variable (low birth weight or small-for-dates).

In addition, it has been observed that placental weight was also diminished with maternal alcohol consumption (Kaminski *et al.*, 1976; Olsen *et al.*, 1991), contrary to what is observed with smoking. This observation suggests that alcohol and tobacco affect birth weight through mechanisms that are at least partly different.

From studies on birth weight that have been analyzed after grouping the quantity of alcohol consumed into categories, it is possible to discuss a level of alcohol consumption above which birth weight seems to be affected. The review by Larroque (1992) shows that significant relations between alcohol consumption and birth weight were found in most large prospective studies in which the heavier drinkers consumed at least 2–3 drinks per day, although one very large study found a lower birth weight at 1 drink per day (Mills *et al.*, 1984). This observation does not mean that 1 or 2 drinks per day could be considered a biological threshold. First, underreporting of alcohol consumption, even independently from outcome, may mask a threshold effect or underestimate the value of the threshold (Verkerk, 1992); thus the actual level of risk could be higher than the values mentioned above. Second, if we assume that alcohol affects birth weight (or any other outcome measure) in a dose-dependent manner, we expect the response to be smaller with lower levels of exposure. To detect small effects, very large-scale studies are needed, and yet the effects might be too small to be clinically detectable.

Alcohol affects birth weight to a lesser degree than does smoking. A decrease of 80 g is reported for moderate drinking, and of up to 160 g for heavier drinking (Mills *et al.*, 1984) as compared with about 200 g for smoking (EUROMAC, 1992).

In a few studies, the data collected permitted the changes in alcohol consumption during pregnancy to be monitored, and the comparison of the outcome according to whether or not the heavier drinkers had ceased drinking or had reduced their alcohol consumption at some stage of pregnancy. Such studies have shown that a decrease in alcohol consumption during pregnancy was associated with an average birth weight (and other growth parameters) intermediate between those of babies born to women who drank not at all or only lightly and to women who continued to drink heavily (Rosett *et al.*, 1983; Smith *et al.*, 1986).

One question that is often asked relates to the potential risks of occasional binge drinking in otherwise moderate drinkers. Evidence from the literature is limited for several reasons. First, the information is difficult to collect precisely. Also, binge drinking is more common among regular heavier drinkers than among light drinkers, and thus the two indicators can be highly correlated. However, one recent study found that, among light and moderate drinkers, occasional binge drinking either just before pregnancy or in the first 6 months was not associated with lower birth weight or with any other growth characteristic (Tolo & Little, 1993).

Some studies seem to suggest that beer may have a stronger effect on birth weight than other alcoholic beverages (Kaminski *et al.*, 1976, 1981; Kuzma & Sokol, 1982; Sulaiman *et al.*, 1988). Although beer contains several potentially toxic components, the social characteristics of beer drinkers or a more accurate declaration of beer consumption may play a role in this result.

Most studies found no difference in birth weight between babies born to abstainers and women who were light drinkers during pregnancy. However, in several cases the optimal outcome (for example, the highest average birth weight) was observed not among abstainers but among light drinkers (Marbury *et al.*, 1983; Lumley *et al.*, 1985; EUROMAC, 1992). There are several explanations for such an observation: (1) misclassification of heavy drinkers who deny alcohol consumption as abstainers, (2) diseases in which abstinence from alcohol is advised or psychological characteristics that may put women at risk of complications of pregnancy. Similar results have been observed concerning alcohol consumption before pregnancy, with an even larger difference between abstainers and light drinkers. Biological explanations are discussed by Little & MacGillivray (1995).

In two recent studies, a significant effect of alcohol on birth weight was observed only for babies of smokers (Brooke *et al.*, 1989; Verkerk *et al.*, 1993). Further data from the first of these studies showed similar results for ponderal index, crown–heel length, and head circumference (Haste *et al.*, 1991). Two more studies found a stronger relation of alcohol with birth weight among babies of smokers than nonsmokers (Wright *et al.*, 1983; Olsen *et al.*, 1991). But, in several other instances in which an interaction between smoking and alcohol consumption was said to have been sought, no significant interaction was reported (Kuzma & Sokol, 1982; Mills *et al.*, 1984; Little *et al.*, 1986; Russell & Skinner, 1988; Larroque *et al.*, 1993). When an interaction was observed, the absence of a relation between maternal alcohol consumption and birth weight of babies in non-smokers might be due to the very small number of heavier drinkers among nonsmokers, as in the studies of Wright *et al.* (1983) and Brooke *et al.* (1989), or to a lower level of alcohol consumption by the heavier drinkers who do not smoke than by the heavier drinkers who smoke. Another explanation might be a residual confounding effect of tobacco, i.e., among smokers the number of cigarettes smoked might be higher for the heavier drinkers than for the abstainers or light drinkers. Such hypotheses are supported by the association between alcohol consumption and tobacco use described in the first part of this chapter. Also, the observation made above concerning the differences in the way tobacco and alcohol affect the placenta does not support the hypothesis of a biological interaction of the two substances with regard to intrauterine growth.

Crown–heel length

The literature contains more contradictory evidence regarding the potential effect of prenatal alcohol exposure on length at birth than on birth weight. Although some studies did find a shorter length with heavier alcohol use (Ouellette *et al.*, 1977; Streissguth *et al.*, 1981; Rosett *et al.*, 1983; Little *et al.*, 1986; Smith *et al.*, 1986; EUROMAC, 1992), a larger number of studies did not find such a relation (Tennes & Blackard, 1980; Kaminski *et al.*, 1981; Hingson *et al.*, 1982; Olsen *et al.*, 1983a; Ernhart *et al.*, 1985; Russell &

Skinner, 1988; Day *et al.*, 1989). In all studies in which crown–heel length was significantly linked to maternal alcohol consumption, there was also a significant association with birth weight.

Head circumference

Contrary to the findings for crown–heel length, head circumference at birth was more often than not associated with alcohol consumption. A smaller head circumference was found for children born to women who consumed alcohol during pregnancy, even in some studies in which birth weight was not significantly associated with alcohol consumption (Ouellette *et al.*, 1977; Streissguth *et al.*, 1981; Davis *et al.*, 1982; Little *et al.*, 1986; Smith *et al.*, 1986; Sulaiman *et al.*, 1988; Day *et al.*, 1989). However, no association was found in other studies (Tennes & Blackard, 1980; Kaminski *et al.*, 1981; Hingson *et al.*, 1982; Rosett *et al.*, 1983; Ernhart *et al.*, 1985; Russell & Skinner, 1988; EUROMAC, 1992).

Congenital anomalies

A small number of studies have found a higher rate of nonspecific congenital anomalies among children of women who were heavy alcohol consumers during pregnancy. However, in one study (Ouellette *et al.*, 1977) this excess risk was limited to very heavy drinkers. In the second study (Lumley *et al.*, 1985) and in the third (Rosett *et al.*, 1983) the numbers of heavy drinkers were very small, and in the fourth (Davis *et al.*, 1982) the trend was inconsistent. Several other studies, including large-scale studies, did not find any relation between alcohol consumption and major congenital defects (Kaminski *et al.*, 1976; Hingson *et al.*, 1982; Marbury *et al.*, 1983; Mills & Graubard, 1987; EUROMAC, 1992; McDonald *et al.*, 1992b).

In contrast, most studies that have investigated specific anomalies similar to the characteristics observed in FAS have found that the frequency of these anomalies was higher and they were more numerous among children of heavier drinkers than among children of abstainers or light drinkers. Hanson *et al.* (1978) and Coles *et al.* (1985) found that the proportion of children affected by anomalies compatible with a prenatal effect of alcohol on growth and morphogenesis tended to be higher among heavier drinkers. In the first of these studies alcohol consumption just before pregnancy was a stronger predictor than alcohol consumption in midpregnancy. Similar results were found by Day *et al.* (1989) for alcohol consumption during the first month of pregnancy. Two studies did not find a similar relation; however, one involved a small sample with few 'heavy' drinkers (Tennes & Blackard, 1980) and the second was very restrictive in identifying children affected by signs compatible with a prenatal alcohol effect (Hingson *et al.*, 1982).

In two studies (Ernhart *et al.*, 1985; Rostand *et al.*, 1990) standardized morphological assessments were carried out to collect systematic information for a list of anomalies compatible with prenatal alcohol effects; scores were calculated from these lists of anomalies. The first study included all types of anomalies, whereas the second included only craniofacial anomalies. Both studies found an association between maternal alcohol consumption and the scores; however, in the first study the association was stronger for the sub-score of craniofacial anomalies (Ernhart *et al.*, 1987), which is consistent with the results of the second study. When intrauterine growth retardation and craniofacial anomalies were considered together, the association with alcohol exposure *in utero* was even stronger (Rostand *et al.*, 1990). Both studies suggest a dose–response relationship. Ernhart *et al.* (1987) believed that these anomalies were linked more strongly to prepregnancy and first trimester alcohol consumption than to consumption later in pregnancy. In contrast, Rostand *et al.* (1990) showed that among women who were heavy drinkers before pregnancy, the children of those who became abstainers or light drinkers during pregnancy had a score for anomalies significantly lower than the children of women who remained heavy drinkers during pregnancy.

In summary, moderate to heavy alcohol consumption during pregnancy in non-alcoholic women does not increase the risk of major congenital malformation but is associated with an increase in the number of specific craniofacial minor anomalies.

Neonatal neurobehavioral status

The Brazelton Neonatal Behavioural Assessment Scale (NBAS) has been used in several studies to investigate whether and how moderate prenatal alcohol exposure affects the behavior of the newborn. One study did not find any relation between maternal alcohol consumption and NBAS scores, except for one case that contradicted the hypothesis (Ernhart *et al.*, 1985). In all other studies at least one dimension of behavior was significantly affected by prenatal alcohol exposure; however, there was no consistency between studies in the aspects of behavior found to be associated with alcohol exposure. Streissguth *et al.* (1983*a*) observed that maternal alcohol consumption during pregnancy was associated with poorer habituation to repetitive stimuli and with low arousal. Another study (Jacobson *et al.*, 1984), which included only a very small number of moderate drinkers, found that alcohol consumption in pregnancy affected the 'range of state' dimension of the NBAS, with the

children of alcohol users showing a greater placidity than other children. In
the study by Smith *et al.* (1986), children of mothers who consumed alcohol
during pregnancy showed decreased scores on orientation, i.e., ability to
attend to auditory and visual stimuli, and on autonomic regulation, i.e., stability in responses. The same study also showed an association of prenatal
alcohol exposure with alterations in reflexive behavior, less mature motor
behavior, and increased level of activity (Coles *et al.*, 1985). These results
are in line with clinical observations made previously by Ouellette *et al.*
(1977) and Landesman-Dwyer *et al.* (1978).

Another assessment method was used by Walpole *et al.* (1991), i.e., the
Einstein Neonatal Behavioural Assessment Schedule. In this study only a
weak association of alcohol with muscle tonus was observed. Coles and
Smith (Coles *et al.*, 1985; Smith *et al.*, 1986) also compared women who
were all heavy drinkers during the second trimester of pregnancy but who
either stopped drinking before the end of the pregnancy or continued
throughout the pregnancy, with women who did not drink at all. Their
findings show that, for most of the behavioral and motor indicators analyzed,
the children of the women who stopped drinking had intermediate outcomes
between those of children whose mothers did not drink at all and children
whose mothers continued drinking alcohol throughout pregnancy, independent of the quantity of alcohol consumed.

Experiments conducted on newborn conditioning showed that children of
both heavier drinkers and heavier smokers had poorer operant learning on a
head-turning and an operant-sucking task (Martin *et al.*, 1977).

A clinical observation of poor sucking and decreased ability to suck was
made by Ouellette *et al.* (1977) in children of heavy drinkers. This was confirmed in an experimental study by Martin *et al.* (1979). This study found
that the time to initiate sucking and the intensity of sucking pressure were
correlated with alcohol consumption before pregnancy: the children of heavier alcohol drinkers were found to be poorer suckers.

Sleep disturbances have also been reported in association with prenatal
alcohol exposure. Rosett *et al.* (1979) observed that children of heavy drinkers
had a shorter duration of sleep, a poorer quality of quiet sleep, were more
often restless, and had more body movements. Electroencephalogram (EEG)
analyses have shown increased integrated EEG power in at-term children of
women who were heavy drinkers (at least 4 drinks per day) during pregnancy.
These observations were recorded for quiet, intermediate, and active sleep,
but the difference compared with children of nondrinkers was especially
marked in the active sleep phase (Chernick *et al.*, 1983). The same study
was repeated with children of gestational age 30–40 weeks who were born

to more moderate alcohol drinkers; the same results were observed at all gestational ages for both active and quiet sleep. Furthermore, 'binge' drinking seemed to affect the EEG more than chronic moderate drinking (Ioffe & Chernick, 1988). Another group (Scher *et al.*, 1988) found that lower levels of alcohol consumption (at least 1 drink per day) during the first and second trimester were associated with an increased number of arousals, whereas alcohol consumption in the first trimester was associated with disruptions in sleep state cycling.

All the above results are indications that prenatal alcohol exposure can affect the development and maturation of the central nervous system. Consistent with these results, a recent study has shown that, in the population of very premature babies of less than 31 weeks gestation, the risk of brain hemorrhage and white matter damage was significantly increased with prenatal alcohol exposure at relatively low levels (at least 1 drink per day or 3 or more drinks per occasion) (Holzman *et al.*, 1995). This higher risk of brain injury in premature babies of alcohol drinkers might be explained by the role of alcohol in delayed maturation of the brain and/or by the effect of alcohol on cerebral blood circulation.

For valid analysis, the assocation between alcohol consumption and any outcome variable must be studied after controlling for confounding variables. Many of the outcome variables we have described have several known determinants, such as maternal age, parity, social class, and tobacco, all of which are often related to alcohol consumption. In several studies, crude associations disappeared or decreased in size after confounding variables were controlled for (Marbury *et al.*, 1983; Russell & Skinner, 1988; Sulaiman *et al.*, 1988). Tobacco use, which is the main confounder for growth characteristics, has usually been controlled for.

On the other hand, there is a need to avoid overadjustment. Overadjustment can occur when controlling for birth weight in the association between prenatal alcohol exposure and neonatal neurological or behavioral variables (Scher *et al.*, 1988; Walpole *et al.*, 1991). Alcohol can affect birth weight as well as neurobehavioral status and, if the neurobehavioral status varies according to birth weight, controlling for birth weight may erroneously lead to the conclusion of an absence of effect of alcohol on neonatal neurobehavior (Kiely, 1991).

Conclusion

The literature reviewed shows that moderate to heavy alcohol consumption in nonalcoholic pregnant women is associated with an increased risk of adverse pregnancy outcome, intrauterine growth retardation (especially regarding birth weight), morphological anomalies (in particular minor craniofacial anomalies), and neurobehavioral signs of central nervous system dysfunction. Such associations were found, in most cases, for an equivalent average daily consumption of at least 1–2 drinks. There is good evidence from epidemiological as well as experimental studies that this association is causal (see Chapters 4–6). Yet, many questions remain unanswered because of insufficient scientific knowledge. We will conclude this chapter by discussing the most crucial of these questions.

The first question is the actual threshold of risk. Many methodological difficulties make it very difficult to answer this question. There are no valid biological markers of moderate alcohol consumption and, in spite of the risk of underreporting, especially among heavier drinkers, detailed questionnaires remain the best instrument for measuring alcohol exposure (Waterson & Murray-Lyon, 1989*a*). However, Da Costa Pereira *et al.* (1993) have shown how the reported consumption varied with the stage of pregnancy and the type of questionnaire used. Whereas some women may have a regular pattern of alcohol consumption, others may experience wide variations from day to day or from week to week (Goddard, 1991).

Moreover, as the risks of moderate alcohol consumption in pregnancy are better known in the population, one can expect an increase in feelings of guilt and unease among pregnant alcohol consumers, leading to an increase in underreporting. However, there is evidence of an actual decrease in alcohol consumption over recent years (Kaminski *et al.*, 1995). If one adds the need for very large studies to detect small effects to all these sources of misclassification and, thus, of bias in the estimation of risk, one can see why the identification of a threshold is so difficult.

Another question concerns the period of greatest susceptibility, i.e., the stage of pregnancy at which alcohol consumption would be particularly dangerous. There is currently no clear answer to this question. We have seen above that ceasing to drink during the second part of pregnancy was associated with better outcomes, thus showing that alcohol can affect growth and development during all stages of pregnancy. Other studies have found that alcohol consumption prior to pregnancy, which can be considered as a proxy for alcohol consumption around the time of conception, was more strongly associated with morphological or neurological anomalies than was alcohol consumption during midpregnancy. These results are not contradictory, as the period of highest susceptibility may vary according to the type of anomaly or delay in development. Again, irregularity in the patterns of alcohol consumption makes it difficult for epidemiological studies to answer this question precisely.

There has been little research concerning how alcohol interacts with other factors such as other toxic agents, malnutrition, and maternal diseases that are linked to or independent of heavy alcohol consumption. One exception to this concerns the potential interaction of alcohol and tobacco on growth characteristics, the evidence for which, as we have seen above, is not conclusive.

The last question we will raise is that of the individual variability of effects in response to similar levels of exposure to alcohol. One explanation might be found in variations of genetic origin in the susceptibility of the mother and/or the child to alcohol effects, a field that has not yet been seriously investigated.

These issues are the ones we think further research should try to confront in a multidisciplinary approach. Animal experiments are necessary to complement epidemiological studies when the multiple factors involved in human alcohol consumption cannot be controlled, although we know that extrapolation from animals to humans is not easy. Progress in identification of biological indicators of alcohol consumption and of markers of genetic susceptibility to alcohol effects would be very valuable for future epidemiological research.

Acknowledgments

The authors thank Blandine Yemmou for her help in the preparation of the manuscript.

References

Anokute, C.C. (1986). Epidemiology of spontaneous abortions: the effects of alcohol consumption and cigarette smoking. *Journal of the National Medical Association*, **78**, 771–5.

Armstrong, B.G., McDonald, A. & Sloan, M. (1992). Cigarette, alcohol and coffee consumption and spontaneous abortion. *American Journal of Public Health*, **82**, 85–7.

Berkowitz, G.S. (1981). An epidemiologic study of preterm delivery. *American Journal of Epidemiology*, **113**, 81–92.

Brooke, O.G., Anderson, H.R., Bland, J.M., Peacock, J.L. & Stewart, C.M. (1989). Effects on birth weight of smoking, alcohol, caffeine, socioeconomic factors, and psychosocial stress. *British Medical Journal*, **298**, 795–801.

Chernick, V., Childiaeva, R. & Ioffe, S. (1983). Effects of maternal alcohol intake and smoking on neonatal electroencephalogram and anthropometric measurements. *American Journal of Obstetrics and Gynecology*, **146**, 41–7.

Coles, C.D., Smith, I.,Fernhoff, P.M. & Falek, A. (1985). Neonatal neurobehavioral characteristics as correlates of maternal alcohol use during gestation. *Alcoholism: Clinical and Experimental Research*, **9**, 454–60.

Da Costa Pereira, A., Olsen, J. & Ogston, S. (1993). Variability of self-reported measures of alcohol consumption: implications for the association between drinking in pregnancy and birth weight. *Journal of Epidemiology and Community Health*, **47**, 326–30.

Davis, P.J., Partridge, J.W. & Storrs, C.N. (1982). Alcohol consumption in pregnancy. How much is safe? *Archives of Disease in Childhood*, **57**, 940–3.

Day, N.L., Jasperse, D., Richardson, G., Robles, N., Sambamoorthi, U., Taylor, P., Scher, M., Stoffer, D. & Cornelius, M. (1989). Prenatal exposure to alcohol: effect on infant growth and morphologic characteristics. *Pediatrics*, **84**, 536–41.

Ernhart, C.B., Sokol, R.J., Martier, S., Moron, P., Nadler, D., Ager, J.W. & Wolf, A. (1987). Alcohol teratogenicity in the human: a detailed assessment of specificity, critical period and threshold. *American Journal of Obstetrics and Gynecology*, **156**, 33–9.

Ernhart, C.B., Wolf, A.W., Linn, P.L., Sokol, R.J., Kennard, M.J. & Filipovich, H.F. (1985). Alcohol related birth defects: syndromal anomalies, intrauterine growth retardation, and neonatal behavioral assessment. *Alcoholism: Clinical and Experimental Research*, **9**, 447–53.

EUROMAC (1992). A European Concerted Action: maternal alcohol consumption and its relation to the outcome of pregnancy and child development at 18 months, ed. C. du V. Florey, D. Taylor, F. Bolumar, M. Kaminski & J. Olsen. *International Journal of Epidemiology*, **21**, Suppl. 1.

Fox, S.H., Brown, C., Koontz, A.M. & Kessel, S.S. (1987). Perception of risks of smoking and heavy drinking during pregnancy: 1985 NHS findings. *Public Health Reports*, **102**, 73–8.

Goddard, E. (1991). *Drinking in England and Wales in the Late 1980s*. OPCS, Social Survey Division. London: HMSO.

Goujard, J., Kaminski, M., Rumeau-Rouquette, C. & Schwartz, D. (1978). Maternal smoking, alcohol consumption, and abruptio placentae. *American Journal of Obstetrics and Gynecology*, **130**, 738–9.

Grodstein, F., Goldman, M.B. & Cramer, D.W. (1994). Infertility in women and moderate alcohol use. *American Journal of Public Health*, **84**, 1429–32.

Guignon, N. (1994). Les consommations d'alcool, de tabac et de psychotropes en France en 1991–92. *Solidarité-Santé*, **1**, 171–85.

Halmesmaki, E., Raivio, K.O. & Ylikorkala, O. (1987). Patterns of alcohol consumption during pregnancy. *Obstetrics and Gynecology*, **69**, 594–7.

Hanson, J.W., Streissguth, A.P. & Smith, D.W. (1978). The effects of moderate alcohol consumption during pregnancy on fetal growth and morphogenesis. *Pediatrics*, **62**, 457–60.

Harlap, S. & Shiono, P.H. (1980). Alcohol, smoking and incidence of spontaneous abortion in the first and second trimesters. *Lancet*, **ii**, 173–5.

Haste, F., Anderson, H., Brooke, O., Bland, J. & Peacock, J. (1991). The effects of smoking and drinking on the anthropometric measurements of neonates. *Paediatric and Perinatal Epidemiology*, **5**, 83–92.

Heller, J., Anderson, H.R., Bland, J.M., Brooke, O.G., Peacock, J.L. & Stewart, C.M. (1988). Alcohol in pregnancy; patterns and association with socio-economic, psychological and behavioral factors. *British Journal of Addiction*, **83**, 541–51.

Hingson, R., Alpert, J.J., Day, N., Dooling, E., Kaine, H., Morelock, S., Oppenheimer, E. & Zuckerman, B. (1982). Effects of maternal drinking and marijuana use on fetal growth and development. *Pediatrics*, **70**, 539–46.

Holzman, C., Paneth, N., Little, R., Pinto-Martin, J. & the Neonatal Brain Hemorrhage Study Team (1995). Perinatal brain injury in premature infants born to mothers using alcohol in pregnancy. *Pediatrics*, **95**, 66–73.

Ioffe, S. & Chernick, V. (1987). Maternal alcohol ingestion and the incidence of respiratory distress syndrome. *American Journal of Obstetrics and Gynecology*, **156**, 1231–5.

Ioffe, S. & Chernick, V. (1988). Development of the EEG between 30 and 40 weeks gestation in normal and alcohol exposed infants. *Developmental Medicine and Child Neurology*, **30**, 797–807.

Jacobson, S.W., Fein, G.G., Jacobson, J.L., Schwartz, P.M. & Dowler, J.K. (1984). Neonatal correlates of prenatal exposure to smoking, caffeine, and alcohol. *Infant Behavior and Development*, **7**, 253–65.

Joesoef, M.R., Beral, B., Aral, S.O., Rolfs, R.T. & Cramer, D.W. (1993). Fertility and use of cigarettes, alcohol, marijuana and cocaine. *Annals of Epidemiology*, **3**, 592–4.

Johnson, S.F., McCarter, R.J. & Ferencz, C. (1987). Changes in alcohol, cigarette, and recreational drug use during pregnancy: implications for intervention. *American Journal of Epidemiology*, **126**, 695–702.

Kaminski, M., Franc, M., Lebouvier, M., Du Mazaubrun, C. & Rumeau-Rouquette, C. (1981). Moderate alcohol use and pregnancy outcome. *Neurobehavioral Toxicology and Teratology*, **3**, 173–81.

Kaminski, M., Lelong, N., Bean, K., Chwalow, J. & Subtil, D. (1995). Change in alcohol, tobacco and coffee consumption in pregnant women: evolution between 1988 to 1992 in an area of high consumption. *European Journal of Obstetrics, Gynecology and Reproductive Biology*, **60**, 121–8.

Kaminski, M., Rostand, A., Lelong, N., Dehaene, P., Delestret, I., Klein-Bertrand, C., Querleu, D. & Crépin, G. (1989). Consommation d'alcool pendant la grossesse et caractéristiques néonatales. *Journal d'Alcoologie*, **1**, 35–46.

Kaminski, M., Rumeau-Rouquette, C. & Schwartz, D. (1976). Consommation d'alcool chez les femmes enceintes et issue de la grossesse. *Revue d'Epidémiologie et de Santé Publique*, **24**, 27–40.

Kiely, J.L. (1991). Some conceptual problems in multivariable analyses of perinatal mortality. *Paediatric and Perinatal Epidemiology*, **5**, 243–57.

Kline, J., Shrout, P., Stein, Z., Susser, M. & Warburton, D. (1980). Drinking during pregnancy and spontaneous abortion. *Lancet*, **ii**, 176–80.

Kuzma, J.W. & Sokol, R.J. (1982). Maternal drinking behavior and decreased uterine growth. *Alcoholism: Clinical and Experimental Research*, **6**, 396–402.

Landesman-Dwyer, S., Keller, L.S. & Streissguth, A.P. (1978). Naturalistic observations of newborns: effects of maternal alcohol intake. *Alcoholism: Clinical and Experimental Research*, **2**, 171–7.

Larroque, B. (1992). Alcohol and the fetus. *International Journal of Epidemiology*, **21**, Suppl. 1, 8–16.

Larroque, B., Kaminski, M., Lelong, N., Subtil, D. & Dehaene, P. (1993). Effects on birth weight of alcohol and caffeine consumption during pregnancy. *American Journal of Epidemiology*, **137**, 941–50.

Lelong, N., Kaminski, M., Chwalow, J., Bean, K. & Subtil, D. (1995). Attitudes and behavior of pregnant women and health professionals towards alcohol and tobacco consumption. *Patient Education and Counseling*, **25**, 39–49.

Little, R.E. (1977). Moderate alcohol use during pregnancy and decreased infant birth weight. *American Journal of Public Health*, **67**, 1154–6.

Little, R.E., Asker, R.L., Sampson, P.D. & Renwick, J.H. (1986). Fetal growth and moderate drinking in early pregnancy. *American Journal of Epidemiology*, **123**, 270–8.

Little, R.E. & Hook, E.B. (1979). Maternal alcohol and tobacco consumption and their association with nausea and vomiting during pregnancy. *Acta Obstetrica Scandinavica*, **58**, 15–17.

Little, R.E. & MacGillivray, J. (1995). Abstinence from alcohol before pregnancy and reproductive outcome. *Paediatric and Perinatal Epidemiology*, **9**, 105–8.

Little, R.E., Streissguth, A.P. & Guzinski, G.M. (1981). Public awareness and knowledge about the risks of drinking during pregnancy in Multiomah county. *American Journal of Public Health*, **71**, 312–14.

Lumley, J., Correy, J.F., Newman, N.M. & Curran, J.T. (1985). Cigarette smoking, alcohol consumption and fetal outcome in Tasmania 1981–82. *Australia and New Zealand Journal of Obstetrics and Gynaecology*, **25**, 33–40.

Marbury, M.C., Linn, S., Monson, R., Schoenbaum, S., Stubblefield, P.G. & Ryan, K.J. (1983). The association of alcohol consumption with outcome of pregnancy. *American Journal of Public Health*, **73**, 1165–8.

Martin, D.C., Martin, J.C., Lund, C.A. & Streissguth, A.P. (1979). Sucking frequency and amplitude in newborns as a function of maternal drinking and smoking. In *Currents in Alcoholism*, vol. V, ed. M. Galanter, pp. 359–65. New York: Grune and Stratton.

Martin, J., Martin, D.C., Lund, C.A. & Streissguth, A.P. (1977). Maternal alcohol ingestion and cigarette smoking and their effects on newborn conditioning. *Alcoholism: Clinical and Experimental Research*, **1**, 243–7.

McDonald, A.D., Armstrong, B.G. & Sloan, M. (1992a). Cigarette, alcohol and coffee consumption and prematurity. *American Journal of Public Health*, **82**, 87–90.

McDonald, A.D., Armstrong, B.G. & Sloan, M. (1992b). Cigarette, alcohol and coffee consumption and congenital defects. *American Journal of Public Health*, **82**, 91–3.

Midanik, L.T. & Clark, W.B. (1994). The demographic distribution of US drinking patterns in 1990: description and trends from 1984. *American Journal of Public Health*, **84**, 1218–22.

Mills, J.L. & Graubard, B.I. (1987). Is moderate drinking during pregnancy associated with an increased risk for malformations? *Pediatrics*, **80**, 309–14.

Mills, J.L., Graubard, B.I., Harley, E.E., Rhoads, G.G. & Berendes, H.W. (1984). Maternal alcohol consumption and birth weight. How much drinking during pregnancy is safe? *JAMA*, **252**, 1875–9.

Olsen, J., da Costa Pereira, A. & Olsen, F. (1991). Does maternal tobacco smoking modify the effect of alcohol on fetal growth? *American Journal of Public Health*, **81**, 69–73.

Olsen, J., Frische, G., Poulsen, A.O. & Kirchheiner, H. (1989). Changing smoking, drinking and eating behaviour among pregnant women in Denmark. *Scandinavian Journal of Social Medicine*, **17**, 277–80.

Olsen, J., Rachootin, P. & Schiodt, A.V. (1983a). Alcohol use, conception time, and birthweight. *Journal of Epidemiology and Community Health*, **37**, 63–5.

Olsen, J., Rachootin, P., Schiodt, A.V. & Damsbo, N. (1983b). Tobacco use, alcohol consumption and infertility. *International Journal of Epidemiology*, **12**, 179–84.

Ouellette, E., Rosett, H.L. & Rosman, N.P. (1977). Adverse effects on offspring of maternal alcohol abuse during pregnancy. *New England Journal of Medicine*, **297**, 528–30.

Parazzini, F., Bocciolone, L.A., La Vecchia, C., Negri, E. & Fedele, L. (1990). Maternal and paternal daily alcohol consumption and unexplained miscarriages. *British Journal of Obstetrics and Gynaecology*, **97**, 618–22.

Plant, M. (1987). *Women, Drinking, and Pregnancy*. London: Tavistock Publications.

Plant, M.L. (1990). *Women and Alcohol: A Review of International Literature on the Use of Alcohol by Females*. WHO, Regional Office for Europe.

Rosett, H., Snyder, P., Sander, P., Lee, A., Cook, P., Weiner, L. & Gould, J. (1979). Effect of maternal drinking on neonate state regulation. *Developmental Medicine and Child Neurology*, **21**, 467–73.

Rosett, H.L., Weiner, L., Lee, A., Zuckerman, B., Dooling, E. & Oppenheimer, E. (1983). Patterns of alcohol consumption and fetal development. *Obstetrics and Gynecology*, **61**, 539–46.

Rostand, A., Kaminski, M., Lelong, N., Dehaene, P., Delestret, I., Klein-Bertrand, C., Querleu, D. & Crépin, G. (1990). Alcohol use in pregnancy, craniofacial features, and fetal growth. *Journal of Epidemiology and Community Health*, **44**, 302–6.

Russell, M. & Skinner, J.B. (1988). Early measures of maternal alcohol use as predictors of adverse pregnancy outcome. *Alcohol: Clinical and Experimental Research*, **12**, 824–30.

Scher, M.S., Richardson, G.A., Coble, P.A., Day, N.L. & Stoffer, D.S. (1988). The effects of prenatal alcohol and marijuana exposure: disturbances in neonatal sleep cycling and arousal. *Pediatric Research*, **24**, 101–5.

Shiono, P.H., Klebanoff, M.A. & Rhoads, G.G. (1986). Smoking and drinking during pregnancy: their effects on preterm birth. *JAMA*, **255**, 82–4.

Smith, I.E., Coles, C.D., Lancaster, J., Fernhoff, P.M. & Falek, A. (1986). The effects of volume and duration of prenatal ethanol exposure on neonatal physical and behavioral development. *Neurobehavioral Toxicology and Teratology*, **8**, 375–81.

Smith, I.E., Lancaster, J.S., Moss-Wells, S., Coles, C.D. & Falek, A. (1987). Identifying high risk pregnant drinkers: biological and behavioral correlates of continuous heavy drinking during pregnancy. *Journal of Studies on Alcohol*, **48**, 304–9.

Smyth, M. & Browne, F. (1992). *General Household Survey*. OPCS Series GH5 no. 21. London: HMSO.

Streissguth, A.P., Barr, H.M. & Martin, D.C. (1983a). Maternal alcohol use and neonatal habituation assessed with the Brazelton Scale. *Child Development*, **54**, 1109–18.

Streissguth, A.P., Darby, B.L., Barr, H.M., Smith, J.R. & Martin, D.C. (1983b). Comparison of drinking and smoking patterns during pregnancy over a six year interval. *American Journal of Obstetrics and Gynecology*, **145**, 716–24.

Streissguth, A.P., Martin, D.C., Martin, J.C. & Barr, H.M. (1981). The Seattle longitudinal prospective study on alcohol and pregnancy. *Neurobehavioral Toxicology and Teratology*, **3**, 223–33.

Sulaiman, N.D., Florey, C. du V., Taylor, D.J. & Ogston, S.A. (1988). Alcohol consumption in Dundee primigravidas and its effects on outcome of pregnancy. *British Medical Journal*, **296**, 1500–3.

Tennes, K. & Blackard, C. (1980). Maternal alcohol consumption, birthweight, and minor physical anomalies. *American Journal of Obstetrics and Gynecology*, **138**, 774–80.

Tolo, K.A. & Little, R.E. (1993). Occasional binges by moderate drinkers: implications for birth outcomes. *Epidemiology*, **4**, 415–20.

Verkerk, P.H. (1992). The impact of alcohol misclassification on the relationship between alcohol and pregnancy outcome. *International Journal of Epidemiology*, **21**, Suppl. 1, 33–7.

Verkerk, P.H., Van Noord-Zaadstra, B.M., du V. Florey, C., de Jonge, G.A. & Verloove-Vanhorick, S.P. (1993). The effect of moderate alcohol consumption on birth weight and gestational age in a low risk population. *Early Human Development*, **32**, 121–9.

Walpole, I., Zubrick, S. & Pontré, J. (1989). Confounding variables in studying the effects of maternal alcohol consumption before and during pregnancy. *Journal of Epidemiology and Community Health*, **43**, 153–61.

Walpole, I., Zubrick, S., Pontré, J. & Lawrence, C. (1991). Low to moderate maternal alcohol use before and during pregnancy and neurobehavioral outcome in the newborn infant. *Developmental Medicine and Child Neurology*, **33**, 875–83.

Waterson, E.J., Evans, C. & Murray-Lyon, I.M. (1990). Is pregnancy a time of changing drinking and smoking patterns for fathers as well as mothers? An initial investigation. *British Journal of Addiction*, **85**, 389–96.

Waterson, E.J. & Murray-Lyon, I.M. (1989*a*). Screening for alcohol related problems in the antenatal clinic: an assessment of different methods. *Alcohol and Alcoholism*, **24**, 21–30.

Waterson, E.J. & Murray-Lyon, I.M. (1989*b*). Drinking and smoking patterns amongst women attending an antenatal clinic. II. During pregnancy. *Alcohol and Alcoholism*, **24**, 163–73.

Waterson, E.J. & Murray-Lyon, I.M. (1990). Preventing alcohol related birth damage: a review. *Social Science and Medicine*, **30**, 349–64.

Williams, G.D. & Debakey, S.F. (1992). Changes in levels of alcohol consumption: United States. 1983–88. *British Journal of Addiction*, **87**, 643–8.

Windham, G.C., Fenster, L. & Swan, S.H. (1992). Moderate maternal and paternal alcohol consumption and the risk of spontaneous abortion. *Epidemiology*, **3**, 264–70.

Wright, J.T., Waterson, E.J., Barrison, I.C., Toplis, P.J., Lewis, I.G., Gordon, M.G., MacRae, K.D., Morris, N.F. & Murray-Lyon, I.M. (1983). Alcohol consumption, pregnancy and low birthweight. *Lancet*, **i**, 663–5.

Part II

Pathogenesis and neuropathology

4

Risk factors and pathogenesis

ERNEST L. ABEL AND JOHN H. HANNIGAN

Introduction

Fetal alcohol syndrome (FAS) is a cluster of growth-related physical and behavioral problems in children born to alcoholic women (Abel, 1984). Alcohol exposure *in utero* may give rise to a spectrum of adverse effects ranging from spontaneous abortion, through individual alcohol-related birth defects (ARBDs), to FAS to newborn mortality (Abel, 1984). However, none of these effects, other than FAS, is pathognomonic, and therefore attribution of specific ARBDs to alcohol is problematic.

The latest conservative estimate for the incidence of FAS in the Western world is 1.02 per 1000 live births (Abel, 1995). However, most of the cases contributing to this estimate have been diagnosed in the United States. The majority of FAS cases in the United States (1.95 per 1000) were identified in inner city hospitals where the population was characterized by low socio-economic status and was predominantly African-American or Native American. At sites where the population was primarily middle class and Caucasian, the rate is much lower at 0.26 per 1000 (Abel, 1995). The estimated incidence of FAS among alcoholics is 43 cases per 1000 live births (Abel, 1995). Although reported rates for FAS are believed to represent the proverbial 'tip of the iceberg' as far as the 'true' rate is concerned (Little *et al.*, 1990), this argument is unsubstantiated. In fact, it is just as likely that FAS is now being overdiagnosed as that it is underdiagnosed (J. Nanson, personal communication).

Risk factors

Since there is little evidence FAS is underdiagnosed, one inference from its relatively low rate of occurrence, even among alcoholic women, is that *while alcohol is clearly the etiological case of FAS, permissive and provocative factors affect its expression.* By 'permissive', we mean predisposing behavioral, social or environmental factors, such as patterns of alcohol consumption, socio-economic status and poor nutrition, that initiate the 'provocative' conditions that contribute to FAS. Provocative factors are those biological conditions that create an internal milieu that increases fetal vulnerability to alcohol at the cellular level.

Permissive factors

Clinical, epidemiological and experimental studies consistently point to per-missive factors as contributing to the occurrence of FAS. We discuss three such factors – pattern of alcohol consumption, poverty, and smoking beha-vior – as major risk factors in FAS.

Pattern of alcohol consumption

Experiments in neonatal rats have found that the threshold blood alcohol level (BAL) for abnormal brain development is about 150 mg% (150 mg/dl) (Pierce & West, 1986; Bonthius *et al.*, 1988). This BAL would result from ingestion of about 7 'drinks' in a 2 hour period by a 140 lb (63.5 kg) woman (U. Michigan, n.d.). A woman who sips 7 drinks throughout a 12 hour day, or one who consumes 2 drinks a day at mealtime, would not exceed that threshold, whereas a woman who consumes 7 drinks during a particularly short time on a particular day of the week could equal or exceed this thresh-old. Since exceeding the critical threshold depends not so much on alcohol consumption as the way it is consumed, teratogenicity is dependent on pat-terns of consumption. Whereas the average consumption per week might be the same, the higher BALs associated with weekend drinking compared with lower sustained drinking would be a risk factor for FAS (Pierce & West, 1986; Bonthius *et al.*, 1988). Summarizing drinking patterns in terms of drinks or amount of absolute alcohol per week during pregnancy is not meaningful, given that BAL is a critical factor; a much more meaningful measure is consumption during drinking episodes. Since peak BAL is a key risk factor for FAS, group differences in drinking behavior may explain group differences in the incidence of FAS.

In general, there are stronger relationships between indicators of problem drinking and deleterious effects in offspring than between maternal alcohol consumption levels and offspring outcomes (Majewski, 1981; Russell *et al.*, 1991). A positive Michigan Alcohol Screening Test (MAST) score, indicative of problem drinking and, by inference, high levels of drinking, is a major predictor for FAS (Sokol *et al.*, 1986) and the main factor contributing to formulas relating low levels of alcohol consumption to adverse fetal outcome (Ernhart *et al.*, 1985).

Racial differences in susceptibility to alcohol have been proposed as the reason for the higher incidence of FAS among African-Americans compared with Caucasians (e.g., Sokol *et al.*, 1986, 1989). Although individuals may have some undefined embryo/fetal genotype that may render them more susceptible to alcohol's teratogenic effects (Christoffel & Salafsky, 1975; Santolaya *et al.*, 1978), we are unaware of any biological conditions capable of accounting for the large disparities in the incidence of FAS among racial groups. On the other hand, there are data indicating racial differences in drinking patterns. For example, African-American alcoholic women drink more heavily on weekends compared with Caucasian alcoholic women, who are more likely to drink constantly (Dawkins & Harper, 1983).

Epidemiological studies suggesting African-Americans have a lower threshold for FAS than Caucasians are based entirely on self-report data, and are subject to underestimation, especially among problem drinkers (Ernhart *et al.*, 1988). The possibility that women from different racial backgrounds differ in denial or distortion has not been examined. Since drinking is much less common among African-American women than among Caucasian (Russell, 1989), there may be much more social pressure for denial with respect to alcohol in the African-American community.

Poverty

A second major permissive factor contributing to FAS is poverty, which is a global indicator for poor maternal nutrition and health, and increased stress (e.g., marital instability, unemployment, decreased access to prenatal care), any of which can independently affect pregnancy adversely (Feinleib, 1989). Each may also interact with alcohol to affect pregnancy outcome (Dreosti, 1993). For example, whereas as few as 2 drinks per week were found to pose a risk for spontaneous abortion among women on public assistance, this relationship between drinking and spontaneous abortion was not present when the study was repeated with private patients (Kline *et al.*, 1980; Kolata, 1981).

The poor nutritional status associated with alcohol consumption may also act additively or synergistically with alcohol on the embryo/fetus (Dreosti, 1993). Despite diligent attempts using animal models to unravel the role of nutritional factors in ARBDs, questions remain about the role secondary nutritional effects (e.g., reduced protein levels) have on fetal growth and development (Wunderlich *et al.*, 1979; see Hannigan & Abel, this volume; Kennedy, 1984).

Studies in animals have created a misleading impression that nutrition does not contribute to alcohol's teratogenicity. For instance, in controlling for differences in food intake between alcohol-treated and control animals, a 'pair-feeding' technique is typically employed, in which control animals are given the same relative amount of diet as the alcohol-treated group with some other carbohydrate, usually sucrose or maltose-dextrin, substituted isocalorically for ethanol-derived calories (EDC). Whereas the caloric intake for experimental and control groups may be similar, the alcohol-treated group experiences both alcohol treatment and undernourishment. Differences between this group and animals solely undernourished may be due to the interactive effects of alcohol plus undernutrition. If anomalies occur more often in alcohol-exposed animals than in the control pair-fed animals, this does not eliminate the likelihood that nutritional factors contribute to occurrence of those defects.

Poverty is associated with stress, which results in increased adrenal release of corticosterone and epinephrine, and with living in the inner city, which increases exposure to environmental pollutants such as lead. Prenatal stress and lead exposure can independently produce many of the effects associated with perinatal alcohol exposure (Pasamanick & Lilienfield, 1955; Weller *et al.*, 1988; Ernhart, 1992; Edwards *et al.*, 1994).

Smoking

It is now very uncommon to find women who abuse alcohol only (Coles *et al.*, 1985). Statistical techniques (e.g., multiple regression) can be used to separate the influences of individual factors in complex systems, but important interactive effects between alcohol and other drugs can also occur, leading to additive and/or synergistic teratogenic effects. The combination of alcohol ingestion and smoking is particularly of interest because a large percentage of all alcoholics are also smokers (Abel, 1984; Sokol *et al.*, 1986). The combination of maternal alcohol consumption and cigarette smoking increases the risk for low birth weight, smaller head circumference, learning difficulties, and febrile convulsions compared with alcohol alone (Wright *et al.*, 1983; Halmesmaki, 1988; Cassano *et al.*, 1990; Olsen *et al.*, 1991).

Mechanisms

Ultimately, all embryo/fetal damage will involve perturbations in cellular growth, differentiation, proliferation, migration and/or regulation. The absence of a specific pathognomonic feature or, conversely, the number of ubiquitous anomalies associated with FAS, implies alcohol is acting through a relatively general mechanism or one which has wide-ranging impact. We hypothesize that two of these mechanisms are hypoxia and free radical formation.

Hypoxia

Since cellular oxygenation is critical for all physiological processes, any factors which reduce cellular oxygenation can be expected to affect living organisms adversely, especially those in an embryological or fetal state of development.

Decreased embryo/fetal oxygenation can arise as a result of many factors, such as decreased blood flow to tissues, decreased oxygen content in the blood, decreased oxygen saturation of red blood cells, and impaired dissociation of oxygen from red blood cells, all of which are associated with maternal alcohol ingestion. Since hepatic metabolism of alcohol removes considerable amounts of oxygen from blood (Ugarte & Valenzuela, 1971), the result is reduced availability of oxygen for other tissues. During pregnancy, such alcohol-related decreases in tissue oxygenation are manifested in placental hyperplasia (Fisher *et al.*, 1985; Sanchis & Guerri, 1986). Decreased placental oxygenation may in turn affect energy-dependent placental transport of nutrients to the fetus (Fisher *et al.*, 1981, 1984, 1986). High BALs may also induce a transient collapse of human umbilical arteries (Mukherjee & Hodgen, 1982), thereby depriving the fetus of blood flow altogether. Spasms in human uterine tissue at low alcohol concentrations may also occur (Savoy-Moore *et al.*, 1989). In addition to decreasing blood flow to tissues, alcohol may also decrease availability of oxygen to tissues because it impairs the unloading of oxygen from red blood cells by acidifying blood (Yang *et al.*, 1986).

Alcohol-related hypoxia can lead to intrauterine growth retardation via several different but related mechanisms. Since cell proliferation and differentiation are dependent on protein synthesis, decreased substrate availability could lead to intrauterine growth retardation (Fisher *et al.*, 1984; Fisher, 1988). The nutrient substrate may initially be less than optimal because alcohol-abusing mothers consume less than the required amounts of nutrients for support of normal fetal growth, and because alcohol itself may interfere with gastrointestinal absorption of these nutrients into the blood. Decreased substrate availability could arise from alcohol-related impairment of essential amino acids (Henderson *et al.*, 1982; Fisher *et al.*, 1985), glucose (Snyder *et al.*, 1986), or vitamins and minerals (Schenker *et al.*, 1992) due to a combination of decreased placental blood flow (Falconer, 1990) and impairment of oxygen-dependent Na^+K^+-ATPase membrane transport processes (Fisher *et al.*, 1986).

Impairment of membrane transport processes may not only reduce placental transport of nutrients, it may also inhibit protein synthesis throughout the body, as shown in *in vitro* studies and in models that circumvent placental transport, such as chicks and embryos grown in culture (Brown *et al.*, 1979; Dreosti *et al.*, 1981; Pennington *et al.*, 1983). The resulting growth retardation could also result in minor physical anomalies and developmental delays by altering the timing and interplay between different organ systems (Kennedy, 1984).

As Michaelis (1990) has argued, alcohol's impact on the developing brain can also be understood in terms of hypoxia. In the adult brain, episodes of hypoxia have their greatest impact on pyramidal neurons in the CA_1 area of the hippocampus and on Purkinje cells in the cerebellum (Jorgensen & Diemer, 1982; Auer *et al.*, 1989). These are the same areas that are most affected by gestational or neonatal alcohol exposure in animals (e.g., Barnes & Walker, 1981; Dewey & West, 1985). The hippocampus may be more vulnerable because it is richly vascularized and densely populated with excitatory amino acid neurotransmitters such as glutamate and aspartate, and these transmitters are released selectively during periods of hypoxia (Bosley *et al.*, 1983). Hypoxia directly induces down-regulation of glutamate receptors in the fetal rat brain (Kater *et al.*, 1988), an effect that also occurs in brains exposed prenatally to alcohol (Farr *et al.*, 1988). Excess release of L-glutamate can have neurotoxic effects on postsynaptic glutamate receptors, especially *N*-methyl-*D*-asparate-sensitive glutamate receptors (i.e., NMDA sites) (Rothman & Olney, 1987; Michaelis, 1990). The excessive, sustained neuroexcitation is believed ultimately to become neurotoxic due to subsequent release of lipid peroxides (Riley & Behrman, 1991) and fatty acids such as prostaglandins, and accumulation of calcium (Ca^{2+}) which ultimately results in cell death.

Free radicals

Alcohol's teratogenic effects may also arise as a result of damage to cells through generation of free oxygen radicals such as superoxide anion (O_3^-), hydroxyl radical (OH^-), and highly potent hydrogen peroxide (H_2O_2). Such oxygen radicals are continuously generated in the course of normal cellular respiration when electrons escape from their carriers and are taken up by oxygen. These ephemeral molecular entities are highly reactive within cells, and cause peroxidation of cell membranes (Riley & Behrman, 1991).

To protect themselves from oxygen-related free radicals, cells normally rely on various antioxidants and enzymes (e.g., vitamins C and E, glutathione), but these resources can be depleted by alcohol and by reduced nutrient supply. One of these enzyme systems, superoxide dismutase, uses zinc as a cofactor. Zinc is also an essential trace element for fetal growth and a cofactor in alcohol dehydrogenase, the enzyme involved in metabolism of alcohol. Decreased zinc levels are commonly associated with alcoholism (McClain & Su, 1983) and zinc deficiency has frequently been implicated in FAS (Flynn *et al.*, 1981; Halmesmaki *et al.*, 1985; Assadi & Ziai, 1986). Alcohol may also impair placental transport of zinc and fetal uptake of zinc (Grishan *et al.*, 1982; Zeidenberg-Cherr *et al.*, 1988). When alcohol is administered in combination with a low zinc diet, the combination has a much greater impact on fetal weight reduction than either alcohol or zinc deficiency alone (Keppen *et al.*, 1985).

In addition to undernutrition, tobacco smoke not only directly increases the body's burden of free radicals, it also depletes cellular reserves of antioxidants and zinc, and contributes to primary undernutrition by reducing food consumption, especially intake of antioxidants such as vitamins A, C and E, and zinc. As a result, the body's cellular defense mechanisms against free oxygen radicals are further weakened by smoking, increasing vulnerability to alcohol-generated radicals.

Drugs such as indomethacin, aspirin and ibuprofen, which have been found to counteract the effects of alcohol exposure *in utero* on fetal breathing movements (Smith *et al.*, 1989, 1990*a,b*), and to reduce the fetal mortality, litter weight reductions, brain hypoplasia, and limb and kidney malformations seen in mouse and chick embryos exposed to alcohol (Randall & Anton, 1984; Randall *et al.*, 1991*a,b*), may also act by affecting free radicals. Although the mechanism of action of these drugs is generally discussed in terms of their inhibition of prostaglandins, they are also oxygen free radical scavengers (Kennedy *et al.*, 1990) and their mechanism of action may just as readily be interpreted in terms of these scavenging actions.

An integrative hypothesis: risk and mechanisms

We hypothesize a link between the differential susceptibility to FAS/ARBDs among certain populations and the hypoxia/free radical mechanism of alcohol teratogenesis.

We contend that 'permissive' sociobehavioral factors such as binge drinking, poverty, and smoking, are major risk factors for FAS. Dose for dose, binge drinking, for example, creates higher toxic peak BALs than sustained levels of alcohol consumption. Poverty is a risk factor because it is associated with decreased nutritional intake, stress, and exposure to environmental pollutants because of living in inner cities. These 'permissive' factors lead to internal biological conditions which are 'provocative' in that they provoke cellular changes that exacerbate alcohol's toxic effects. These provocative changes include altered blood flow, decreased reserves of antioxidants, generation of stress hormones, and increased body burdens of free radicals. The cellular hypoxia from decreased blood flow, stress-related respiratory alkalosis, and/or from smoking (which independently decreases uterine blood flow and blood oxygenation) combine with alcohol-induced cellular hypoxia in an additive or synergistic manner. When an undefined critical level of hypoxia is exceeded, cellular changes occur which manifest themselves in various aspects of FAS/ARBDs such as altered facial morphology or lower birth weight. Increased free radical formation likewise contributes to cell damage and may account for the physical as well as behavioral damage associated with FAS/ARBDs.

Conclusion

Prenatal alcohol exposure can result in FAS and other physical and behavioral anomalies. Alcohol is clearly an etiological factor in FAS/ARBDs. However, permissive risk factors must also contribute to the occurrence of these anomalies because only a relatively small proportion of children exposed prenatally to even high levels of alcohol are born with FAS. Among these permissive factors are the pattern of alcohol consumption, low socioeconomic status, smoking, and as yet unspecified maternal constitutional factors. Several possible mechanisms have been proposed for alcohol's teratogenic effects and it is unlikely that there is any single causative process. The hypothesis we have proposed integrates known risk factors with biological mechanisms known to affect embryo/fetal development. Research in the coming decade should be directed at: identifying objective biological markers for alcohol abuse in women and fetal risk for FAS in women or fetuses; clarifying presently identified and additional risk factors contributing to or permitting the varied expression of FAS/ARBDs; improving our understanding of mechanisms of alcohol teratogenesis; and developing methods for the prevention, treatment, and amelioration of FAS/ARBDs.

References

Abel, E.L. (1984). *Fetal Alcohol Syndrome and Fetal Alcohol Effects.* New York: Plenum Press.

Abel, E.L. (1995). An update on incidence of FAS: FAS is not an equal opportunity birth defect. *Neurobehavioral Toxicology*, **17**, 437–43.

Assadi, F.K. & Ziai, M. (1986). Zinc status of infants with fetal alcohol syndrome. *Pediatric Research*, **20**, 551–4.

Auer, R.N., Jensen, M.L. & Whishaw, I.Q. (1989). Neurobehavioral deficit due to ischemic brain damage limited to half of the CA_1 sector of the hippocampus. *Journal of Neuroscience*, **9**, 1641–7.

Barnes, D.E. & Walker, D.W. (1981). Prenatal ethanol exposure permanently reduces the number of pyramidal neurons in rat hippocampus. *Developmental Brain Research*, **1**, 333–40.

Bonthius, D.J., Goodlett, C.R. & West, J.R. (1988). Blood alcohol concentration and severity of microencephaly in neonatal rats depend on the pattern of alcohol administration. *Alcohol*, **5**, 209–14.

Bosley, T.M., Woodhams, P.L., Gordon, R.D. & Balazs, R. (1983). Effects of anoxia on the stimulated release of amino acid neurotransmitters in the cerebellum *in vitro*. *Journal of Neurochemistry*, **40**, 189–201.

Brown, N.A., Goulding, E.H. & Fabro, S. (1979). Ethanol embryotoxicity: direct effects on mammalian embryos *in vitro*. *Science*, **206**, 573–5.

Cassano, P.A., Koepsell, T.D. & Farwell, J.R. (1990). Risk of febrile seizure in childhood in relation to prenatal cigarette smoking and alcohol intake. *American Journal of Epidemiology*, **132**, 462–73.

Christoffel, K.K. & Salafsky, I. (1975). Fetal alcohol syndrome in dizygotic twins. *Pediatrics*, **87**, 963–7.

Coles, C.D., Smith, I.E., Fernhoff, P.M. & Falek, A. (1985). Neonatal neurobehavioral characteristics as correlates of maternal alcohol use during gestation. *Alcoholism: Clinical and Experimental Research*, **9**, 454–60.

Dawkins, M.P. & Harper, F.D. (1983). Alcoholism among women: a comparison of black and white problem drinkers. *International Journal of the Addictions*, **18**, 333–49.

Dewey, S.L. & West, J.R. (1985). Perforant pathway lamination in the dentate gyrus is unaffected by prenatal ethanol exposure. *Alcohol*, **2**, 221–5.

Dreosti, I.E. (1993). Nutritional factors underlying the expression of the fetal alcohol syndrome. *Annals of the New York Academy of Sciences*, **678**, 193–204.

Dreosti, I.E., Ballard, J., Belling, B., Record, I.R., Manuel, S.J. & Hetzel, B.S. (1981). The effect of ethanol and acetaldehyde on DNA synthesis in growing cells and on fetal development in rat. *Alcoholism: Clinical and Experimental Research*, **5**, 355–62.

Edwards, C.H., Cole, O.J., Oyemade, J., Knight, E.M., Johnson, A.A., Westney, D.E., Laryea, H., West, W., Jones, S. & Westney, L.S. (1994). Maternal stress and pregnancy outcome in a prenatal clinic population. *Journal of Nutrition*, **124**, S1006–21.

Ernhart, C.B. (1992). A critical review of low-level prenatal lead exposure in the human. I. Effects on the fetus and newborn. *Reproductive Toxicology*, **6**, 9–19.

Ernhart, C.B., Morrow-Tlucak, M., Sokol, R.J. & Martier, S. (1988). Underreporting of alcohol use in pregnancy. *Alcoholism: Clinical and Experimental Research*, **12**, 506–11.

Ernhart, C.B., Wolf, A.W., Sokol, R.J., Brittenham, G.M. & Erhard, P. (1985). Fetal lead exposure: antenatal factors. *Environmental Research*, **38**, 54–66.

Falconer, J. (1990). The effect of maternal ethanol infusion on placental blood flow and fetal glucose metabolism in sheep. *Alcohol and Alcoholism*, **25**, 413–16.

Farr, K.L., Montano, C.Y., Paxton, L.L. & Savage, D.D. (1988). Prenatal ethanol exposure decreases hippocampal ³H-glutamate binding in 45-day-old rats. *Alcohol*, **5**, 125–33.

Feinleib, M. (1989). Advance report on final mortality statistics, 1987. *Monthly Vital Statistics Report*, **38**, Suppl.

Fisher, S.E. (1988). Selective fetal malnutrition: the fetal alcohol syndrome. *Journal of the American College of Nutrition*, **7**, 101–6.

Fisher, S.E., Atkinson, M. & Van Thiel, D.H. (1984). Selective fetal malnutrition: the effect of nicotine, ethanol and acetaldehyde upon *in vitro* uptake of alpha-aminoisobutryric acid by human term placental villous slices. *Developmental Pharmacology*, **7**, 229–38.

Fisher, S.E., Barnicle, M.A., Steis, B., Holzman, I. & Van Thiel, D.H. (1981). Effects of acute ethanol exposure upon *in vivo* leucine uptake and protein synthesis in the fetal rat. *Pediatric Research*, **13**, 335–9.

Fisher, S.E., Duffy, L. & Atkinson, M. (1986). Selective fetal malnutrition: effect of acute and chronic ethanol exposure upon rat placental Na,K-ATPase activity. *Alcoholism: Clinical and Experimental Research*, **10**, 150–3.

Fisher, S.E., Inselman, L.S., Duffy, L., Atkinson, M., Spencer, H. & Chang, B. (1985). Ethanol and fetal nutrition: effects of chronic ethanol exposure on rat placental growth and membrane-associated folic acid receptor binding activity. *Journal of Pediatric Gastroenterology and Nutrition*, **4**, 645–9.

Flynn, A., Martier, S.S., Sokol, R.J., Miller, S.I., Golder, N.L. & Del Villano, B.C. (1981). Zinc status of pregnant alcoholic women: a determinant of fetal outcome. *Lancet*, **i**, 572–4.

Grishan, F.K., Patwardhan, R. & Greene, H.L. (1982). Fetal alcohol syndrome: inhibition of placental transport as a potential mechanism for fetal growth retardation in the rat. *Journal of Laboratory and Clinical Medicine*, **100**, 45.

Halmesmaki, E. (1988). Alcohol counselling of 85 pregnant problem drinkers: effect on drinking and fetal outcome. *British Journal of Obstetrics and Gynaecology*, **95**, 243–7.

Halmesmaki, E., Ylikorkala, O. & Alfthan, G. (1985). Concentration of zinc and copper in pregnant problem drinkers and their newborn infants. *British Medical Journal*, **291**, 1470–1.

Henderson, G.I., Patwardhan, R.V., McLeroy, S. & Schenker, S. (1982). Inhibition of placental amino acid uptake in rats following acute and chronic ethanol. *Alcoholism: Clinical and Experimental Research*, **6**, 495–505.

Jorgensen, M.B. & Diemer, N.H. (1982). Selective neuron loss after cerebral ischemia in the rat: possible role of transmitter glutamate. *Acta Neurologica Scandinavica*, **66**, 536–46.

Kater, S.B., Mattson, M.P., Cohan, C. & Connor, J. (1988). Calcium regulation of the neuronal growth cone. *Trends in Neurosciences*, **11**, 315–21.

Kennedy, L.A. (1984). The pathogenesis of brain abnormalities in the fetal alcohol syndrome: an integrating hypothesis. *Teratology*, **29**, 363–8.

Kennedy, T.P., Rao, N.V., Noah, W., Michael, J.R., Jafri, M.H., Gurtner, G.H. & Hoidal, J.R. (1990). Ibuprofen prevents oxidant lung injury and *in vitro* lipid peroxidation by chelating iron. *Journal of Clinical Investigation*, **86**, 1565–73.

Keppen, L.D., Pysher, T. & Rennert, O.M. (1985). Zinc deficiency acts as a co-teratogen with alcohol in fetal alcohol syndrome. *Pediatric Research*, **19**, 944–7.

Kline, J., Shrout, P., Stein, A., Susser, M., Warburton, D. (1980). Drinking during pregnancy and spontaneous abortion. *Lancet*, **ii**, 176–80.

Kolata, G.B. (1981). Fetal alcohol advisory debated. *Science*, **214**, 642.

Little, B.B., Snell, L.M., Rosenfeld, C.R., Gilstrap, L.C. & Grant, N.F. (1990). Failure to recognize fetal alcohol syndrome in newborn infants. *American Journal of Diseases of Children*, **144**, 1142–6.

McClain, C.J. & Su, L.C. (1983). Zinc deficiency in the alcoholic. *Alcoholism: Clinical and Experimental Research*, **7**, 5.

Majewski, F. (1981). Alcohol embryopathy: some facts and speculations about pathogenesis. *Neurobehavioral Toxicology and Teratology*, **3**, 129–44.

Michaelis, E.K. (1990). Fetal alcohol exposure: cellular toxicity and molecular events involved in toxicity. *Alcoholism: Clinical and Experimental Research*, **14**, 819–26.

Mukherjee, A.B. & Hodgen, G.D. (1982). Maternal ethanol exposure induces transient impairment of umbilical circulation and fetal hypoxia in monkeys. *Science*, **218**, 700–1.

Olsen, J., Pereira, A. da C. & Olsen, S.F. (1991). Does maternal tobacco smoking modify the effect of alcohol on fetal growth? *American Journal of Public Health*, **81**, 69–73.

Pasamanick, B. & Lilienfield, A.M. (1955). Association of maternal and fetal factors with development of mental deficience. I. Abnormalities in the prenatal and perinatal periods. *JAMA*, **159**, 155–60.

Pennington, J., Boyd, W., Kalmus, G. & Wilson, R.W. (1983). The molecular mechanism of fetal alcohol syndrome (FAS). I. Ethanol-induced growth suppression. *Neurobehavioral Toxicology and Teratology*, **5**, 259–62.

Pierce, D.R. & West, J.R. (1986). Alcohol-induced microencephaly during the third trimester equivalent: relationship to dose and blood alcohol concentration. *Alcohol*, **3**, 185–91.

Randall, C.L. & Anton, R.F. (1984). Aspirin reduces alcohol-induced prenatal mortality and malformations in mice. *Alcoholism: Clinical and Experimental Research*, **8**, 513–15.

Randall, C.L., Anton, R.F., Becker, H.C., Hale, R. & Ekblad, U. (1991a). Aspirin dose-dependently reduces alcohol-induced birth defects and prostaglandin E levels in mice. *Teratology*, **44**, 521–9.

Randall, C.L., Becker, H.C. & Anton, R.F. (1991b). Effect of ibuprofen on alcohol-induced teratogenesis in mice. *Alcoholism: Clinical and Experimental Research*, **15**, 673–7.

Riley, J.C.M. & Behrman, H.R. (1991). Oxygen radicals and reactive oxygen species in reproduction. *Proceedings of the Society for Experimental Biology and Medicine*, **198**, 781–91.

Rothman, S.M. & Olney, J.W. (1987). Excitotoxicity and the NMDA receptor. *Trends in Neurosciences*, **10**, 299–302.

Russell, M. (1989). Alcohol use and related problems among black and white gynecologic patients. In *Alcohol Use Among US Ethnic Minorities*, NIAA Research Monograph no. 18, ed. D.L. Spiegler, D.A. Tate, S.S. Aitken &

C.M. Christian, pp. 75–94. Washington, DC: US Government Printing Office.

Russell, M., Czarneci, D.M., Cowan, R., McPherson, E. & Mudar, P.J. (1991). Measures of maternal alcohol use as predictors of development in early childhood. *Alcoholism: Clinical and Experimental Research*, **15**, 991–1000.

Sanchis, R. & Guerri, C. (1986). Alcohol-metabolizing enzymes in placenta and fetal liver: effect of chronic ethanol intake. *Alcoholism: Clinical and Experimental Research*, **10**, 39–44.

Santolaya, J.M., Martinez, G., Gorostiza, E., Alzpiri, J. & Hernandez, M. (1978). Alcoholismo fetal. *Drogalcohol*, **3**, 183–93.

Savoy-Moore, R.T., Dombrowski, M.P., Cheng, A., Abel, E.A. & Sokol, R.J. (1989). Low dose alcohol contracts the human umbilical artery *in vitro*. *Alcoholism: Clinical and Experimental Research*, **13**, 40–2.

Schenker, S., Johnson, R.F., Mahuren, J.D., Henderson, G.I. & Coburn, S.P. (1992). Human placental vitamin B_6 (pyridoxal) transport: normal characteristics and effects of ethanol. *American Journal of Physiology*, **262**, R966–74.

Smith, G.N., Brien, J.F., Homan, J., *et al.* (1989). Indomethacin antagonizes the ethanol-induced suppression of breathing activity, but not the suppression of brain activity in the near-term fetal sheep. *Journal of Developmental Physiology*, **12**, 69–75.

Smith, G.N., Brien, J.F., Homan, J., Carmichael, J., Treissman, D. & Patrick, J. (1990*a*). Effect of ethanol on ovine fetal and maternal plasma prostaglandin E_2 concentrations and fetal breathing movements. *Journal of Developmental Physiology*, **14**, 23–8.

Smith, G.N., Brien, J.F., Homan, J. *et al.* (1990*b*). Indomethacin reversal of ethanol-induced suppression of ovine fetal breathing movements and relationship to prostaglandin E_2. *Journal of Developmental Physiology*, **14**, 28–36.

Snyder, A.K., Singh, S.P. & Pullen, G.L. (1986). Ethanol-induced intrauterine growth retardation: correlation with placental glucose transfer. *Alcoholism: Clinical and Experimental Research*, **10**, 167–70.

Sokol, R.J., Ager, J., Martier, S., Debanne, S., Ernhart, C., Kuzma, J. & Miller, S.I. (1986). Significant determinants of susceptibility to alcohol teratogenicity. *Annals of the New York Academy of Sciences*, **477**, 87–102.

Sokol, R.J., Smith, M., Ernhart, C.B., Baumann, R., Martier, S.S., Ager, J.W. & Morrow-Tlucak, M. (1989). A genetic basis for alcohol-related birth defects (ARBD)? *Alcoholism: Clinical and Experimental Research*, **13**, 343A.

Ugarte, G. & Valenzuela, J. (1971). Mechanisms of liver and pancreas damage in man. In *Biological Basis of Alcoholism*, ed. Y. Israel & J. Mardones, pp. 133–61. New York: Wiley.

Weller, A., Glaubman, H., Yehuda, S., Caspy, T. & Ben-uria, Y. (1988). Acute and repeated gestational stress affect offspring learning and activity in rats. *Physiology and Behavior*, **43**, 139–43.

Wright, J.T., Waterson, E.J., Barrison, I.G., Toplis, P.J., Lewis, I.G., Gordon, M.G., MacRae, K.D., Morris, N.F. & Murray-Lyon, I.M. (1983). Alcohol consumption, pregnancy, and low birth weight. *Lancet*, **i**, 663–5.

Wunderlich, S.M., Surendra, B. & Munro, H.N. (1979). Rat placental protein synthesis and peptide hormone secretion in relation to malnutrition from protein deficiency or alcohol administration. *Journal of Nutrition*, **109**, 1534–41.

Yang, H.Y., Shum, A.Y.C., Ng, H.T. & Chen, C.F. (1986). Effect of ethanol on human umbilical artery and vein *in vitro. Gynecologic and Obstetric Investigation*, **21**, 131–5.

Zidenberg-Cherr, S., Judith, R. & Keen, C.L. (1988). Influence of ethanol consumption on maternal–fetal transfer of zinc in pregnant rats on day 14 of pregnancy. *Journal of Nutrition*, **118**, 865–70.

5

Animal models for the study of alcohol-related birth defects

JOHN H. HANNIGAN AND ERNEST L. ABEL

Introduction: overview of animal models

Soon after fetal alcohol syndrome (FAS) was defined in children in Seattle in the early 1970s by Smith and Jones and their colleagues (Jones & Smith, 1973), laboratories began to develop animal models to help address initial skepticism about the impact of maternal alcohol consumption during pregnancy (Chernoff, 1977; Randall & Taylor, 1979; reviews in Abel, 1984; Randall, 1987). In the 20 years since, many models have been developed which have proven that prenatal alcohol rather than other factors associated with alcoholism and alcohol abuse (e.g., smoking, poor maternal diet, or some 'constitutional' susceptibility) is the proximate cause of alcohol-related birth defects (ARBDs), including FAS. These studies were valuable not only for verifying alcohol's teratogenicity, but also for providing insights into other ARBDs not entirely appreciated in case studies (cf., Church, 1987; DeBeukelar et al., 1977; but see Taylor et al., 1994). This chapter will describe some of the advantages and disadvantages of several of these animal models of ARBDs, as well as some of the methodological issues that define and limit their utility in helping to resolve important questions that remain about FAS (Abel & Hannigan, 1995a).

In most ways, the issues we discuss here have not changed substantially since they were first elucidated (e.g., Abel, 1984; Riley & Meyer, 1984; Abel & Riley, 1986), but interpretations can change (Meyer & Riley, 1986; West, 1986; Randall, 1987). In this chapter, certain principles of research in animal models will be described and specific protocols will illustrate how the effects of alcohol exposure on development can be studied effectively in animal models. In this way we hope to show how our understanding of biobehavioral outcome, biological markers, risk factors, mechanisms of alcohol teratogenesis, prevention, and treatment of FAS/ARBDs in humans can be advanced and given new direction by basic research with *in vivo* and *in vitro* animal models.

There are two general points to be emphasized at the start. First, there is currently no animal model of FAS, other than the non-human primate perhaps, and likely never will be. This is because FAS is a human condition defined by three cardinal diagnostic features: growth retardation (e.g., low birth weight), a characteristic facial dysmorphology (e.g., midface hypoplasia, indistinct philtrum), and central nervous system (CNS) involvement (e.g., mental retardation or other motor and/or sensory and/or cognitive deficits) (Sokol & Clarren, 1989; Hannigan *et al.*, 1992). Although there are certainly several effective ways to approximate some of these effects in animals (Driscoll *et al.*, 1990; Hannigan *et al.*, 1992), there is no rodent FAS *per se* because no model expresses all features of clinical ARBDs/FAS. Also, there is no single 'best' animal model of ARBDs although each model may express some features more reliably and in a way more accessible to study than others. A corollary to this point is that this is no ideal control group against which to evaluate the specific effects of alcohol. The choice of model and experimental design depends in large part on the specific questions being asked. Specific ARBDs in animals may be evident as biobehavioral responses to early alcohol exposure under one particular set of circumstances and not others (Meyer & Riley, 1986; Becker *et al.*, 1994). This chapter will describe some of these experimental circumstances.

The value of animal models

There are clearly important questions about the effects of alcohol on developing embryos and fetuses that can be studied effectively in whole animals or various *in vitro* animal models. Because of ethical considerations or simple feasibility, questions about cellular and molecular mechanisms cannot be studied in humans. Descriptions of biobehavioral outcome and explorations of potential treatments, detection schemes, risk factors, or prevention strategies can be studied in people, but such activities can benefit from preliminary investigations and confirmation using animal models.

Advantages of animal models

The general advantages of animal models are found in the closely related features of (1) experimental design, (2) simplification and control, and (3) replicability and statistical power.

An experiment with animals can be designed specifically to control, measure, and/or randomize the many factors other than alcohol itself that are intimately associated with alcohol drinking and also influence fetal development. For example, the role of poor nutrition associated with alcoholism is very complex and can profoundly affect fetal development independently of and interactively with alcohol (see below). Considerable effort has gone into devising ways to assure that alcohol-treated dams are adequately nourished (Weinberg, 1984). Experiments designed to control the influences of nutrition can address the problem. Animal models are powerful tools because they afford the opportunity to assess up to hundreds of subjects in repeatable experiments. This is important because FAS can be quite rare in the overall human population (Abel & Hannigan, 1995a, b; this volume), because individual ARBDs are as yet difficult to identify reliably in people, and because some of the effects of fetal alcohol exposure can be subtle, requiring very large study populations for reliable detection. Finally, well-defined genetic differences among and within animal species can be used as tools in studying susceptibility and mechanisms of alcohol teratogenesis (see below).

Disadvantages of animal models

Animals are not humans and despite the sometimes extraordinary similarity in normal physiology or alcohol metabolism or behavior, species differences cannot be ignored. While skillful experimental design can maximize the likelihood of detecting an effect of perinatal alcohol that may be subtle and/or infrequent in humans, interpretation of animal results should avoid overstating the implications for humans. The obverse of this potential for exaggeration is that the control, removal or measurement of associated risk factors such as poor nutrition or smoking (Abel & Hannigan, 1995a) could reduce the interactive effects of alcohol in animal models and so underestimate alcohol's teratogenic impact in human populations that are at increased risk precisely because of these factors.

Animal models

Species are not interchangeable: the use of more than one species, strain or line of animals confers clear advantages for both genetic analyses and increasing the generalizability of results for different studies within and across laboratories. Several species have been used to study *in utero* alcohol.

Rodents

The most commonly used animal species in fetal alcohol research is the pregnant rat or mouse. The preponderance of research on rodents is because they are relatively inexpensive compared with 'higher' mammals, although it should be noted that the continuing escalation of animal care costs in the United States is making all developmental studies with animals more expensive. Rodents are valuable because of the extensive research literature describing rodent development, physiology and biochemistry, anatomy and behavior. Rodents are also appropriate and valid species with which to model the effects of alcohol consumption in humans because there are substantial similarities with humans in alcohol metabolism and in responses to toxic and/ or teratogenic substances. That testing in rats and mice is a required standard in toxicology and teratology testing for new drugs attests to this (Adams, 1986).

In the typical rodent model, alcohol is administered during pregnancy and the effects are measured on offspring, either as fetuses or as pups. Mice and rats have relatively short gestation periods (20–21 days), reach sexual maturity about 8 weeks after birth, and typically have litters of 8–15 pups. These features make rodents quite efficient animals for assessing gestational shifts in sensitivity and for producing many affected offspring to assess postnatal effects. Although rats are more expensive than mice, their larger size lends itself to studies that require cannulation (e.g., Subramanian *et al.*, 1990; Subramanian, 1994) or electrode implantation (e.g., Shen *et al.*, 1995).

Mice and rats differ, however, in sensitivity to morphological anomalies. Mice appear to show more renal (Randall & Taylor, 1979) and craniofacial dysmorphology than rats (Sulik & Johnston, 1983; Kotch & Sulik, 1992). However, the same types of defects are seen in rats, either at lower frequencies or more subtly (e.g., Edwards & Dow-Edwards, 1991). Different susceptibility to teratology may occur because strains and lines of rodents vary in characteristics related to alcohol responsivity (e.g., LS vs SS, DBA vs C57B/ 6J mice; and P vs NP rats). Such species differences are proving valuable in assessing hypotheses about the potential genetic bases for differential susceptibility to the teratogenic effects of alcohol (e.g, Melcer *et al.*, 1995*a, b*). However, it is not always obvious exactly what phenotype is being selected for evaluation. For example, rats may drink more alcohol because reduced gustatory function increases palatability. To date, no animals have been bred specifically for sensitivity to any teratogenic outcome, although there is evidence that sensitivity in one measure can be correlated with susceptibility to fetal alcohol effects (Gilliam *et al.*, 1987, 1990; Gilliam & Irtenkauf, 1990). If selected phenotypes later prove to be associated with different susceptibilities to fetal alcohol effects, then the mechanism(s) of alcohol teratogenesis would be expected to be related to the biological bases for the phenotypic difference (e.g., in alcohol metabolism or CNS sensitivity). Studies examining genotypic risk factors in human FAS are also in progress (e.g., Sokol *et al.*, 1989; Faustman *et al.*, 1992).

Non-human primates

The monkey has been viewed as a more appropriate animal model because non-human primates are the species most similar to humans in many respects (e.g., Altshuler & Shippenberg, 1981; Clarren & Bowden, 1982). Like humans, monkeys have very long gestation periods and typically produce singleton births. The maturational course of their brain development and the levels of cognitive functioning are also quite comparable to humans. However, use of non-human primates in fetal alcohol research has been infrequent because they are very expensive to house and the numbers of subjects used in experiments have been relatively small. Attempts to coordinate use of the offspring of monkeys exposed to alcohol during gestation for a multidisciplinary assessment by several laboratories may help maximize results for the extra investment in primates.

Other mammals

Research on sheep has contributed to our understanding of placental transport systems and endocrinology of the maternal/fetal unit (e.g., Falconer, 1990). Because of their large size and extended gestation period of 147 days, the ewe and fetus can be monitored and treated separately and for long periods in chronic preparations. For example, changes in ovine thyroid hormone release and metabolism were measured directly in cannulated fetuses while the ewe was infused with alcohol (Castro *et al.*, 1986; Rose *et al.*, 1981; Smith *et al.*, 1990; Sinervo *et al.*, 1992). Dogs, cats and pigs have also been studied. Guinea pigs (Catlin *et al.*, 1993; Clarke *et al.*, 1986) and the so-called 'spiny mouse' (*Acomys*) would be valuable because, as precocious species, more of their CNS development occurs *in utero*, as it does in humans, than is the case in mice and rats (see Sensitive or 'Critical' Periods below). Porcine models (e.g., Dexter *et al.*, 1976, 1980) are valuable because of their very large size and because the pig may be unique in apparently liking alcohol, preferring it to plain water in choice situations.

Avian models

Birds have been used effectively to assess effects of alcohol on growth and trophic factors (e.g., Pennington, 1990, 1992). Chick embryos have the distinct advantages of being very inexpensive because dozens of eggs, with singleton embryos, can be treated directly, simply, and with little more in the way of requirements than warmth. Since there is no mother, the intervening influences of differential maternal stress, food consumption and other behaviors, and of placental transport, are eliminated. Eggs are very easy to manipulate and excellent control can be maintained over alcohol concentration.

Other species

Specific biological questions of interest can also be addressed in other animals, and the options are limited only by an investigator's inventiveness. For example, tadpoles have been developed as a model to study how alcohol disrupts hormonal control of development (cf., Uray *et al.*, 1987). Depending on concentration, tadpoles raised with alcohol in their water can continue to grow well but not metamorphose into frogs. Because alcohol decreases thyroxine levels, very large tadpoles are produced with CNS abnormalities similar to those found in rats, perhaps due to analogous endocrine mechanism.

Methodological considerations

A key pharmacological predictor of fetal alcohol effects is peak blood alcohol level (BAL). Peak BAL depends upon several factors especially dose, route of administration, and pattern of consumption, and other factors affecting alcohol absorption, distribution and metabolism, including food consumption, alcohol tolerance and genetics.

Dose

The total amount of alcohol consumed during pregnancy is clearly a most important risk factor for ARBDs and FAS in humans (Brown *et al.*, 1979; Coles, 1994; Abel & Hannigan, 1995*a*) and in animals (Pierce & West, 1986*a*, *b*) and, of course, a determinant of peak BAL (West *et al.*, 1989, 1990*b*; West & Goodlett, 1990; Bonthius & West, 1988). Dose must be carefully defined as the relative amount of alcohol administered per unit body weight. Estimates of total daily alcohol intake among pregnant alcoholic women giving birth to alcohol-affected infants can vary substantially (Abel, 1984; Coles, 1994; Jacobson & Jacobson, 1994). It is important to note that different species of animals, and humans, may respond differently to the same relative daily dose, in grams per kilogram body weight, because of species differences based on metabolic rate, alcohol metabolism, and alcohol sensitivity.

While it may be satisfying to design alcohol consumption and BALs in animals that look like those in humans, it is important that the chosen doses be within a species-relevant range. Ideally, doses should include a no alcohol group (0 g/kg), some very high dose defined as a threshold dose for maternal toxicity, and one or two doses in between. It is often useful in teratology to define the highest dose near a threshold for maternal toxicity, both to max-imize the likelihood that the fetuses will be affected by some dose (i.e., to optimize a dose–response curve) and to address the possibility that fetal effects may be secondary to maternally mediated toxic responses rather than a teratogenic action on the fetus itself. Maternal toxicity is an overt sign that fetuses may be at risk and doses at less-than-maternal toxicity may not obviously be a risk for fetuses. In practice, however, fetal alcohol research in animal models often uses only one dose of alcohol because the designs of the experiments are otherwise so large and expensive. If single doses must be used, the investigator must take care to justify why the specific dose was chosen. The investigator should also be aware that when any single dose is administered, positive results need not be specific to alcohol. Any perturbation may have the same general effect. Generation of a dose–response relationship is more convincing evidence that an effect is specific to alcohol.

Route of administration

Oral administration is preferred in animal models because it is obviously the route used by humans drinking alcohol. Other routes (e.g., subcutaneous or intraperitoneal) are not advised because subcutaneous injections can be irri-tating to dermal membranes and intraperitoneal injections run the risk of direct injection to the uterus or other organ. Intravenous administration is impractical with smaller animals, in chronic administration routines, and in large experiments, but can afford exquisite dose control and maintenance of BALs in some acute preparations (e.g., Rose *et al.*, 1981). Inhalation models are valuable particularly in studying hazards of environmental exposure to alcohol, an industrial solvent. Inhalation models require special housing and ventilation systems to control inspired alcohol and protect research staff from exposure, but have the advantage of allowing a rapid rise to relatively stable BALs (cf. Nelson *et al.*, 1985, 1990).

Oral administration is achieved in several ways. Voluntary consumption of alcohol in drinking water (e.g., 10% ethanol) has been used more often in Europe (e.g., Ledig *et al.*, 1988; Portoles *et al.*, 1988; Guerri *et al.*, 1989) and has the advantage of relative ease. However, animals tend to avoid alcohol in this form so that peak BALs higher than 100 mg/dl (100 mg%) are difficult to obtain. Oral consumption is 'voluntary' in that animals choose between drinking alcohol and not drinking anything.

Oral alcohol administration via free-feeding of an alcohol-adulterated nutritionally complete liquid diet is one of the most common methods of giving ethanol to pregnant animals (Abel, 1984; Meyer & Riley, 1986). Liquid diets are made palatable by adding chocolate or sugars to mask the taste of alcohol. There are several base formulae for liquid diets, including commercial human dietary supplements (e.g., Sustacal, Mead-Johnson) that are fortified with additional vitamins and minerals, and several products designed specifically for rats (e.g., BioServ products).

Mankes *et al.* (1992) assessed several liquid diets and evaluated them on the basis of alcohol intake. For example, animals fed a commercial rat diet (BioServ) consumed more alcohol and had higher BACs than those fed fortified Sustacal diet and had smaller decreases in birth weight, although each diet could be appropriate by other criteria (specific nutrients, etc.). Liquid diet procedures give animals only one source of food and can produce relatively stable, low peak BALs throughout the day. The procedure can be simple but has the disadvantage that alcohol intake can vary considerably among individual animals. For example, in a 'retrospective' analysis of 221 dams administered a liquid diet with 6.1% ethanol from gestation days 6 (GD6) through GD20, the average daily ethanol consumption was 12.95 g/kg (± 1.32), but ranged between about 4 and 18 g/kg per day, with consumption for 95% of the dams between 10.36 and 15.54 g/kg per day. Such fluctuation in the actual dose of alcohol is a disadvantage of the model because it can increase the variability in the alcohol-exposed groups regardless of outcome, making it more difficult to detect systematic effects due to alcohol. Within nominally uniform alcohol groups, alcohol consumption was correlated inversely with birth weight (Hannigan *et al.*, 1993*a*).

Oral administration via intragastric intubation can achieve much greater control of dose and peak BAL than alcohol in diets or drinking water, by delivering the alcohol solution directly into the dam's stomach. Oral intubation procedures allow the investigator to determine precisely when, how much and how frequently alcohol will be consumed. In this protocol, a smooth curved or sometimes flexible tube is inserted into the esophagus and a bolus of dilute alcohol is injected quickly. This procedure can be done relatively easily and requires some training and skill to do so. The disadvantages of this procedure are that the animals need to be handled and are stressed by the intubation procedure itself, even with the most skillful intubation.

It has been our experience that dams given intubations or liquid diets *without* ethanol frequently produce offspring that are different on various biobehavioral measures from the offspring of non-intubated control dams. Intubation or restricted diet effects can be independent of fetal alcohol effects. Animals fed liquid diets containing alcohol distribute intake of the less palatable solution evenly across each day, whereas the pair-fed dams tend to drink all available diet quickly, remaining hungry and perhaps stressed most of the day. It appears also that animals given both the intubation treatment and alcohol may be stressed differentially by the intubation procedure. Interactions between prenatal stress and prenatal alcohol exposure have been demonstrated (e.g., McGivern, 1989; Ward & Wainwright, 1991; Tritt *et al.*, 1993). These interactions and the effects of intubations *per se* mean that the statistical detection of selective prenatal alcohol effects can be more difficult.

Patterns of administration

Peak BAL is profoundly affected by the pattern of alcohol consumption. Women who drink in binges during pregnancy are more likely to have infants born with cognitive fetal alcohol effects (Streissguth *et al.*, 1994). Animal models have demonstrated more severe effects of early neonatal alcohol exposure (Bonthius & West, 1990) on growth and brain maturation when alcohol was given in four daily feedings than when the same amount of total daily alcohol was distributed over 12 daily feedings. The 'binging' pattern in both humans (Jacobson & Jacobson, 1994) and animals (Bonthius & West, 1990; Goodlett *et al.*, 1991) clearly increased the severity and extent of fetal alcohol effects.

Sensitive or 'critical' periods of exposure

Closely related to patterns of administration, is the specification of when the animal is given alcohol: before, during and/or after pregnancy (Clode *et al.*, 1987; Brodie & Vernadikis, 1990). One of the primary tenets of teratology is that specific outcomes depend critically on when during the developmental period teratogenic exposure occurs (Vorhees, 1986). Animal models can be used effectively to discriminate when specific developmental processes will be sensitive to the teratogenic effects of alcohol by restricting alcohol exposure to discrete developmental periods. A disadvantage of this approach is that such restricted exposure may not reflect the timing of human alcohol consumption. Alcoholic women do not begin their alcohol abuse only after they are 2 or 3 months pregnant. It may be argued that animal models of ARBDs that do not test dams that are tolerant to some of the effects of alcohol may not be evaluating the potential risk to the fetuses fairly (cf. Coles, 1994). Risk to fetuses may be *exaggerated* if a mechanism of alcohol teratogenesis is related to an effect of alcohol to which tolerance develops in the dams. Risk to fetuses may be *under*estimated in offspring of tolerant dams if teratogenesis is due to an effect of alcohol that does not show tolerance because alcohol consumption increases following the development of tolerance. In either case, maternal tolerance is clearly a potential contributor to the effects of alcohol on developing fetuses. However, effects on behavior, physiology, growth, neurochemistry and endocrinology have been found in offspring born to rat dams that had drunk 10% alcohol in their drinking water for several months before mating, as well as in offspring where the first alcohol exposure did not occur until the second or third week of gestation (cf., Meyer & Riley, 1986; Ledig *et al.*, 1988; Portoles *et al.*, 1988; Guerri *et al.*, 1989). A related point is that the age of the rat dam can also influence the impact of alcohol (Vorhees, 1988), even without prior pregnancies or experience with alcohol.

The 'pup-in-the-cup' artificial rearing procedure is a version of direct oral intubation that allows alcohol to be administered during the CNS developmental period in the rat that is equivalent to the third trimester of human gestation (West, 1993). Alcohol is delivered through an indwelling intragastric canula to neonatal pups. In this artificial rearing procedure, a plastic tube is inserted surgically through the abdominal and stomach walls of a young rat pup and secured. Liquid diets are infused via a programmable pump at regular intervals, with or without alcohol. The pups are maintained this way typically from postnatal days 4 (PN4) through PN10 in a small plastic cup with nesting material, and floating in a warm bath. The floating cups, and a daily handling to stimulate bladder elimination, are designed to mimic warm nest conditions and some maternal interactions. Control groups include cannulated animals that do not receive alcohol, and untreated pups, called suckled controls, raised by foster dams. However, one of the clear disadvantages of this procedure is that animals are isolated and have no real maternal or litter contact. These disadvantages must be weighed against the clear advantages of gaining precise control of alcohol administration at a developmentally important period modelling the CNS maturational equiva-lent of the human third trimester.

Design considerations

Nutritional control groups

After alcohol, nutritional factors are perhaps the most influential contributor to fetal alcohol effects (Weinberg, 1984; Fisher *et al.*, 1986; Fisher, 1988; Dreosti, 1993; Abel & Hannigan, 1995*a*). Alcoholism in humans is accom-panied by a host of primary and secondary metabolic and nutritional com-promises that exacerbate the impact of alcohol abuse. There are several recent reviews that detail the relationship between alcohol and nutrition (Watson & Watzl, 1992). Each of the changes in nutrients can affect fetal development in the pregnant alcoholic, and some have been implicated as specific mechanisms of alcohol teratogenesis (Dreosti, 1993; Abel & Hannigan, 1995*a*). Considerable effort has gone into devising methods to assure that alcohol-exposed groups are nourished equivalently to controls so that any effects of alcohol on fetuses could be attributed to prenatal alcohol exposure *per se* (Weinberg, 1984; Fisher *et al.*, 1986; Fisher, 1988). These methods are needed because alcohol provides calories to the diet (Lieber, 1991), and maternal caloric intake is clearly a factor that can affect fetal development.

Pair-feeding is the primary method for equating caloric intake between groups. This technique involves measuring the daily food intake of alco-hol-treated animals and allocating that same amount to control dams on a relative body weight basis. Pair-fed liquid diets are made isocaloric to the alcohol diets usually with added carbohydrates such as sucrose or maltose/dextrin. Pair-feeding can also equate calories with protein or lipids, and can be used to equate food intake for oral intubation administrations as well. Pair-feeding can help match the daily pattern of food intake of control animals to the pattern in alcohol-fed dams, which tend to distribute intake of the non-preferred alcohol across the day rather than to eat in a normal prandial pattern.

Pair-feeding regimes equating calorie intake and limiting food access are one way to control for differential nutrients. Other protocols address nutri-tional issues by supplementing diets of alcohol-exposed dams with various nutrients. Alcohol depletes levels of many specific nutrients – from vitamin A to zinc – by decreasing nutrient intake, altering gastrointestinal absorption, and compromising metabolism (e.g., Fisher *et al.*, 1988). By supplementing diets, alcohol's effects can be studied independently of these nutrient deficiencies. Supplementation studies can indicate whether fetal alcohol effects are due directly to the alcohol rather than to the secondary effects of nutrition and can also determine whether alcohol-related nutritional compromise is integral to mechanism(s) of fetal alcohol effects (Dreosti, 1993). Depending on the investigator's perspective, the same results of a dietary supplementation study might have different interpretations. Supplementation of animals' diets with specific nutrients has attenuated fetal alcohol effects. For example, increasing the protein contents of diets reduced alcohol-induced fetal growth retardation (Weiner *et al.*, 1981). Addition of Ω-3 fatty acids (Wainwright *et al.*, 1989, 1995) or ganglioside GM_1(Hungund *et al.*, 1991, 1994) similarly improved fetal outcome and behavioral competence. On the other hand, whereas nutrient deficiencies (e.g., reduced zinc levels: Fisher *et al.*, 1988) have been associated with increased fetal vulnerability to alcohol, supplementation beyond normally adequate dietary levels of nutrients for pregnant rats may not eliminate ARBDs (e.g., Tanaka *et al.*, 1983, 1988). Such studies emphasize the importance of pre-existing nutritional deficiency to the teratogenic potential of alcohol (cf., Abel & Hannigan, 1995*a*) and to the design of valid animal models.

Prenatal stress

In the same way that nutritional factors must be considered in animal models of ARBDs, handling pregnant animals and the procedures for administering alcohol also have to be considered because these procedures can produce general stress reactions in dams and their fetuses (Archer & Blackman, 1971; Ward & Wainwright, 1991; Tritt *et al.*, 1993). For example, we noted above that the offspring of pair-fed dams and dams intubated without alcohol appear to be different from control (unhandled) rats. The liquid diet pairfeeding procedure may be intrinsically stressful to pair-fed controls because these dams consume a relatively small amount of diet all at once when it is presented, compared with the alcohol-treated dams who measure out their intake of the unpalatable alcohol-adulterated solution across the day. The pair-fed dams therefore spend much of the day hungry. This potential confound can be rectified by 'yoking' the availability of diet for the pair-fed dam to the actual consumption pattern of an alcohol-treated dam. For example, the use of yoked, water-jacketed Richter tubes can automatically control the pattern of diet availability. The control oral intubation procedure itself is stressful and can affect fetuses. Alcohol, on the other hand, may reduce the stressful component of intubation, but this has not been tested. These aspects of the alcohol administration procedures themselves imply that there should also be an untreated *ad libitum*-fed or nonintubated control group included in the design of these experiments. Interpretation of the results from these animal models should include recognition that these inter-actions between stress and alcohol operate in people as well (Bingol *et al.*, 1987; Blomberg, 1980).

Postnatal development

In terms of CNS maturation, the early postnatal period is continuous with the fetal period and models studying the impact of postgestational alcohol are an important component of fetal alcohol research. We noted above how the first postnatal week in rats is the CNS developmental equivalent of the human third trimester of gestation. The 'pup-in-the-cup' procedures allow alcohol to be administered in high concentrations and in specific patterns during this time (West, 1993). Other models begin or continue alcohol admin-istration to the dam during the lactation period (Portoles *et al.*, 1988; Gottesfeld & LeGrue, 1990; Subramanian *et al.*, 1990; Subramanian, 1994). Maternal alcohol at this time does not produce high BALs in offspring but can influence neonatal development by altering lactation and milk let-down and/or by altering maternal–pup interactions critical to normal maturation.

It is necessary to cull litters to a constant number of pups per dam (e.g., 8 or 10) to limit the postnatal impact of differential nursing. Prenatal alcohol can reduce litter size and increase intralitter variability in several measures (e.g., birth weight: Hannigan *et al.*, 1993a). The increased heterogeneity within alcohol-exposed litters means that random culling could eliminate some of the more affected pups from the experiment, reducing the apparent impact of alcohol. Conversely, if the most affected pups are selected inten-tionally (e.g., on the basis of birth weight), they may not survive to testing.

The influence of gestational alcohol exposure can profoundly affect what happens during the early postnatal period. Prenatal alcohol exposure can also affect maternal behavior, even when alcohol administration has stopped prior to birth, due in part to withdrawal from alcohol. Depending upon the method of alcohol administration, compromised maternal behavior can include cannibalism (Abel, 1979). If the focus of the study is the persistent postnatal effects of alcohol exposure during the fetal period, then it may be necessary to control for differential maternal behavior by fostering. In sur-rogate fostering, untreated lactating dams are given the alcohol-exposed or

pair-fed pups soon after birth to replace their own. The rationale is to eliminate postnatal differences in maternal interactions with pups due to maternal
alcohol treatment, although it is possible that rat pups exposed prenatally to
alcohol may react differently to fostering than do control pups (Rockwood &
Riley, 1990). Fostering can also be used to assess the contribution of maternal behavior. In cross-fostering, offspring from each prenatal treatment
group are raised by dams from each of the other groups (Meyer & Riley,
1986). A factorial design would allow detection of any maternal–fetal treatment interactions.

Surrogate and cross-fostering more than double the number of animals
needed and so are very expensive procedures. Vorhees (1989) has shown that
such procedures are not always necessary since fostering had little effect on
rat behavioral maturation after liquid diet administration of alcohol to dams.
However, Abel (1979) showed that following oral intubation offspring of
alcohol-intubated dams were profoundly affected by being raised with their
birth dams and benefited from surrogate fostering.

Few studies have assessed the role of the postweaning environment on the
expression of fetal alcohol effects. Earlier reports (e.g., Osbourne *et al.*, 1980)
found no differential effect of enriched environments. More recent work has
shown that behavioral performance can be significantly improved by rearing
fetal alcohol-exposed rats or mice in enriched environments (Wainwright *et
al.*, 1993; Hannigan *et al.*, 1993*b*) although the brains of alcohol-exposed
offspring may not retain the same level of plasticity in response to the environment as controls (Wainwright *et al.*, 1993; Berman *et al.*, 1996). It is
necessary to recognize that there are no standard living conditions among
laboratories and that the details of the environment and how animals are
handled and reared at all developmental phases can influence the expression
of fetal alcohol effects and must be specified (cf., Holson *et al.*, 1991).

Age at testing

Related to postnatal factors is age of testing. It has been argued that testing
at younger ages is a more sensitive assessment of fetal alcohol effects because
these can diminish over time due to recovery of function and/or withdrawal
(Riley *et al.*, 1985; West *et al.*, 1990*a*). Assessments can also be made prenatally, including the many studies of fetal chemistry, growth, anatomy, and
physiology assessing directly the sensitive periods of response to alcohol.
Fetal behavior has also been assessed in an elegant model where the uterus
is exteriorized from a pregnant rat dam given local (spinal) anesthesia. The
fetus is freed from the uterine membranes and allowed to float in a warm

bath still connected to the dam via the umbilical cord. With this model, Smotherman *et al.* (1986, 1987) directly observed the effects of alcohol given to the dam on fetal behavior. Other applications of this acute preparation, including other species, could help measure how alcohol affects fetuses.

Effects detected at one age may not be present in another. For example, deficits in learning a Morris maze are evident in younger but not older animals (e.g. Blanchard *et al.*, 1990), while dysmetric gait is found in older but not younger animals (e.g., Hannigan & Riley, 1988; Meyer *et al.*, 1990). Prior postnatal experience also influences effects at testing. Hall *et al.* (1995) reported radial arm maze deficits in young rats or in adult rats when tested the first time, but not in adult rats that had been in the maze before. Similar dependence on outcome is also seen for neuroanatomical and neurochemical measures. It is difficult to generalize that fetal alcohol effects are transitory since some deficits are revealed only at later maturational stages (Abel *et al.*, 1993; Riley, 1990; West *et al.*, 1990a). Researchers must be aware of the importance of age of testing and be able to justify the ages chosen.

Paternal influences

Women alcoholics tend to consort with male alcoholics. In addition to the social facilitation in the pattern and amount of alcohol that these associations afford (Cicero, 1994), animal models have been able to eliminate social factors to show that there are biological contributions of paternal alcohol consumption to fetal outcome (Abel, 1992). Offspring sired by alcohol-treated male rats show deficits in sexual maturation, altered endocrine and immune function, and behavioral differences from control offspring (Abel, 1989; Gottesfeld & Abel, 1991; Wozniak *et al.*, 1991) even after a single, acute injection with alcohol (Cicero *et al.*, 1994). This means that animal models in which only the pregnant females are given alcohol may not be evaluating the full risk. The mechanism(s) of this paternal influence are not known, but likely involve some change to sperm integrity, selection or activity (Cicero, 1994).

Analytic considerations

Sample size

Determination of sample size depends upon the statistical considerations (e.g., effect size, alpha level, desired power) as well as the outcome measures. We have demonstrated in an analysis of historical data on birth weight in rats exposed prenatally to alcohol, that 7 litters are needed reliably to detect differences between offspring of *ad libitum* chow-fed control dams and of alcohol-treated dams ($\alpha = 0.05$, $1-\beta = 0.90$), and 12 litters are needed reliably to detect the same magnitude differences between the pair-fed and alcohol-exposed offspring (Hannigan *et al.*, 1993a). For behavioral teratogenesis effects, it has been argued that because of the relatively greater variability in fetal response to prenatal alcohol than, for example, in an acute pharmacological response, more subjects are needed. Abel & Riley (1986) recommended 15 subjects per cell in the design of experiments assessing behavioral outcome.

Unit of analysis

The affected fetus is the subject of interest although analyses of data from species with multiple-offspring litters require special considerations. Because it is the pregnant dam that is treated, the litter should be the unit of analyses. This means that either the litter means for dependent variables, or the measure from a single representative from each litter, should be included in any cell of an experimental design. Because interlitter variability can be much greater than intralitter variability for rodents, using more than one subject from the same litter would weight analyses in favor of that one litter (Abbey & Howard, 1973). Using as few as 2 rats per litter as independent measurements can inflate apparent significance, increase within-treatment error and actually reduce power (Holson & Pearce, 1992). It has been recommended that the preferred analyses would measure just one pup per litter, although litter means can be used if possible (Holson & Pearce, 1992). In practical terms, unit litter analyses with multiparous species remains an advantage because littermates can be distributed among several experiments, or used in different conditions (e.g., dose of a challenge drug, age at testing) in the same experiment. It does not appear to be the case that chance sampling from litters can influence detection of significant effects. For example, prenatal alcohol exposure via liquid diets in rats affected birth weight of whole litters equivalently (Hannigan *et al.*, 1993a). That is, since the intralitter variability in birth weight was not altered by alcohol, any pup selected at random would be as valid a representative of the litter's response to alcohol as would any other pup or the litter mean (Hannigan *et al.*, 1993a).

Gender as a repeated factor

Male and female offspring responded differently to the teratogenic effects of alcohol (e.g., Hannigan & Pilati, 1991; Weinberg, 1992; McGivern & Riley,

1993). Recognition of gender differences may make it difficult to justify assessing one gender only on either historic or economic grounds. Including both sexes is strongly recommended. An issue related to units of analysis in multiple offspring litters and offspring gender concerns statistical analyses. Using males and females from the same litter is essentially using more than one subject per litter. Analyzing 'gender' as a between-subjects factor does distribute the influence of the litter across cells in the design. While it may be more appropriate to treat 'gender' as a repeated measure (i.e., a within-litter factor), our preliminary analyses suggest there is little difference in outcome compared with between-litter analysis (Abel, unpublished data). This issue requires further study.

Cofactors

While control of potential 'confounding' factors is a clear advantage of animal models, including those factors as specifically manipulated variables can greatly enhance the value of experiments. As noted, the potential interactions of poor nutrition (Keppen *et al.*, 1985; Weinberg *et al.*, 1990), environmental toxins (e.g., Grasnick & Huel, 1985) or drugs (e.g., Henderson *et al.*, 1991; Church *et al.*, 1991; Randall *et al.*, 1994; Hannigan, 1995) with prenatal alcohol have been assessed with factorial designs. The feasibility of including these cofactors depends upon the availability of resources and the specific hypotheses under consideration, and certainly all factors will not always be included.

In vitro systems

In addition to the whole animal models described above, *in vitro* models are being used with increasing sophistication to assess potential mechanisms of alcohol teratogenesis. The extraordinary control of these simple systems is particularly amenable to cell biological and molecular biological approaches. These models include whole mouse or chick embryos ranging from blastulae to early fetal stages (Brown *et al.*, 1979; Clode *et al.*, 1987; Brodie & Vernadikis, 1990; Davis *et al.*, 1990; Pennington, 1990, 1992; Leach *et al.*, 1993; Stachecki *et al.*, 1994*a, b*) and primary cultures of neurons and/or glial cells harvested from rat and mouse fetal brains, livers and hearts (e.g., Fletcher & Shain, 1993; Henderson *et al.*, 1982, 1991). Cell cultures of rodent (e.g., pheocytochrome cells: PC-12) or human tumor lines (e.g., neuroblastoma cells: LA-N-5) have also been used to assess alcohol's interference in early cellular developmental processes (e.g., Pantazis *et al.*, 1992; Saunders *et* *al.*, 1995). Finally, *in vitro* systems using human tissues (e.g., neuroblastoma cells or placenta) are quite valuable for directly assessing potential mechanisms in humans (Fisher *et al.*, 1983, 1986; Henderson *et al.*, 1982, 1991; Schenker *et al.*, 1990; Devi *et al.*, 1993).

Enhancing the complexity of animal models: parsimony versus power

Little is known about why only some of the infants born to frankly alcoholic women are diagnosed as having FAS and it is currently not possible to predict which alcoholic women give birth to children with FAS (cf., Abel, 1990; Abel & Hannigan, 1995*a*), except that women who have previously had one FAS child are fairly certain to have another (e.g., Abel, 1990). Animal models and basic research can substantially facilitate our understanding of risk factors and mechanisms by allowing a degree of control of the many 'confounding' factors influencing alcohol teratogenesis not possible in epidemiological or clinical studies (Schenker *et al.*, 1990). We believe that fetal alcohol research has reached a stage where it should build 'confounders' back into the experimental designs in systematic ways, to assess directly how factors such as co-drug use or abuse, and maternal undernutrition or stress are influencing susceptibility to prenatal alcohol exposure. For all their disadvantages, animal models will continue to be in the vanguard of fetal alcohol research because of their advantages.

Acknowledgments

Preparation of this chapter was supported in part by the Fetal Alcohol Research Center grant (P50-AA07606) and research grant R01-06721 from NIAAA.

References

Abbey, H. & Howard, E. (1973). Statistical procedures in developmental studies on species with multi-offspring. *Developmental Psychobiology*, **6**, 329–36.

Abel, E.L. (1979). Effects of alcohol withdrawal and under-nutrition in cannibalism of rat pups. *Behavioral Neurology and Biology*, **25**, 411–13.

Abel, E.L. (1984). *Fetal Alcohol Syndrome and Fetal Alcohol Effects*. New York: Plenum Press.

Abel, E.L. (1989). Paternal and maternal alcohol consumption: effects on offspring in two strains of rats. *Alcoholism: Clinical and Experimental Research*, **13**, 533–41.

Abel, E.L. (1990). *Fetal Alcohol Syndrome*. New Jersey: Medical Economic Press.

Abel, E.L. (1992). Paternal exposure to alcohol. In *Perinatal Substance Abuse: Research Findings and Clinical Implications*, ed. T.B. Sonderegger, pp. 132–62. Baltimore: Johns Hopkins University Press.

Abel, E.L., Berman, R.F. & Church, M.W. (1993). Prenatal alcohol exposure attenuates pentylenetetrazol-induced convulsions in rats. *Alcohol*, **10**, 155–7.

Abel, E.L. & Hannigan, J.H. (1995*a*). Maternal risk factors in fetal alcohol syndrome: provocative and permissive influences. *Neurobehavioral Teratology and Toxicology*, **17**, 445–62.

Abel, E.L. & Hannigan, J.H. (1995*b*). J-shaped relationship between drinking during pregnancy and birth weight: reanalysis of prospective epidemiological data. *Alcohol and Alcoholism*, **30**, 345–55.

Abel, E.L. & Riley, E.P. (1986). Studies of prenatal alcohol exposure: methodological considerations. In *Alcohol and Brain Development*, ed. J.R. West, pp. 105–19. New York: Oxford University Press.

Adams, J. (1986). Methods in behavioral teratology. In *Handbook of Behavioral Teratology*, ed. E.P. Riley & C.V. Vorhees, pp. 67–99. New York: Plenum Press.

Altshuler, H.L. & Shippenberg, T.S. (1981). A subhuman primate model for fetal alcohol syndrome research. *Neurobehavioral Toxicology and Teratology*, **3**, 121–6.

Archer, J.E. & Blackman, D.E. (1971). Prenatal psychological stress and offspring behavior in rats and mice. *Developmental Psychobiology*, **4**, 193–248.

Becker, H.C., Randall, C.L., Salo, A.L., Saulnier, J.L. & Weathersby, R.T. (1994). Animal research: charting the course of FAS. *Alcohol Health and Research World*, **18**, 10–16.

Berman, R.F., Hannigan, J.H., Sperry, M.A. & Zajac, C.S. (1996). Prenatal alcohol exposure eliminates the effects of environmental enrichment as hippocampal dendritic spine density. *Alcohol*, in press.

Bingol, N., Scuster, C., Fuchs, M., Iosub, S., Turner, G., Stone, R.K. & Gromisch, D.S. (1987). The influence of socioeconomic factors on the occurrence of fetal alcohol syndrome. *Advances in Alcoholism and Substance Abuse*, **6**, 105–18.

Blanchard, B.A., Pilati, M.L. & Hannigan, J.H. (1990). The role of stress and age in spatial navigation deficits following prenatal exposure to ethanol. *Psychobiology*, **18**, 48–54.

Blomberg, S. (1980). Influence of maternal distress during pregnancy on fetal malformations. *Acta Psychiatrica Scandinavica*, **62**, 315–30.

Bonthius, D.J. & West, J.R. (1988). Blood alcohol concentration and microencephaly: a dose–response study in the neonatal rat. *Teratology*, **37**, 223–31.

Bonthius, D.J. & West, J.R. (1990). Alcohol-induced neuronal loss in developing rats: increased brain damage with binge exposure. *Alcoholism: Clinical and Experimental Research*, **14**, 107–18.

Brodie, C. & Vernadikis, A. (1990). Critical periods to ethanol exposure during early neuroembryogenesis in the chick embryo: cholinergic neurons. *Developmental Brain Research*, **56**, 223–8.

Brown, N.A., Goulding, E.H. & Fabro, S. (1979). Ethanol embryotoxicity: direct effects on mammalian embryos *in vitro*. *Science*, **206**, 573–5.

Castro, M.I., Koritnik, D.R. & Rose, J.C. (1986). Fetal plasma insulin and thyroid hormone levels during acute *in utero* ethanol exposure in a maternal–fetal sheep model. *Endocrinology*, **118**, 1735–42.

Catlin, M.C., Abdollah, S. & Brien, J.F. (1993). Dose-dependent effects of prenatal ethanol exposure in the guinea pig. *Alcohol*, **10**, 109–15.

Chernoff, G.F. (1977). The fetal alcohol syndrome in mice: an animal model. *Teratology*, **15**, 223–30.

Church, M.W. (1987). Chronic *in utero* alcohol exposure affects auditory function in rats and humans. *Alcohol*, **4**, 231–9.

Church, M.W., Holmes, P.A., Overbeck, G.W., Tilak, J.P. & Zajac, C.S. (1991). Interactive effects of prenatal alcohol and cocaine exposure on postnatal mortality, development and behavior in the Long-Evans rat. *Neurotoxicology and Teratology*, **13**, 377–86.

Cicero, T.J. (1994). Effects of paternal exposure to alcohol on offspring development. *Alcohol Health and Research World*, **18**, 37–41.

Cicero, T.J., Nock, B., O'Connor, L.H., Sewing, B.N., Adams, M.L. & Meyer, E.R. (1994). Acute paternal alcohol exposure impairs fertility and fetal outcome. *Life Sciences*, **55**, 33–6.

Clarke, D.W., Stenaart, N.A., Slack, C.J. & Brien, J.F. (1986). Pharmacokinetics of ethanol and its metabolite, acetaldehyde, and fetolethality in the third-trimester pregnant guinea pig for oral administration of acute, multiple-dose ethanol. *Canadian Journal of Physiology and Pharmacology*, **64**, 1060–7.

Clarren, S.K. & Bowden, D.M. (1982). Fetal alcohol syndrome: a new primate model for binge drinking and its relevance to human ethanol teratogenesis. *Journal of Pediatrics*, **101**, 819–24.

Clode, A.M., Pratten, M.K. & Beck, F. (1987). A stage-dependent effect of ethanol on 9.5-day rat embryos grown in culture and the role played by the concomitant rise in osmolality. *Teratology*, **35**, 395–403.

Coles, C.D., (1994). Critical periods for prenatal alcohol exposure. *Alcohol Health and Research World*, **18**, 22–9.

Davis, W.L., Crawford, L.A., Cooper, O.J., Farmer, G.R., Thomas, D.L. & Freeman, B.L. (1990). Ethanol induces the generation of reactive free radicals by neural crest cells *in vitro*. *Journal of Craniofacial Genetics and Development Biology*, **10**, 277–93.

DeBeukelar, M.M., Randall, C.L. & Stond, D.R. (1977). Renal anomalies in the fetal alcohol syndrome. *Journal of Pediatrics*, **91**, 759–60.

Devi, B.G., Henderson, G.I., Frosto, T.A. & Schenker, S. (1993). Effect of ethanol on rat fetal hepatocytes: studies on cell replication, lipid peroxidation and glutathione. *Hepatology*, **18**, 648–59.

Dexter, J.D., Tumbleson, M.E., Hutcheson, D.P. & Middleton, C.C. (1976). Sinclair (S-1) miniature swine as a model for the study of human alcoholism. *Annals of the New York Academy of Sciences*, **273**, 188–93.

Dexter, J.D., Tumbleson, M.E., Decker, J.D. & Middleton, C.C. (1980). Fetal alcohol syndrome in Sinclair (S-1) miniature swine. *Alcoholism: Clinical and Experimental Research*, **4**, 146–51.

Dreosti, I.E. (1993). Nutritional factors underlying the expression of the fetal alcohol syndrome. *Annals of the New York Academy of Sciences*, **678**, 193–204.

Driscoll, C.D., Streissguth, A.P. & Riley, E.P. (1990). Prenatal alcohol exposure: comparability of effects in humans and animal models. *Neurotoxicology and Teratology*, **12**, 231–7.

Edwards, H.G. & Dow-Edwards, D.L. (1991). Craniofacial alterations in adult rats prenatally exposed to ethanol. *Teratology*, **44**, 373–8.

Falconer, J. (1990). The effect of maternal ethanol infusion on placental blood flow and fetal glucose metabolism in sheep. *Alcohol and Alcoholism*, **25**, 413–16.

Faustman, E.M., Streissguth, A.P., Stevenson, L.M., Omenn, G.S. & Yoshida, A. (1992). Role of maternal and fetal alcohol metabolizing genotypes in fetal alcohol syndrome. *The Toxicologist*, **12**, 1562.

Fisher, S.E. (1988). Selective fetal malnutrition: the fetal alcohol syndrome. *Journal of the American College of Nutrition*, **7**, 101–6.

Fisher, S.E., Atkinson, M., Jacobson, S., Shegal, P., Burnap, J., Holmes, E., Teichberg, S., Kahn, E., Jaffe, R. & Van Thiel, D.H. (1983). Selective fetal malnutrition: the effect of *in vivo* ethanol exposure upon *in vitro* placental uptake of amino acids in the non-human primate. *Pediatric Research*, **17**, 704–7.

Fisher, S.E., Duffy, L. & Atkinson, M. (1986). Selective fetal malnutrition: effects of acute and chronic ethanol exposure upon rat placental Na,K-ATPase activity. *Alcoholism: Clinical and Experimental Research*, **10**, 150–3.

Fisher, S.E., Alcock, N.W., Amirian, J. & Altshuler, H.L. (1988). Neonatal and maternal hair zinc levels in a non-human primate model of the fetal alcohol syndrome. *Alcoholism: Clinical and Experimental Research*, **12**, 417–21.

Fletcher, T.L. & Shain, W. (1993). Ethanol-induced changes in astrocyte gene expression during rat central nervous system development. *Alcoholism: Clinical and Experimental Research*, **17**, 993–1101.

Gilliam, D.M., Dudek, B.C. & Riley, D.P. (1990). Responses to ethanol challenge in long- and short-sleep mice prenatally exposed to alcohol. *Alcohol*, **7**, 1–5.

Gilliam, D.M. & Irtenkauf, K.I. (1990). Maternal genetics effects on ethanol teratogenesis and dominance of relative embryonic resistance to malformations. *Alcoholism: Clinical and Experimental Research*, **14**, 539–45.

Gilliam, D.M., Stillman, A., Dudek, B.C. & Riley, E.P. (1987). Fetal alcohol effects in long- and short-sleep mice: activity, passive avoidance, and *in utero* ethanol levels. *Neurotoxicology and Teratology*, **9**, 349–57.

Goodlett, C.R., Thomas, J.D. & West, J.R. (1991). Long-term deficits in cerebellar growth and rotorod performance of rats following binge-like alcohol exposure during the neonatal brain growth spurt. *Neurotoxicology and Teratology*, **13**, 69–74.

Gottesfeld, Z. & Abel, E.L. (1991). Mini-review. Maternal and paternal alcohol use: effects on the immune system of the offspring. *Life Sciences*, **48**, 1–8.

Gottesfeld, Z. & LeGrue, S.J. (1990). Lactational alcohol exposure elicits long-term immune deficits and increased noradrenergic synaptic transmission in lymphoid organs. *Life Sciences*, **47**, 457–65.

Grasnick, C. & Huel, G. (1985). The combined effect of tobacco and alcohol consumption on the level of lead and cadmium in blood. *Science of the Total Environment*, **41**, 207–17.

Guerri, C., Marques, A., Sancho-Tello, M. & Renau-Piqueras, J. (1989). Effect of prenatal exposure to alcohol on membrane-bound enzymes during astrocyte development *in vivo* and in primary culture. *International Journal of Developmental Biology*, **33**, 239–44.

Hall, J.L., Church, M.W. & Berman, R.F. (1994). Radial-arm maze deficits in rats exposed to alcohol during midgestation. *Psychobiology*, **22**, 181–5.

Hannigan, J.H. (1995). The effects of prenatal exposure to alcohol plus caffeine in rats: pregnancy outcome and early offspring development. *Alcoholism: Clinical and Experimental Research*, **19**, 238–46.

Hannigan, J.H., Abel, E.L. & Kruger, M.L. (1993*a*). 'Population' characteristics of birth weight in an animal model of alcohol-related developmental effects. *Neurotoxicology and Teratology*, **15**, 97–105.

Hannigan, J.H., Berman, R.F., & Zajac, C.S. (1993*b*). Environmental enrichment and the behavioral effects of prenatal exposure to alcohol in rats. *Neurotoxicology and Teratology*, **15**, 261–6.

Hannigan, J.H. & Pilati, M.L. (1991). The effects of chronic postweaning amphetamine on rats exposed to alcohol *in utero*: weight gain and behavior. *Neurotoxicology and Teratology*, **13**, 649–56.

Hannigan, J.H. & Riley, E.P. (1988). Prenatal ethanol alters gait in rats. *Alcohol*, **5**, 451–4.

Hannigan, J.H., Welch, R.A. & Sokol, R.J. (1992). Recognition of fetal alcohol syndrome and alcohol-related birth defects. In *Medical Diagnosis and Treatment of Alcoholism*, ed. J. Mendelson & N. Mellow, pp. 639–67. New York: McGraw-Hill.

Henderson, G.I., Baskin, G.S., Frosto, T.A. & Schenker, S. (1991). Interactive effects of ethanol and caffeine on rat fetal hepatocyte replication and EGF receptor expression. *Alcohol: Clinical and Experimental Research*, **15**, 175–80.

Henderson, G.I., Patwardhan, R.V., McLeroy, S. & Schenker, S. (1982). Inhibition of placental amino acid uptake in rats following acute and chronic ethanol. *Alcoholism: Clinical and Experimental Research*, **6**, 495–505.

Holson, R.R. & Pearce, B. (1992). Principles and pitfalls in the analysis of prenatal treatment effects in multiparous species. *Neurotoxicology and Teratology*, **14**, 221–8.

Holson, R.R., Scallet, A.C., Ali, S.F. & Turner, B.B. (1991). 'Isolation stress' revisited: isolation-rearing effects depend on animal care methods. *Physiology and Behavior*, **49**, 1107–18.

Hungund, B.L., Gokhale, V.S., Cooper,T.B. & Mahalik, S.P. (1991). Prenatal ganglioside GM1 treatment protects ethanol-induced sleep time in rats exposed to ethanol *in utero* during gestation days 7 and 8. *Drug Development Research*, **24**, 261–7.

Hungund, B.L., Ross, D.C. & Gokhale, V.S. (1994). Ganglioside GM1 reduces fetal alcohol effects in rat pups exposed to ethanol *in utero*. *Alcoholism: Clinical and Developmental Research*, **18**, 1248–51.

Jacobson, J.L. & Jacobson, S.W. (1994). Prenatal alcohol exposure and neurobehavioral development: Where is the threshold? *Alcohol Health and Research World*, **18**, 30–6.

Jones, K.L. & Smith, D.W. (1973). Recognition of the fetal alcohol syndrome in early infancy. *Lancet*, **ii**, 999–1001.

Keppen, L.D., Pysher, T. & Rennert, O.M. (1985). Zinc deficiency acts as a co-teratogen with alcohol in fetal alcohol syndrome. *Pediatric Research*, **19**, 944–7.

Kotch, L.E. & Sulik, K.K. (1992). Experimental fetal alcohol syndrome: proposed pathogenic basis for a variety of associated facial and brain anomalies. *American Journal of Medical Genetics*, **44**, 168–76.

Leach, R.E., Stachecki, J.J. & Armant, D.R. (1993). Development of *in vitro* fertilized mouse embryos exposed to ethanol during the preimplantation period: accelerated embryogenesis at subtoxic levels. *Teratology*, **47**, 57–64.

Ledig, M., Ciesielski, L., Simler, S., Lorentz, J.G. & Mandel, P. (1988). Effect of pre- and postnatal alcohol consumption on GABA levels of various brain regions in the rat offspring. *Alcohol and Alcoholism*, **23**, 63–7.

Lieber, C.S. (1991). Alcohol, liver, and nutrition. *Journal of the American College of Nutrition*, **10**, 602–32.

Mankes, R.M., Battles, A.H., LeFevre, R., van der Hoeven, T. & Glick, S.D. (1992). Preferential alcoholic embryopathy: effects of liquid diets. *Laboratory Animal Science*, **42**, 561–6.

McGivern, R.F. (1989). Low birthweight in rats induced by prenatal exposure to testosterone combined with alcohol, pair-feeding, or stress. *Teratology*, **40**, 335–8.

McGivern, R.F. & Riley, E.P. (1993). Influence of perinatal alcohol exposure on sexual differentiation. In *Alcohol and the Endocrine System*, ed. S. Zakhari, pp. 253–50. NIAAA Research Monograph. Bethesda, MD: NIAAA.

Melcer, T., Gonzalez, D., Somes, C. & Riley, E.P (1995*a*). Postnatal alcohol exposure and early development of motor skills in alcohol-preferring (P) and non-preferring (NP) rats. *Neurotoxicology and Teratology*, **17**, 103–10.

Melcer, T., Gonzalez, D. & Riley, E.P. (1995*b*). Locomotor activity and alcohol preference in alcohol-preferring and non-preferring rats following neonatal alcohol exposure. *Neurotoxicology and Teratology*, **17**, 41–8.

Meyer, L.S. & Riley, E.P. (1986). Behavioral teratology in alcohol. In *Handbook of Behavioral Teratology*, ed. E.P. Riley & C.V. Vorhees, pp. 101–40. New York: Plenum Press.

Meyer, L.S., Kotch, L.E. & Riley, E.P. (1990). Alterations in gait following ethanol exposure during the brain growth spurt in rats. *Alcohol: Clinical and Experimental Research*, **14**, 23–7.

Nelson, B.K., Brightwell, W.S. & Krieg, E.F. Jr (1990). Developmental toxicology of industrial alcohols: a summary of 13 alcohols administered by inhalation to rats. *Toxicology and Industrial Health*, **6**, 373–87.

Nelson, B.K., Brightwell, W.S., MacKenzie, D.R., Khan, A., Burg, J.R., Weigel, W.W. & Goad, P.T. (1985). Teratological assessment of methanol and ethanol at high inhalation levels in rats. *Fundamental and Applied Toxicology*, **5**, 727–36.

Osbourne, G.L., Caul, W.F. & Fernandez, K. (1980). Behavioral effects of prenatal ethanol exposure and differential early experience in rats. *Pharmacology, Biochemistry and Behavior*, **12**, 393–401.

Pantazis, N.J., Dohrman, D.P., Luo, J., Goodlett, C.R. & West, J.R. (1992). Alcohol reduces the number of pheochromocytoma (PC12) cells in culture. *Alcohol*, **9**, 171–80.

Pennington, S.N. (1990). Molecular changes associated with ethanol-induced growth suppression in the chick embryo. *Alcohol: Clinical and Experimental Research*, **14**, 832–7.

Pennington, S.N. (1992). Ethanol-induced teratology and second messenger signal transduction. In *Development of the Central Nervous System*, ed. M.W. Milla, pp. 198–208. New York: Wiley/Liss.

Pierce, D.R. & West, J.R. (1986*a*). Alcohol-induced microencephaly during the third trimester equivalent: relationship to dose and blood alcohol concentration. *Alcohol*, **3**, 185–91.

Pierce, D.R. & West, J.R. (1986*b*). Blood alcohol concentration: a critical factor for producing fetal alcohol effects. *Alcohol*, **3**, 269–72.

Portoles, M., Sanchis, R. & Guerri, C. (1988). Thyroid hormone levels in rats exposed to alcohol during development. *Hormone and Metabolic Research*, **20**, 267–70.

Randall, C.L. (1987). Alcohol as a teratogen: a decade of research in review. *Alcohol and Alcoholism*, Suppl. **1**, 125–32.

Randall, C.L., Salo, A.L., Becker, H.C. & Patrick, K.S. (1994). Cocaine does not influence the teratogenic effects of acute ethanol in mice. *Reproductive Toxicology*, **8**, 341–50.

Randall, C.L. & Taylor, W.J. (1979). Prenatal ethanol exposure in mice. *Teratology*, **19**, 305–12.

Riley, E.P. (1990). The long-term behavioral effects of prenatal alcohol exposure in rats. *Alcohol: Clinical and Experimental Research*, **14**, 670–3.

Riley, E.P., Hannigan, J.H. & Balaz-Hannigan, M.A. (1985). Behavioral teratology on the study of early brain damage: considerations for the assessment of neonates. *Neurobehavioral Toxicology and Teratology*, **7**, 635–8.

Riley, E.P. & Meyer, L.S. (1984). Considerations for the design, implementation and interpretation of animal models of fetal alcohol effects. *Neurobehavioral Teratology and Toxicology*, **6**, 97–101.

Rockwood, G.A. & Riley, E.P. (1990). Nipple attachment behavior in rat pups exposed to alcohol *in utero*. *Neurotoxicology and Teratology*, **12**, 383–9.

Rose, J.C., Meis, P.J. & Castro, M.I. (1981). Alcohol and fetal endocrine function. *Neurobehavioral Toxicology and Teratology*, **3**, 105–10.

Saunders, D.E., Hannigan, J.H., Zajac, C.S. & Wappler, N.L. (1995). Reversal of alcohol's effects on neurite extension and on neuronal GAP43/B50, N-*myc* and C-*myc* protein levels by retinoic acid. *Developmental Brain Research*, **86**, 16–23.

Schenker, S., Becker, H.C., Randall, C.L., Phillips, D.K., Baskin, G.S. & Henderson, G.I. (1990). Fetal alcohol syndrome: current status of pathogenesis. *Alcohol: Clinical and Experimental Research*, **14**, 635–47.

Shen, R.Y., Hannigan, J.H. & Chido, L.A. (1995). The effects of chronic amphetamine treatment on prenatal ethanol-induced changes in dopamine receptor function: electrophysiological findings. *Journal of Pharmacology and Experimental Therapeutics*, **224**, 1054–60.

Sinervo, K.R., Smith, G.N., Bocking, A.D., Patrick, J. & Brien, J.F. (1992). Effect of ethanol on the release of prostaglandins from ovine fetal brain stem during gestation. *Alcohol: Clinical and Experimental Research*, **16**, 443–8.

Smith, G.N., Brien, J.F., Homan, J., Carmichael, J., Treissman, D. & Patrick, J. (1990). Effect of ethanol on ovine fetal and maternal plasma prostaglandin E_2 concentrations and fetal breathing movements. *Journal of Developmental Physiology*, **14**, 23–8.

Smotherman, W.P. & Robinson, S.R. (1987). Stereotypic behavioral response of rat fetuses to acute hypoxia is altered by maternal alcohol consumption. *American Journal of Obstetrics and Gynecology*, **157**, 982–6.

Smotherman, W.P., Woodruff, K.S., Robinson, S.R., Del Real, C., Barron, S. & Riley, E.P. (1986). Spontaneous fetal behavior after maternal exposure to ethanol. *Pharmacology, Biochemistry and Behavior*, **24**, 165–70.

Sokol, R.J. & Clarren, S.K. (1989). Guidelines for use of terminology describing the impact of prenatal alcohol on the offspring. *Alcohol: Clinical and Experimental Research*, **13**, 597–8.

Sokol, R.J., Smith, M., Ernhart, C.B., Baumann, R., Martier, S.S., Ager, J.W. & Morrow-Tlucak, M.A (1989). A genetic basis for alcohol-related birth defects (ARBD)? *Alcohol: Clinical and Experimental Research*, **13**, 343A.

Stacheki, J.J., Yelian, F.D., Leach, R.E. & Armant, D.R. (1994a). Mouse blastocyst outgrowth and implantation rates following exposure to ethanol or A23187 during culture *in vitro. Journal of Reproduction and Fertility*, **101**, 611–17.

Stacheki, J.J., Yelian, F.D., Schultz, J.F., Leach, R.E. & Armant, D.R. (1994b). Blastocyst cavitation is accelerated by ethanol- or ionophore-induced elevation of intracellular calcium. *Biology of Reproduction*, **50**, 1–9.

Streissguth, A.P., Sampson, P.D., Olson, H.C., Bookstein, F.L., Barr, H.M., Scott, M., Feldman, J. & Mirsky, A.F. (1994). Maternal drinking during pregnancy: attention and short-term memory in 14-year-old offspring – a longitudinal prospective study. *Alcohol: Clinical and Experimental Research*, **18**, 202–18.

Subramanian, M.G. (1994). Beta-endorphin-stimulated prolactin release in lactating rats following alcohol administration. *Alcohol*, **11**, 269–72.

Subramanian, M.G., Chen, X.G. & Bergeski, B.A. (1990). Pattern and duration of the inhibitory effect of alcohol administered acutely on suckling-induced prolactin in lactating rats. *Alcohol: Clinical and Experimental Research*, **14**, 771–5.

Sulik, K.K. & Johnston, M.C. (1983). Sequence of developmental alterations following acute ethanol exposure in mice: craniofacial features of the fetal alcohol syndrome. *American Journal of Anatomy*, **166**, 257–69.

Tanaka, H., Inomata, K. & Arima, M. (1983). Zinc supplementation in ethanol-treated pregnant rats increases the metabolic activity in the fetal hippocampus. *Brain Development*, **5**, 549–54.

Tanaka, H., Iwasaki, S., Nakazawa, K. & Inomata, K. (1988). Fetal alcohol syndrome in rats: conditions for improvements of ethanol effects on fetal cerebral development with supplementary agents. *Biology of the Neonate*, **54**, 320.

Taylor, C.L., Jones, K.L., Jones, M.C. & Kaplan, G.W. (1994). Incidence of renal anomalies in children prenatally exposed to ethanol. *Pediatrics*, **94**, 209–12.

Tritt, S.H., Delia, T.L., Brammer, G.L. & Taylor, A.N. (1993). Adrenalectomy but not adrenal demedulation during pregnancy prevents the growth-retarding effects of fetal alcohol exposure. *Alcohol: Clinical and Experimental Research*, **17**, 1281–9.

Uray, N.J., Gona, A.G. & Hauser, K.F. (1987). Autoradiographic studies of cerebellar histogenesis in the premetamorphic bullfrog tadpole. *Journal of Comparative Neurology*, **266**, 234–46.

Vorhees, C.V. (1986). Principles of behavioral teratology. In *Handbook of Behavioral Teratology*, ed. E.P. Riley & C.V. Vorhees, pp. 23–30. New York: Plenum Press.

Vorhees, C.V. (1988). Maternal age as a factor in determining the reproductive and behavioral outcome of rats prenatally exposed to ethanol. *Neurotoxicology and Teratology*, **10**, 23–4.

Vorhees, C.V. (1989). A fostering/cross-fostering analysis of the effects of prenatal ethanol exposure in a liquid diet on offspring development and behavior in rats. *Neurotoxicology and Teratology*, **11**, 115–20.

Wainwright, P.E., Huang, Y.S., Mills, D.E., Ward, G.R. & McCutcheon, D. (1989). Interactive effects of prenatal ethanol and N-3 fatty acid supplementation on brain development in mice. *Lipids*, **24**, 989–97.

Wainwright, P.E., Huang, Y.-S., Simmons, V., Mills, D.E., Ward, R.P., Ward, G.R., Winfield, D. & McCutcheon, D. (1990). Effects of prenatal ethanol and long chain n-3 fatty acid supplementation on development in mice. II. Fatty acid composition of brain membrane phospholipids. *Alcohol: Clinical and Experimental Research*, **14**, 413–20.

Wainwright, P.E., Levesque, S., Krempulec, L. Bulman-Fleming, B. & McCutcheon, D. (1993). Effects of environmental enrichment on cortical depth and Morris-maze performance in B6D2F2 mice exposed prenatally to ethanol. *Neurotoxicology and Teratology*, **15**, 11–20.

Ward, G.R. & Wainwright, P.E. (1991). Effects of prenatal stress and ethanol on cerebellar fiber tract maturation in B6D2F2 mice: an image analysis study. *Neurotoxicology*, **12**, 655–76.

Watson, R.R. & Watzil, B. (1992). *Nutrition and Alcohol*. Boca Raton, FL: CRC Press.

Weinberg, J. (1984). Nutritional issues in perinatal alcohol exposure. *Neurobehavioral Toxicology and Teratology*, **6**, 261–9.

Weinberg, J. (1992). Prenatal ethanol effects: sex differences in offspring stress responsiveness. *Alcohol*, **9**, 219–23.

Weinberg, J., D'Alquen, G. & Bezio, S. (1990). Interactive effects of ethanol intake and maternal nutritional status on skeletal development of fetal rats. *Alcohol*, **7**, 383–8.

Weiner, S.G., Shoemaker, W.J., Koda, L.Y. & Bloom, F.E. (1981). Interactions of ethanol and nutrition during gestation: influence on maternal and offspring development in the rat. *Journal of Experimental Pharmacology and Therapeutics*, **216**, 572–9.

West, J.R. (1986). *Alcohol and Brain Development*. New York: Oxford University Press.

West, J.R. (1993). Use of the pup in cup model to study brain development. *Journal of Nutrition*, **123**, 382–5.

West, J.R. & Goodlett, C.R. (1990). Teratogenic effects of alcohol on brain development. *Annals of Medicine*, **22**, 319–25.

West, J.R., Goodlett, C.R., Bonthius, D.J. & Pierce, D.R. (1989). Manipulating peak blood alcohol concentrations in neonatal rats: review of an animal model for alcohol-related developmental effects. *Neurotoxicology*, **10**, 347–65.

West, J.R., Goodlett, C.R. & Brandt, J.P. (1990*a*). New approaches to research on the long-term consequences of prenatal exposure to alcohol. *Alcohol: Clinical and Experimental Research*, **14**, 684–9.

West, J.R., Goodlett, C.R., Bonthius, D.J., Hamre, K.M. & Marcussen, B.L. (1990*b*). Cell population depletion associated with fetal alcohol brain damage: mechanisms of BAC-dependent cell loss. *Alcohol: Clinical and Experimental Research*, **14**, 813–18.

Wozniak, D.F., Cicero, T.J., Kettinger, L. & Meyer, E.R. (1991). Paternal alcohol consumption in the rat impairs spatial learning performance in male offspring. *Psychopharmacology*, **105**, 289–302.

6

Neuropathology in experimental fetal alcohol syndrome

LINDA C. BAND AND JAMES R. WEST

Introduction

Fetal alcohol syndrome (FAS) is a leading cause of mental retardation in the Western world (Abel & Sokol, 1986, 1987, 1991; Centers for Disease Control and Prevention, 1993*a*, *b*; Cordero *et al.*, 1994). For this reason, abatement of alcohol effects on the central nervous system (CNS) is a critically important direction in the development of preventive strategies. This effort is best served by precise information concerning damage to the CNS produced by alcohol and by insight into underlying mechanisms. Experimental models of FAS are useful in achieving both these objectives.

Humans with FAS provide a kind of naturally occurring experiment in the impact of alcohol on the CNS. In the past, assessment of brain damage in children or infants with FAS was limited to those instances where maternal alcohol abuse resulted in fatality, or death ensued from other causes. It was not possible to examine neural structures at discrete intervals from the point of alcohol exposure or to vary levels of prenatal alcohol intake experimentally.

Experimental models of FAS

Magnetic resonance imaging

Magnetic resonance imaging (MRI) has revolutionized the study of FAS in humans. Using self-report techniques and MRI, it is now possible to examine the relationship between maternal and paternal drinking patterns and abnormalities in brain structures of prenatally exposed children. This non-invasive procedure also enables investigators to screen children at various time points following prenatal exposure, thereby determining the severity and duration of effects. Using these techniques, Mattson and colleagues (1994) found that FAS children had a reduction in size of basal ganglia and corpus callosum relative to the reduction in total brain mass. In comparing non-FAS children of heavy drinkers with FAS children, these investigators found that basal ganglia and corpus callosum were more sensitive to damage than diencephalon.

A key methodological issue concerns the contribution that animal models may make when techniques such as MRI permit examination of brain structures in humans with FAS. Animal model systems continue to offer more precise control over the quantity and timing of alcohol administration and the ability to detect neurological change at microscopic and molecular levels. In addition, some experimental paradigms permit control over environmental and nutritional cofactors influencing the expression of FAS.

Animal models

Prenatal exposure

Many toxicological models employ administration of toxins to animals *ad libitum*. Alcohol administered in a liquid diet to pregnant animals offers the advantage of being relatively nonstressful and the oral route represents a 'natural' alcoholic environment. Disadvantages of this method include the inability to control precisely alcohol intake and delivery to fetuses. These limitations make examination of relationships between maternal or fetal blood alcohol levels and neuropathology difficult. This model furnishes some information concerning chronic alcohol effects, but does not elucidate the influence of episodic maternal alcohol intake, or 'binge drinking', on the developing nervous system. In addition, this approach makes it difficult to distinguish possible interactive effects of alcohol consumption and nutritional status on neuronal growth and differentiation.

Controlled, rather than *ad libitum*, alcohol administration enables investigators to assess drinking pattern effects in more detail. In the rat, alcohol injected or administered orally via gavage allows the amount and timing of alcohol exposure to be controlled experimentally. Blood alcohol levels approaching those of acute intoxication in humans can be obtained and related to features of FAS originating prenatally in rodents or other species.

Comparative aspects

When using animal model systems, it is important to take into consideration species differences in maturity at birth. The period of most rapid brain growth occurs during the third trimester in humans and in early postnatal life in the rat (Dobbing & Sands, 1979). Increased teratogenesis in a given organ system has been associated with the introduction of damaging agents as the system undergoes intensified development (Randall, 1987; Webster, 1989; Becker *et al.*, 1994). Consistent with this principle, the 'brain growth spurt' is characterized by heightened susceptibility to alcohol-induced micro-encephaly (reduced brain size in relation to body size) (Samson, 1986) and damage to specific structures and neuronal pathways (Kelly *et al.*, 1989; Goodlett *et al.*, 1990).

Artificial rearing

Because the brain growth spurt occurs postnatally in the rat, it would be problematic to compare the effects of alcohol delivered in the human pre-natal environment with alcohol received via suckling in the neonatal rat. The use of artificial rearing was adapted to fetal alcohol studies in order to circumvent some of these difficulties (Samson & Diaz, 1982; West *et al.*, 1984). Using this procedure, rat pups are separated from dams and surgically implanted with intragastric tubes for the infusion of a liquid diet. Pups are then housed singly in an environment which allows the level and timing of the alcohol dose delivered in the diet, nutritional status, and external stimuli to be manipulated experimentally. The strengths and weaknesses of various animal models of FAS are discussed in the previous chapter (Hannigan & Abel, this volume). However, methods permitting direct administration of alcohol to neonatal animals have yielded useful information concerning neu-ropathological outcomes of human prenatal alcohol exposure. In particular, the degree of experimental control attainable through use of these models has made it possible to compare the CNS effects of binge drinking versus chronic alcohol intake during the third trimester equivalent.

Effects of fetal alcohol exposure on the brain

Relative vulnerability of CNS elements

Experimental models of FAS have revealed several important relationships between analogs of human prenatal exposure and subsequent neurological impairment. A number of studies have shown that CNS structures are not uniformly vulnerable to alcohol teratogenesis. Microencephaly is observed consistently following alcohol exposure during the human third trimester equivalent (Samson, 1986). Enlargement of the lateral ventricles and altera-tions in the cerebellum are seen in rats receiving acute alcohol treatment during this time frame, postnatal days (PD) 4 through 9 (Bonthius &

West, 1991*a*). The cerebellum appears particularly sensitive to damage, in that size reduction and loss of lobular shape can occur following only 1 or 2 days of binge-like alcohol exposure (Goodlett *et al.*, 1990; Hamre & West, 1990).

Neuronal populations

In addition to gross morphological change, alcohol exposure selectively affects certain cell types within brain regions, as described below.

Neocortex. Prenatal alcohol treatment has resulted in increased numbers of unmyelinated axons, reduced dendritic domain, and aberrant interneuronal connections in layer V of somatosensory cortex (Rabiai & Miller, 1989). Ethanol has also been shown to have differential effects in two neocortical proliferative zones. Ethanol increased cell cycle length without affecting the proportion of proliferating cells in the ventricular zone and had the reverse effect in the subventricular zone (Miller & Nowakowski, 1991).

Hippocampus. Hippocampal pyramidal CA1 cells were significantly depleted following acute alcohol administration, whereas CA3 pyramidal neurons were relatively unaffected in the same animals (Pierce & West, 1987; Bonthius & West, 1990, 1991*a*). Similar results were obtained with chronic prenatal alcohol administration (Barnes & Walker, 1981; Wigal & Amsel, 1990). These results indicate that intrastructural location as well as cell type determine vulnerability to alcohol.

Cerebellum. Cerebellar Purkinje and granule cells are depleted by binge-like alcohol exposure, and loss within the two populations is positively correlated at several postnatal intervals observed in rats (Hamre *et al.*, 1991). Cerebellar Purkinje cells are particularly sensitive to alcohol effects: a single day of alcohol exposure has produced depletion of this population (Goodlett *et al.*, 1990). The relative vulnerability of Purkinje cells to alcohol on PD4 through 9 is correlated with their anatomical location and stage of development (Goodlett & West, 1992). Purkinje cells in later maturing lobules (e.g., VI and VII) are less vulnerable to damage than those cells in lobules that mature earlier (lobules I and X) (Bonthius & West, 1990).

Olfactory bulb. Olfactory bulb mitral cells express a high degree of vulnerability to alcohol damage, while the population of olfactory granule cells shows recovery over time. The observation that the area of the subependymal zone containing mitral and granule cells is unaffected by alcohol treatment suggests that compensatory changes may occur in complementary neuronal subsets (Bonthius & West, 1991; Bonthius *et al.*, 1992).

Aberrant neuronal projections and migration

Other abnormalities induced by fetal alcohol exposure include abnormal connections between CNS regions. Alcohol administered throughout gestation results in a permanent aberration in hippocampal mossy fiber projections: fibers originating from dentate gyrus granule cells of the midtemporal hippocampal formation reach the intrapyramidal zone of subfield CA3a, an area which does not normally receive these afferents (West & Hodges-Savola, 1983; West & Pierce, 1984). Alcohol exposure from PD1 through PD10 produces more extensive aberrant mossy fiber projections than does alcohol exposure through gestation (West & Hamre, 1985).

Abnormalities in migration of neuronal cell bodies have been demonstrated following prenatal alcohol exposure. Acute alcohol exposure on gestational days 14 and 15 result in clusters of ectopic neurons, 'brain warts', occurring in supragranular cortex (Kotkoskie & Norton, 1988). The distribution of specific populations of cortical neurons is also affected by alcohol administered prenatally. The cell bodies of rat corticospinal neurons normally found exclusively in layer Vb are found throughout the cortex (i.e., layers II through layer VI) in alcohol-treated animals (Miller, 1987, 1989). Autoradiographic studies have revealed that these abnormal distributions are the result of delayed migration and effects on migratory rate and termination (Miller, 1993).

Reactive gliosis

Alcohol exposure on PD4 through PD9 in neonatal rats resulted in increased size and number of astrocytes labelled with an antibody for glial fibrillary acidic protein (GFAP) (West & Goodlett, 1990; Goodlett *et al.*, 1993). Increased GFAP staining is associated with a variety of neuropathological phenomena. The alcohol dose that produced the highest blood alcohol concentrations (BACs) resulted in a 3-fold increase in GFAP staining in cerebral cortex (Goodlett *et al.*, 1993). GFAP-positive astrocytes were found primarily in two locations: cortical layer V and areas bordering blood vessels. The observed gliosis was transient and could not be detected after PD12 (Goodlett *et al.*, 1993).

A potential explanation for increased numbers of astrocytes is derived from mouse embryo *in vitro* preparations and corresponding *in vivo* data. These studies revealed that alcohol prematurely transformed radial glial cells, which normally serve as guides for migrating neurons, into astrocytes; the postmigratory cortex lacked vertical columnization (Gressens *et al.*, 1992). Recent evidence indicated that gestational and early postnatal alcohol exposure induced delays in the development of optic nerve glia without long-term effects on these cells (Phillips & Krueger, 1992). However, maturational delays in glial cells are thought to disrupt myelination and may underlie neurological dysfunction (Phillips & Krueger, 1992).

Dendritic changes

Neurons exposed to alcohol during development are often aberrant. In addition to stunting (Smith *et al.*, 1986), these neurons exhibit abnormality in intercellular connections (West & Hodges-Savola, 1983), dendrites and dendritic spines (Hammer & Scheibel, 1981; Stoltenburg-Didinger & Spohr, 1983), and synapses (Volk, 1984). Such changes may have profound consequences for subsequent brain development and function.

Threshold of effects

Alcohol permanently alters neurochemical reactions at lower levels of exposure than those required to produce morphological change or neurodegeneration. Only in one case have reductions in cell numbers been documented at BACs below 100 mg/dl (Napper & West, 1995), and, as mentioned previously, microencephaly occurs at even higher BACs. In contrast, much lower BACs produce a variety of more subtle CNS changes.

Neurological changes seen at peak BACs averaging 40–60 mg/dl include: (1) decreased N-methyl-D-aspartate (NMDA) displacement of glutamate binding in the hippocampal formation of offspring measured at PD45 (Savage *et al.*, 1991*a*), (2) reactive astrocytic gliosis as measured by increased GFAP staining in cortex (Goodlett & West, 1992) and (3) lowered hippocampal mossy fiber zinc densities (Savage *et al.*, 1991*b*).

Such findings demonstrate that BACs attainable with light to moderate drinking in humans can permanently alter neurochemical activity in offspring. The data further suggest that currently there is no known practical threshold (i.e. safe level) of alcohol consumption during pregnancy.

Temporal windows of vulnerability

Fetal alcohol-induced CNS damage occurs within a specific temporal framework; alcohol exposure either prior or subsequent to the critical point is less damaging than exposure during the period of greatest susceptibility. The dimensions and position of the temporal window vary with neural substrate and alcohol dose.

Microencephaly

Microencephaly has been reported following heavy alcohol exposure during the third trimester equivalent exclusively; severity is dose and BAC dependent (Samson, 1986). In rats, the window of effects has been further defined as resulting from binge-like alcohol exposure during PD4 through PD9, producing peak BACs of approximately 190 mg/dl or greater (Bonthius & West, 1988). However, reduction in size of whole brain, forebrain, and cerebellum has been observed on PD10 following a single day of alcohol exposure occurring on PD4 that resulted in BACs of 360 mg/dl (Goodlett *et al.*, 1990).

Purkinje cells

The same regimen of alcohol exposure on PD4 only, produced selective loss of cerebellar Purkinje cells (Goodlett *et al.*, 1990). Significant cerebellar cell loss occurred only when alcohol treatment was begun before PD7, and Purkinje cell loss was greatest at the earliest treatments reported, i.e., PD4 and PD5 (Goodlett & West, 1992). In the case of Purkinje cells, the window of vulnerability includes the onset of cellular differentiation. These cells were less susceptible to alcohol damage during the proliferative and migratory stages (Goodlett & West, 1992; Marcussen *et al.*, 1994).

NMDA binding

The binding of the excitatory amino acid glutamate to hippocampal membranes displays a developmental point of increased vulnerability to relatively low levels of alcohol exposure. When administered at intervals throughout the prenatal and the early postnatal period, comparable alcohol doses reduced hippocampal NMDA-agonist binding only when administered during the last third of gestation in rats (Savage *et al.*, 1991*b*).

Diverse alcohol effects on neurotransmission have been reported. Findings include evidence for increased muscarinic cholinergic receptors when alcohol is administered during the third trimester equivalent (Kelly *et al.*, 1989). In contrast, prenatal exposure resulted in reductions in D1 dopaminergic sites in the striatum (Druse *et al.*, 1990) and NMDA-sensitive glutaminergic sites in hippocampus (Savage *et al.*, 1991*a*). Potential explanations for differences in results include change in the impact of alcohol as a function of the point in development at which exposure occurs.

Blood alcohol levels

As previously discussed, artificial rearing and binge-like alcohol exposure have been used to demonstrate a powerful relationship between BACs and certain aspects of CNS damage. A range of alcohol doses administered in a small number of daily feedings resulted in BACs linearly correlated with brain weights (Bonthius & West, 1988). These studies illustrate that alcohol, like other pharmacologically active substances, produces dose-dependent effects provided the schedule of administration remains constant. However, subsequent work has shown that the effect of alcohol dose per unit time may be separated from the effect of acute versus chronic administration. To illustrate this principle more clearly, a higher dose of alcohol per day administered throughout the day is less effective in reducing brain weight than a lower dose delivered in two to four feedings (Bonthius & West, 1990). The latter regime results in much higher peak BACs. Peak BACs, more than any other single factor investigated to date, account for alcohol-induced CNS damage; however, other dimensions of peak BAC effects, including the rate at which the peak is attained or degraded, may modulate the impact of BACs.

Blood alcohol levels during gestation have not been well studied. Most prenatal alcohol studies have employed alcohol in a liquid diet and have not included information on BACs; notable exceptions include the demonstration that an *ad libitum* liquid diet containing 6.7% (v/v) alcohol administered to pregnant rats results in mean peak maternal BACs of 130–150 mg/dl (Miller, 1988, 1992). Because ethanol readily crosses the placental barrier, maternal BACs are thought to represent fetal alcohol levels (Ho *et al.*, 1972; Kesaniemi & Sippel, 1975; Guerri & Sanchis, 1985). The characterization of gestational BACs is complicated by possible alcohol effects on food intake, absorption, and other factors. Further work incorporating necessary controls will help to clarify the neuropathological influence of alcohol exposure during the first and second trimester equivalents. An animal model based on a large maternal/fetal unit (e.g., sheep), which would permit both fetal and maternal blood sampling, would help to resolve this issue.

Mechanisms of damage

How elevated blood alcohol levels during pregnancy produce permanent CNS alteration in offspring is not known. Many mechanisms for alcoholic neurotoxicity have been postulated; we will highlight several that have been the focus of intensive investigation.

Oxygen transport and metabolism

Several proposed mechanisms for aspects of FAS are based on oxygen-related phenomena. These effects include the impact of alcohol on oxygen availability, subsequent neurotransmitter activity, and the production of free radicals.

Hypoxia

Several aspects of FAS parallel neuropathology resulting from diminished oxygen supply; both phenomena are characterized by damage to the cerebellum and hippocampus. A striking commonality is the selective loss of CA1 hippocampal pyramidal neurons and cerebellar Purkinje cells (Barnes & Walker, 1981; Jorgensen & Diemer, 1982; Pierce & West, 1987; Auer *et al.*, 1989; Bonthius & West, 1991*a*, *b*). The specificity of this shared effect suggests that the same mechanism may underlie hypoxia and certain FAS features.

Alcohol impairs oxygen transport prenatally by constricting placental, umbilical, and fetal blood vessels (Mukherjee & Hodgen, 1982). Alcohol may constrict vessels by enhancing the release of prostaglandins locally (Anton *et al.*, 1990), or endothelins synthesized in vascular walls of the placenta and umbilical cord (Tsuji *et al.*, 1992). The increased activity of either substance could impair circulation and induce fetal hypoxia (Michaelis & Michaelis, 1994).

Oxygen depletion can trigger the synthesis of prostaglandin from arachidonic acid (Kukreja & Hess, 1992), further reducing oxygen levels. Anti-inflammatory drugs, such as aspirin, indomethacin, and ibuprofen, inhibit this chemical conversion and have been shown to counteract certain aspects of alcohol teratogenesis (Randall & Anton, 1984; Randall *et al.*, 1987, 1991*b*). However, the pattern of alcohol intake may determine the efficacy of these agents in preventing FAS. Acute and chronic alcohol exposure are associated with increased and lowered prostaglandin levels, respectively. Pretreatment with aspirin has been shown to prevent fetal alcohol-induced damage in animals subsequently treated with a single, concentrated alcohol dose (Randall *et al.*, 1984, 1991*a*). Aspirin treatment worsens FAS in neonatal animals given alcohol chronically (Bonthius & West, 1989). Separate mechanisms may mediate these contrasting effects. Whereas aspirin may prevent hypoxic damage resulting from excess prostaglandin levels seen in acute alcohol treatment, it may further reduce prostaglandin levels lowered by chronic alcohol administration. The latter regimen may hinder normal prostaglandin activity, including regulation of CNS neurotransmission and differentiation (Wolfe, 1989).

Glutamate

The observation that brain areas most susceptible to hypoxic damage – cerebellum and hippocampus – coincide with those exhibiting high levels of excitatory amino acid neurotransmission (Jorgensen & Diemer, 1982), has led to the hypothesis that glutamate modulates the observed damage. Supporting evidence includes reports that hypoxia increases glutamate activity *in vitro* (Bosley *et al.*, 1983); furthermore, hypoxic neurotoxicity is attenuated by the NMDA antagonists MK-801 and dextromethorphan (McDonald *et al.*, 1987; George *et al.*, 1988).

Free radicals

As summarized by Michaelis & Michaelis (1994), both hypoxia and alcohol metabolism generate free radicals. These toxic metabolic by-products are associated with a variety of damaging effects. Alcohol induced the formation of the reactive oxygen intermediates superoxide, hydrogen peroxide, and hydroxyl anion and reduced cellular viability in a neural crest cell population associated with craniofacial malformations seen in FAS (Davis *et al.*, 1990); these effects were reversed by the addition of a free-radical scavenging enzyme, superoxide dismutase (Davis *et al.*, 1990). Insight into free radical formation and protective mechanisms may be useful in the prevention of FAS.

Glutathione

Glutathione (GSH) is an endogenous peptide long recognized as providing protection against lipid peroxidation produced by free radicals (Little & O'Brien, 1968, McCay *et al.*, 1976; Selden *et al.*, 1980). GSH is thought to protect cells from an array of harmful factors including radiation, toxins, and teratogens inducing oxidative stress (Yu *et al.*, 1984). GSH metabolism reaches peak levels prenatally (Igarashi *et al.*, 1981), suggesting that its presence plays a developmental role. Finally, disruption of the synthesis and utilization of GSH has been linked to mental retardation (Konrad *et al.*, 1972; Meister, 1985; Reyes *et al.*, 1993), a characteristic associated with FAS.

An alcohol-containing diet fed to pregnant rats throughout gestation lowered brain GSH levels and brain weight in offspring (Reyes *et al.*, 1993). Analysis of fetal brain tissue revealed that ethanol administration increased levels of γ-glutamyltranspeptidase (Reyes *et al.*, 1989) and reduced γ-glutamylcysteine synthetase (Reyes *et al.*, 1993), enzymes involved in GSH degradation and synthesis, respectively.

The GSH precursor *N*-acetyl-L-cysteine (NAC) administered together with alcohol in liquid diet antagonized alcohol effects on body weight (Reyes *et al.*, 1991); however, a clear relationship between replenished GSH levels and reversal of microencephaly has not been shown. Hepatic GSH levels and brain GSH synthesis were reduced for pair-fed controls as well as alcohol-treated groups, underlining the need to consider nutritional status in evaluating glutathione effects (Bondy & Pearson, 1993). In addition, NAC is reported to be a potent antioxidant/detoxicant (Flanagan, 1987), able to inactivate free radicals directly (Moldeus *et al.*, 1986). NAC has been shown to lower blood alcohol levels in chronically treated animals (C.R. Waltenbaugh, personal communication), thereby directly reducing alcohol toxicity.

Acetaldehyde versus ethanol

As recently reviewed by our laboratory (Chen *et al.*, 1996), controversy exists concerning the relative roles of ethanol and its metabolite acetaldehyde in alcohol-induced brain injury. Aldehyde dehydrogenase inhibitors, which prevent the oxidation of acetaldehyde to acetate, have been shown to worsen alcohol teratogenicity. Furthermore, direct administration of acetaldehyde has resulted in fetal malformation (O'Shea & Kaufman, 1979; Ali & Persaud, 1988). Toxic free radicals are formed during the oxidation of acetaldehyde (Fridovich, 1989), which would then suggest that acetaldehyde is a component of the oxygen-related mechanisms discussed previously.

Several lines of evidence suggest that ethanol alone is directly responsible for alcohol teratogenicity. Coadministration of alcohol and 4-methylpyrazole, an alcohol dehydrogenase inhibitor preventing the conversion of alcohol to acetaldehyde, increased BACs and worsened ethanol reductions of brain weight (Chen *et al.*, 1994); greater embryonic lethality and teratogenicity have also been reported (Blakly & Scott, 1984). Ethanol may act on the nervous system through disruption of gangliosides as discussed below. At present, insufficient evidence exists to resolve the relative neuropathological impact of alcohol and acetaldehyde.

Gangliosides

The lipid component of cellular membrane is important to the structural integrity and function of neurons. Changes in lipid composition may influence membrane permeability, neurotransmission, and cell survival. Gangliosides are a class of membrane lipids known to have neuroprotective properties, and are therefore of interest in fetal alcohol research. Exogenous gangliosides have attenuated neural damage from trauma, ischemia/hypoxia, and toxins (Mahadik & Karpiak, 1988). Gangliosides are thought to protect neuronal function by restoring normal plasma membrane structure and permeability.

Acute alcohol administration has been shown to decrease endogenous CNS ganglioside levels in adult animals (Klemm & Foster, 1986). In contrast, protracted chronic administration of alcohol has increased total brain ganglioside levels, increasing trisialoganglioside 1b and decreasing disialoganglioside 1a (Vrabaski *et al.*, 1984). Increased brain ganglioside effects in adults are consistent with the finding that a genetic mouse strain susceptible to alcohol effects have elevated ganglioside levels in cerebellum (Ullman *et al.*, 1987). Chronic prenatal alcohol exposure has been shown to increase brain gangliosides (Prasad, 1989, 1992, 1993). Prasad (1993) reported elevated ganglioside activity in cerebrum, cerebellum, and brainstem, which was due in part to reduced catabolic enzyme activity. Changes in ganglioside composition were region specific and partially reversed by abstinence. Maternal undernutrition also increases brain ganglioside content in offspring (Prasad, 1989), and this factor must be considered in determining ethanol effects.

Exogenous monosialoganglioside GM1 administered prenatally prevented the development of alcohol tolerance in adult rats associated with *in utero* alcohol exposure (Hungund *et al.*, 1991). The mechanism underlying this effect is unknown; however, the lowering of blood alcohol levels by ganglioside GM1 treatment, preventing intoxication and tolerance in adult rats (Hungund *et al.*, 1990), must be included as a possible reason for GM1 attenuation of prenatal alcohol effects.

Increased endogenous gangliosides in response to alcohol challenge seems incompatible with the protective effects of exogenously administered gangliosides. The reason for this apparent contradiction has not been demonstrated. Increased ganglioside activity in response to alcohol challenge is consistent with sites provided by gangliosides as alcohol competes with water for hydrogen bonds to cell surface molecules – the 'dehydration theory' (Klemm, 1990). In contrast, exogenous gangliosides may interact with cells in a different manner (Hungund & Mahadik, 1993) or may replenish gangliosides altered by alcohol and assume their role in maintaining cell structure and function. Systematic studies are needed to elucidate ganglioside protection against alcohol insult during development.

Conclusion

The past decade of fetal alcohol research has provided a detailed description of the effects of fetal alcohol exposure on the nervous system. Information relating the developmental time frame of exposure and drinking pattern to the degree of CNS damage in offspring has considerable clinical relevance, as does information concerning the threshold of alcohol effects. These findings enable those segments of the population who can easily control their alcohol consumption to make prudent choices. The pharmacological protection that may be needed in other situations requires an understanding of the means by which alcohol produces damage.

The search for mechanisms of alcoholic neurotoxicity can have a number of outcomes. Many efforts are directed toward isolation of a single mechanism accounting for the many facets of neuropathology integral to FAS. Pharmacological prevention of neural damage could be developed directly from the identified mechanism. FAS facial malformation in mice results exclusively from first trimester equivalent alcohol exposure (Sulik *et al.*, 1981); therefore, if a single mechanism underlies the expression of all aspects of FAS, that mechanism is certain to operate early in pregnancy, as well as at later stages. Efforts to identify a singular mechanism could fruitfully include early organogenesis.

An alternative to a single-mechanism interpretation would be the mediation of various aspects of FAS by separate mechanisms. Arguments in favor of this approach include the identification of several temporal windows of vulnerability to alcohol damage. These findings may encourage speculation that different physiological substrates are active at different points of fetal development, and that third trimester phenomena, including microencephaly, are mediated differently from first trimester effects. Effective research strategies are then directed toward specific systems and their point of greatest vulnerability. This approach represents the state of the art in the search for neural mechanisms of alcohol damage and accounts for the focus of attention on the third trimester brain growth spurt. However, counterarguments stem from the observation that alcohol produces some damage at all stages of fetal development and is disruptive to organ systems during organogenesis and the period of most rapid development (e.g., the brain growth spurt). It seems more likely that commonalities in the mediation of alcohol effects can be observed throughout fetal development and will not be distributed conveniently by trimester or other time frame.

A third possibility combines the idea of a singular underlying mechanism and clear separation of mechanisms. Accumulating evidence suggests multiple mechanisms sequentially linked or operating in parallel. Support for this interpretation includes observations that (1) alcohol lacks narrow pharmacological specificity and therefore may act at multiple neural substrates, and (2) manipulation of a variety of systems results in FAS-like teratogenesis or modulation of alcohol teratogenic influence. If multiple mechanisms are connected serially, then interruption at any point in the chain of events might be expected to block alcohol effects. If, however, separate mechanisms operate simultaneously to produce neuropathology, disruption of one will lessen, but not eliminate, the additive impact.

Certain criteria have been defined and have served as the basis for determining the physiological and behavioral function of neural structures; these criteria might well be applied to the search for FAS mechanisms. A given function is attributed to a particular brain region if stimulation of the region is *sufficient* to elicit the behavior or physiological activity. The second criterion requires that stimulation of other brain regions not be equally effective, and that exclusive destruction of the region disrupts the process or behavior. In other words, the region is *necessary* to the execution of the function.

Efforts to reveal substrates of fetal alcohol-induced damage to the CNS have only partially addressed the criteria described above. Many approaches are best suited to the identification of singular mechanisms of action, the existence of multiple mechanisms rendering their application complex. However, experimental manipulation of a physiological system resulting in a pattern of brain damage similar to that produced by fetal alcohol exposure (e.g., hypoxia) approaches demonstration of sufficiency. Evidence that the activity of a substrate (e.g., prostaglandins) diminishes alcohol damage is relevant to the criterion of necessity. At present, no mechanism has met both criteria. Although the need to identify the mechanisms of fetal alcohol-induced neuropathology is urgent, this goal can only be achieved systematically through experimental rigor.

References

Abel, E.L. & Sokol, R.J. (1986). Fetal alcohol syndrome is now leading cause of mental retardation. *Lancet*, **ii**, 1222.

Abel, E.L. & Sokol, R.J. (1987). Incidence of fetal alcohol syndrome and economic impact of FAS-related anomalies. *Drug and Alcohol Dependence*, **19**, 51–70.

Abel, E.L. & Sokol, R.J. (1991). A revised conservative estimate of the incidence of FAS and its economic impact. *Alcoholism: Clinical and Experimental Research*, **15**, 514–24.

Ali, F. & Persaud, T.V.N. (1988). Mechanisms of fetal alcohol effects: role of acetaldehyde. *Experimental Pathology*, **33**, 17–21.

Anton, R.F., Becker, H.C. & Randall, C.L. (1990). Ethanol increases PGE and thromboxane production in mouse pregnant uterine tissue. *Life Sciences*, **46**, 1145–54.

Auer, R.N., Jensen, M.L. & Whishaw, I.Q. (1989). Neurobehavioral deficit due to ischemic brain damage limited to half of the CA1 sector of the hippocampus. *Journal of Neuroscience*, **9**, 1641–7.

Barnes, D.E. & Walker, D.W. (1981). Prenatal alcohol exposure permanently reduces the number of pyramidal neurons in the rat hippocampus. *Developmental Brain Research*, **1**, 333–40.

Becker, H.C., Randall, C.L., Salo, A.L., Saulnier, J.L. & Weathersby, R.T. (1994). Animal research: charting the course for FAS. *Alcohol Health and Research World*, **18**, 10–17.

Blakley, P.M. & Scott, W.J. (1984). Determination of the proximate teratogen of the mouse fetal alcohol syndrome. I. Teratogenicity of ethanol and acetaldehyde. *Toxicology and Applied Pharmacology*, **72**, 355–63.

Bondy, S.C. & Pearson, K.R. (1993). Ethanol-induced oxidative stress and nutritional status. *Alcoholism: Clinical and Experimental Research*, **17**, 651–4.

Bonthius, D.J., Bonthius, N.E., Napper, R.M.A. & West, J.R. (1992). A stereological study of the effect of early postnatal alcohol exposure on the number of granule cells and mitral cells in the rat olfactory bulb. *Journal of Comparative Neurology*, **324**, 557–66.

Bonthius, D.J. & West, J.R. (1988). Blood alcohol concentration and microencephaly: a dose–response study in the neonatal rat. *Teratology*, **37**, 223–31.

Bonthius, D.J. & West, J.R. (1989). Aspirin augments alcohol in restricting brain growth in the neonatal rat. *Neurotoxicology and Teratology*, **11**, 135–43.

Bonthius, D.J. & West, J.R. (1990). Alcohol-induced neuronal loss in developing rats: increased brain damage with binge exposure. *Alcoholism: Clinical and Experimental Research*, **14**, 107–18.

Bonthius, D.J. & West, J.R. (1991a). Permanent neuronal deficits in rats exposed to alcohol during the brain growth spurt. *Teratology*, **44**, 147–63.

Bonthius, D.J. & West, J.R. (1991b). Acute and long-term neuronal deficits in the rat olfactory bulb following alcohol exposure during the brain growth spurt. *Neurotoxicology and Teratology*, **13**, 611–19.

Bosley, T.M., Woodhams, P.L., Gordon, R.D. & Balazs, R. (1983). Effects of anoxia on the stimulated release of amino acid neurotransmitters in the cerebellum *in vitro*. *Journal of Neurochemistry*, **40**, 189–201.

Centers for Disease Control and Prevention (1993a). Fetal alcohol syndrome: United States, 1979–1992. *Morbidity and Mortality Weekly Report*, **42**, 339–41.

Centers for Disease Control and Prevention (1993b). Linking multiple data sources in fetal alcohol syndrome surveillance: Alaska. *Morbidity and Mortality Weekly Report*, **42**, 312–4.

Chen, W.-J.A., Maier, S.E. & West, J.R. (1996). Toxic effects of ethanol on the fetal brain. In *Effects of Ethanol on the Nervous System*, ed. R.A. Deithrich & V.G. Erwin, pp. 343–61. Boca Raton, FL: CRC Press, in press.

Chen, W.-J.A., McAlhany, R.E., Jr & West, J.R. (1994). Alcohol dehydrogenase inhibitor, 4-methylpyrazole, augments ethanol-induced microencephaly in neonatal rats. *Alcoholism: Clinical and Experimental Research*, **17**, 436.

Cordero, J.F., Floyd, R.L., Martin, M.L., Davis, M. & Hymbaugh, K. (1994). Tracking the prevalence of FAS. *Alcohol Health and Research World*, **18**, 82–5.

Davis, W.L., Drawford, L.A., Cooper, O.J., Rarmer, G.R., Thomas, D.L. & Freeman, B.L. (1990). Ethanol induces the generation of reactive free radicals by neural crest cells *in vitro*. *Journal of Craniofacial Genetics and Developmental Biology*, **10**, 277–94.

Dobbing, J. & Sands, J. (1979). Comparative aspects of the brain growth spurt. *Early Human Development*, **3**, 79–83.

Druse, M.J., Tajuddin, N., Kuo, A.P. & Connerty, M. (1990). Effects of *in utero* ethanol exposure on the developing dopaminergic system in rats. *Journal of Neuroscience Research*, **27**, 233–40.

Flanagan, R.J. (1987). The role of acetylcysteine in clinical toxicology. *Medical Toxicology*, **2**, 93–104.

Fridovich, I. (1989). Oxygen radicals from acetaldehyde. *Free Radical Biology and Medicine*, **7**, 557–8.

George, C.P., Goldberg, M.P., Choi, D.W. & Steinberg, G.K. (1988). Dextromethorphan reduces neocortical ischemic neuronal damage *in vivo*. *Brain Research*, **440**, 375–9.

Goodlett, C.R., Leo, J.T., Callaghan, J.P., Mahoney, J.C. & West, J.R. (1993). Transient cortical astrogliosis induced by alcohol exposure during the neonatal brain growth spurt in rats. *Developmental Brain Research*, **72**, 85–97.

Goodlett, C.R., Marcussen, B.L. & West, J.R. (1990). A single day of alcohol exposure during the brain growth spurt induces brain weight restriction and cerebellar Purkinje cell loss. *Alcohol*, **7**, 107–14.

Goodlett, C.R. & West, J.R. (1992). Fetal alcohol effects: rat model of alcohol exposure during the brain growth spurt. In *Maternal Substance Abuse and the Developing Nervous System*, ed. I.S. Zagon & T.A. Slotkin, pp. 45–75. Orlando, FL: Academic Press.

Gressens, P., Lammens, M., Picard, J.J. & Evrard, P. (1992). Ethanol-induced disturbances of gliogenesis and neuronogenesis in the developing murine brain: an *in vitro* and *in vivo* immunohistochemical and ultrastructural study. *Alcohol and Alcoholism*, **27**, 219–26.

Guerri, C. & Sanchis, R. (1985). Acetaldehyde and alcohol levels in pregnant rats and their fetuses. *Alcohol*, **2**, 267–70.

Hammer, R.P., Jr & Scheibel, A.B. (1981). Morphological evidence for a delay of neuronal maturation in fetal alcohol exposure. *Experimental Neurology*, **74**, 587–96.

Hamre, K., Goodlett, C.R. & West, J.R. (1991). Spatial and temporal correlation of Purkinje cell and granule cell loss after postnatal ethanol administration in the rat. *Alcoholism: Clinical and Experimental Research*, **15**, 341.

Hamre, K.M. & West, J.R. (1990). Purkinje cell survival following ethanol exposure during the brain growth spurt depends on the timing of exposure and location the cerebellar vermis. In *Society for Neuroscience Abstracts*, vol. 16, p. 32. Washington: Society for Neuroscience.

Ho, B.T., Fritchie, G.E., Idanpaan-Heikkila, J.E. & McIsaac, W.M. (1972). Placental transfer and tissue distribution of ethanol-1-^{14}C. A radioautographic study in monkeys and hamsters. *Quarterly Journal of Studies on Alcohol*, **33**, 485–94.

Hungund, B.L., Gokhale, V.S., Cooper, T.B. & Mahadik, S.P. (1991). Prenatal ganglioside GM1 treatment protects ethanol-induced sleep time in rats exposed to ethanol *in utero* during gestation days 7 and 8. *Drug Development Research*, **24**, 261–7.

Hungund, B.L. & Mahadik, S.P. (1993). Role of gangliosides in behavioral and biochemical actions of alcohol: cell membrane structure and function. *Alcoholism: Clinical and Experimental Research*, **17**, 329–39.

Hungund, B.L., Reddy, M.V., Bharucha, V.A. & Mahadik, S.P. (1990). Monosialogangliosides (GM1 and AGF2) reduce ethanol intoxication: sleep time, mortality and cerebral cortical Na^+, K^+-ATPase. *Drug Development Research*, **19**, 443–51.

Igarashi, T., Satoh, T., Ueno, K. & Kitagaua, H. (1981). Changes of gamma-glutamyltranspeptidase activity in the rat during development and comparison of the fetal liver, placental and adult liver enzymes. *Life Sciences*, **29**, 483–91.

Jorgensen, M.B. & Diemer, N.H. (1982). Selective neuron loss after cerebral ischemia in the rat: possible role of transmitter glutamate. *Acta Neurologica Scandinavica*, **66**, 536–46.

Kelly, S.J., Black, A.C. & West, J.R. (1989). Changes in the muscarinic cholinergic receptors in the hippocampus of rats exposed to ethyl alcohol during the brain growth spurt. *Journal of Pharmacology and Experimental Therapeutics*, **249**, 798–804.

Kesaniemi, Y.A. & Sippel, H.W. (1975). Placental and fetal metabolism of acetaldehyde in rat. I. Contents of ethanol and acetaldehyde in placenta and fetus of the pregnant rat during ethanol oxidation. *Acta Pharmacologica et Toxicologica*, **37**, 43–8.

Klemm, W.R. (1990). Dehydration: a new alcohol theory. *Alcoholism*, **7**, 49–59.

Klemm, W.R. & Foster, D.M. (1986). Alcohol, in a single pharmacological dose, decreases brain gangliosides. *Life Sciences*, **39**, 897–902.

Konrad, P.N., Richards, F., Valentine, W.N. & Paglia, D.E. (1972). γ-Glutamylcysteine synthetase deficiency: a case of hereditary hemolytic anemia. *New England Journal of Medicine*, **286**, 557–61.

Kotkoskie, L.A. & Norton, S. (1988). Prenatal brain malformations following acute ethanol exposure in the rat. *Alcohol: Clinical and Experimental Research*, **12**, 831–6.

Kukreja, R.C. & Hess, M.L. (1992). The oxygen free radical system: from equations through membrane-protein interactions to cardiovascular injury and protection. *Cardiovascular Research*, **26**, 641–55.

Little, C. & O'Brien, P.J. (1968). An intracellular GSH-peroxidase with a lipid peroxidase substrate. *Biochemical and Biophysical Research Communications*, **31**, 145–50.

Mahadik, S.P. & Karpiak, S.E. (1988). Gangliosides in treatment of neural injury and disease. *Drug Development Research*, **15**, 337–60.

Marcussen, B.L., Goodlett, C.R., Mahoney, J.C. & West, J.R. (1994). Developing rat Purkinje cells are more vulnerable to alcohol-induced depletion during differentiation than during neurogenesis. *Alcohol*, **11**, 147–56.

Mattson, S.N., Jernigan, T.L. & Riley, E.P. (1994). MRI and prenatal alcohol exposure: images provide insight into FAS. *Alcohol Health and Research World*, **18**, 49–52.

McCay, P.B., Gibson, D.D., Fong, K.-L. & Hornbrook, K.R. (1976). Effect of glutathione peroxidase activity on lipid peroxidation in biological membranes. *Biochimica et Biophysica Acta*, **431**, 459–68.

McDonald, J.W., Silverstein, F.S. & Johnston, M.V. (1987). MK-801 protects the neonatal brain from hypoxic–ischemic damage. *European Journal of Pharmacology*, **140**, 359–61.

Meister, A. (1985). The fall and rise of cellular glutathione levels: enzyme-based approaches. *Current Topics in Cellular Regulation*, **26**, 383–94.

Michaelis, E.K. & Michaelis, M.L. (1994). Cellular and molecular bases of alcohol's teratogenic effects. *Alcohol Health and Research World*, **18**, 17–21.

Miller, M.W. (1987). Effect of prenatal exposure to alcohol on the distribution and time of origin of corticospinal neurons in the rat. *Journal of Comparative Neurology*, **257**, 372–82.

Miller, M.W. (1988). Effect of prenatal exposure to ethanol on the development of cerebral cortex. I. Neuronal generation. *Alcoholism: Clinical and Experimental Research*, **12**, 440–49.

Miller, M.W. (1989). Effect of prenatal exposure to ethanol on the development of cerebral cortex: II. Cell proliferation in the ventricular and subventricular zones of the rat. *Journal of Comparative Neurology*, **287**, 326–38.

Miller, M.W. (1992). Circadian rhythm of cell proliferation in the telecephalic ventricular zone: effect of *in utero* exposure to ethanol. *Brain Research*, **595**, 17–24.

Miller, M.W. (1993). Migration of cortical neurons is altered by gestational exposure to ethanol. *Alcoholism: Clinical and Experimental Research*, **17**, 304–14.

Miller, M.W. & Nowakowski, R.S. (1991). Effect of prenatal exposure to ethanol on the cell cycle kinetics and growth fraction in the proliferative zones of fetal rat cerebral cortex. *Alcoholism: Clinical and Experimental Research*, **15**, 229–32.

Moldeus, P., Cotgreave, I.A. & Beggren, M. (1986). Lung protection by a thiol-containing antioxidant: *N*-acetylcysteine. *Respiration*, **50**, (Suppl. 1), 31–42.

Mukherjee, A.B. & Hodgen, G.D. (1982). Maternal ethanol exposure induces transient impairment of umbilical circulation and fetal hypoxia in monkeys. *Science*, **218**, 700–2.

Napper, R.M.A. & West, J.R. (1996). Permanent neuronal deficits in rats induced by low blood alcohol levels during the brain growth spurt: a stereological study. *Journal of Comparative Neurology*, in press.

O'Shea, K.S. & Kaufman, M.H. (1979). The teratogenic effect of acetaldehyde: implications for the study of the fetal alcohol syndrome. *Journal of Anatomy*, **128**, 65–76.

Phillips, D.E. & Krueger, S.K. (1992). Effects of combined pre- and postnatal ethanol exposure (three trimester equivalence) on glial cell development in rat optic nerve. *International Journal of Developmental Neuroscience*, **10**, 197–206.

Pierce, D.R. & West, J.R. (1987). Differential deficits in regional brain growth induced by postnatal alcohol. *Neurotoxicology and Teratology*, **9**, 129–41.

Prasad, V.V.T.S. (1989). Maternal alcohol consumption and undernutrition in the rat: effects on gangliosides and their catabolizing enzymes in the rat CNS of the newborn. *Neurochemical Research*, **14**, 1081–8.

Prasad, V.V.T.S. (1992). Effect of prenatal and postnatal exposure to ethanol on rat central nervous system gangliosides and glycosidases. *Lipids*, **27**, 344–8.

Prasad, V.V.T.S. (1993). Alterations and recovery of rat brain gangliosides and glycosidases following long-term exposure to alcohol and rehabilitation during development. *Brain Research*, **610**, 75–81.

Rabiai, S. & Miller, M.W. (1989). Effect of prenatal exposure to ethanol on the ultrastructure of layer V of mature rat somatosensory cortex. *Journal of Neurocytology*, **18**, 711-29.

Randall, C.L. (1987). Alcohol as a teratogen: a decade of research in review. *Alcohol and Alcoholism*, Suppl. 1, 125–32.

Randall, C.L. & Anton, R.F. (1984). Aspirin reduces alcohol-induced prenatal mortality and malformations in mice. *Alcoholism: Clinical and Experimental Research*, **8**, 513–5.

Randall, C.L., Anton, R.F. & Becker, H.C. (1987). Effect of indomethacin on alcohol-induced morphological anomalies in mice. *Life Sciences*, **41**, 361–9.

Randall, C.L., Anton, R.F., Becker, H.C., Hale, R.L. & Ekblad, U. (1991*a*). Aspirin dose-dependently reduces alcohol-induced birth defects and prostaglandin E levels in mice. *Teratology*, **44**, 521–9.

Randall, C.L., Becker, H.C. & Anton, R.F. (1991*b*). Effect of ibuprofen on alcohol-induced teratogenesis in mice. *Alcoholism: Clinical and Experimental Research*, **15**, 673–7.

Randall, C.L., Becker, H.C. & Anton, R.F. (1984). Aspirin reduces alcohol-induced prenatal mortality and malformations in mice. *Alcoholism: Clinical and Experimental Research*, **8**, 513–15.

Reyes, E., Lucero, M.M., Ott, S. & Coker, H. (1991). Effects of the *in utero* administration of *N*-acetyl-L-cysteine and alcohol on fetal development. *Alcoholism: Clinical and Experimental Research*, **15**, 343.

Reyes, E., Ott, S. & Robinson, B. (1993). Effects of *in utero* administration of alcohol on glutathione levels in brain and liver. *Alcoholism: Clinical and Experimental Research*, **17**, 877–81.

Reyes, E., Wolfe, J. & Marquez, M. (1989). Effects of prenatal alcohol on gamma-glutamyl transpeptidase in various brain regions. *Physiology and Behavior*, **46**, 49–53.

Samson, H.H. (1986). Microcephaly and fetal alcohol syndrome: human and animal studies. In *Alcohol and Brain Development*, ed. J.R. West, pp. 167–83. New York: Oxford University Press.

Samson, H.H. & Diaz, J. (1982). Effects of neonatal ethanol exposure on brain development in rats. In *Fetal Alcohol Syndrome*, vol. 3, ed. E.L. Abel, pp. 131–50. Boca Raton, FL: CRC Press.

Savage, D.D., Montano, C.Y., Otero, M.A. & Paxton, L.L. (1991*a*). Prenatal ethanol exposure decreases hippocampal NMDA-sensitive [^{3}H]glutamate binding-site density in 45-day-old rats. *Alcohol*, **8**, 193–201.

Savage, D.D., Queen, S.A., Paxton, L.L., Goodlett, C.R., Mahoney, J.C. & West, J.R. (1991*b*). Postnatal ethanol exposure decreases hippocampal mossy fiber zinc density in 45-day-old rats. *Alcohol: Clinical and Experimental Research*, **15**, 339.

Savage, D.D., Queen, S.A., Sanchez, C.F., Paxton, L.L., Mahoney, J.C., Goodlett, C.R. & West, J.R. (1991*c*). Prenatal ethanol exposure during the last third of gestation in rat reduces hippocampal NMDA agonist binding site density in 45-day-old offspring. *Alcohol*, **9**, 37–41.

Selden, C., Seymour, C.A. & Peters, T.J. (1980). Activities of some free-radical scavenging enzymes and glutathione concentrations in human and rat liver and their relationship to the pathogenesis of tissue damage in iron overload. *Clinical Science*, **58**, 211–19.

Smith, D.E., Foundas, A. & Canale, J. (1986). Effects of perinatally administered alcohol on the development of the cerebellar granule cell. *Experimental Neurology*, **92**, 491–501.

Stoltenburg-Didinger, G. & Spohr, H.L. (1983). Fetal alcohol syndrome and mental retardation: spine distribution of pyramidal cells in prenatal alcohol-exposed rat cerebral cortex: a Golgi study. *Developmental Brain Research*, **11**, 119–23.

Sulik, K.K., Johnston, M.C. & Webb, M.A. (1981). Fetal alcohol syndrome: embryogenesis in a mouse model. *Science*, **214**, 936–8.

Tsuji, S., Kawano, S., Michaida, T., Masuda, E., Nagano, K., Takei, Y., Fusamoto, H. & Kamada, T. (1992). Ethanol stimulates immunoreactive endothelin-1 and -2 release from cultured human umbilical vein endothelial cells. *Alcoholism: Clinical and Experimental Research*, **16**, 347–9.

Ullman, D.M., Baker, R.C. & Dietrich, R.A. (1987). Gangliosides of long sleep and short sleep mouse cerebellum and hippocampus and cerebellar and whole brain synaptosomal plasma membranes. *Alcohol: Clinical and Experimental Research*, **11**, 158–62.

Volk, B. (1984). Cerebellar histogenesis and synaptic maturation following pre- and postnatal alcohol administration, an electron-microscopic investigation of the rat cerebellar cortex. *Acta Neuropathologica*, **63**, 57–65.

Vrabaski, S.R., Grujic-Injac, B. & Ristic, M. (1984). Phospholipid and ganglioside composition in rat brain after chronic intake of ethanol. *Journal of Neurochemistry*, **42**, 1235–9.

Webster, W.S. (1989). Alcohol as a teratogen: a teratological perspective of the fetal alcohol syndrome. In *Human Metabolism of Alcohol*, vol. 1, ed. K.E. Crow & R.D. Batt, pp. 135–55. Boca Raton, FL: CRC Press.

West, J.R. & Goodlett, C.R. (1990). Teratogenic effects of alcohol on brain development. *Annals of Medicine*, **22**, 319–25.

West, J.R. & Hamre, K.M. (1985). Effects of alcohol exposure during different periods of development: changes in hippocampal mossy fibers. *Developmental Brain Research*, **17**, 280–4.

West, J.R., Hamre, K.M. & Pierce, D.R. (1984). Delay in brain growth induced by alcohol in artificially reared rat pups. *Alcohol*, **1**, 213–22.

West, J.R. & Hodges-Savola, C.A. (1983). Permanent hippocampal mossy fiber hyperdevelopment following prenatal ethanol exposure. *Neurobehavioral Toxicology and Teratology*, **5**, 139–50.

West, J.R. & Pierce, D.R. (1984). The effects of *in utero* ethanol exposure on hippocampal mossy fibers: an HRP study. *Developmental Brain Research*, **15**, 275–9.

Wigal, T. & Amsel, A. (1990). Behavioral and neuroanatomical effects of prenatal, postnatal, or combined exposure to ethanol in weanling rats. *Behavioural Neuroscience*, **104**, 116–26.

Wolfe, L.S. (1989). Eicosanoids. In *Basic Neurochemistry*, ed. G.J. Siegel, B.W. Agranoff, R.W. Alberts & P.B. Molinoff, pp. 399–414. New York: Raven Press.

Yu, N.Y., Bram, J.M. & Phil, D. (1984). Depletion of glutathione *in vivo* as a method of improving the therapeutic ratio of misonidazole and SR2508. *International Journal of Radiation Biology*, **10**, 1265–9.

7

Neuropathology in human fetal alcohol syndrome

GISELA STOLTENBURG-DIDINGER

Introduction

Because of the cardinal symptom of mental retardation in human fetal alcohol syndrome (FAS), the neuropathological investigation of the brain seemed a promising approach to explain the clinically rather uniform picture of statomotor and mental retardation. Neuropathological studies have contributed significantly to this field of research and continue to do so. In this chapter a review will be given by reporting findings from autopsies with special emphasis on central nervous system pathology, gliosis, myelination, and the analyses of the brains of non-human primates. Further topics of this review deal with ocular pathology, skeletal muscle pathology, and placental dysfunction. Finally, some concluding remarks on the pathogenesis of FAS from a neuropathological point of view will be made.

Autopsy findings

Central nervous system pathology

Since the first necropsy on an infant born to a chronic alcoholic mother (Jones & Smith, 1973; Jones, 1975) a number of post-mortem investigations of FAS have been performed (Clarren *et al.*, 1978; Majewski *et al.*, 1978; Peiffer *et al.*, 1979; Wisniewski *et al.*, 1983; Ferrer & Galofré, 1987). According to the autopsy material, no uniform pattern of cerebral malformation could be identified. There is a wide range of severe and minor morphological and structural abnormalities. The spectrum of pathological changes in the central nervous system ranges from severe dysraphic state, arhinencephaly, porencephaly, agenesis of corpus callosum and hydranencephaly to microdysplasias and biochemical abnormalities (Wisniewski & Lupin, 1979).

The post-mortem investigation of Clarren *et al.* (1978) included four brains of infants of different ages: one premature infant died at the age of 6 weeks and was the only one who exhibited microencephaly; one infant born at term died at the age of 10 weeks and showed hydrocephalus and cerebellar and brainstem malformations. An identical pattern of malformations was observed in a fetal brain at the age of 20 gestational weeks. One preterm infant survived 3 days and showed microdysgenetic features with glioneur-onal meningeal heterotopy. The authors stressed particularly the structural abnormalities caused by neuronal and glial migration disorders. Cerebellar dysplasias and heteropic cell clusters were present in all four cases in the study. The migration disorder may be explained by the inhibitory effect of ethanol on neural cell–cell adhesion, which was shown in proliferating neu-roblastoma × glioma hybrid NG108-15 cells with concentrations of ethanol achieved during social drinking (Charness *et al.*, 1994).

In 1978 Majewski *et al.* contributed an observation of a fetal brain of 18 gestational weeks without malformation to the German discussion on induced abortion of alcoholic mothers. Peiffer *et al.* (1979) investigated the brains of 3 infants with FAS and 3 aborted fetuses and have presented the largest number of human post-mortems to date. The morphological picture varied. Malformations with dysraphic state and hydranencephaly repre-sented one side of the spectrum and discrete heterotopies the other. The age of the fetuses ranged between postconceptional week 17 and 20; 2 fetal brains showed microdysplasias only, and the third had severe hydranence-phaly. Two of the infants' brains had minor changes described as microdys-plasias, and the child who died at the age of 9 months showed dysraphic changes and agenesis of the corpus callosum.

The great variability in pathomorphological features may be partly explained by the fact that FAS itself is not a lethal condition, and the infants who die are those with a special combination of additional diseases, malfor-mations, or risk factors, so that among the group with post-mortem investi-gations the number of more serious malformations is disproportionately high. The neuropathological investigations demonstrate that there is no con-stant, specific type of malformation or developmental disorder that can be attributed to ethanol. Nor could an especially vulnerable period of brain development in connection with the harmful effects of ethanol be detected. At present, the evidence of harm to the fetus is much stronger with large amounts of maternal alcohol consumption than with smaller amounts. Moreover, it appears that infants prenatally exposed to the same amount of alcohol will not all be affected to the same degree. Whereas there is continuing controversy about the association between maternal consumption and possible damage to the fetus, current data do not support the notion that alcohol consumption below a certain level is safe for all pregnant women (Committee on Substance Abuse, 1992 to 1993).

In the study by Wisniewski *et al.* (1983) the 5 patients with the diagnosis of FAS had died at the ages of 8 and 4 months and 17, 4 and 2 days. Neuropathological investigation revealed microencephalic brains in all cases, without morphological evidence of maturation delay. One of the brains had agenesis of the corpus callosum and hypoplasia of the cerebellar vermis. Four had only small dysgenetic changes, consisting mainly of glial or glio-neuronal meningeal or parenchymal heterotopias. This study corroborates the finding that microencephaly is the most common affliction of the brain in FAS.

Without doubt, these pioneer neuropathological studies confirmed in principle the devastating effects of ethanol on the developing nervous system. However, they did not contribute to the pathogenesis of the syndrome.

With respect to the pathogenic considerations, the most interesting findings in an autopsy case are those presented by Ferrer & Galofré (1987). The neuropathological findings in this 4-month-old child born to a chronic alcoholic mother were microencephaly, uncovered rostral region of the insula, disordered arrangement of the nerve cells in the cerebral cortex, cerebellar abnormalities, and glial meningeal heterotopias. These findings correspond well to those of all the previous investigators (Jones & Smith, 1973; Clarren *et al.*, 1978; Peiffer *et al.*, 1979; Wisniewski *et al.*, 1983). In addition, Golgi staining of neurons showed decreased numbers of dendritic spines and a predominance of spines with long, thin pedicles on cortical pyramidal cells. The reduced numbers and abnormal geometry of spines observed in this child suggest that an abnormal maturation of nerve cells may occur in children as has been demonstrated to occur in rodents (Hammer & Scheibel, 1981; Reyes *et al.*, 1983; Stoltenburg-Didinger & Spohr, 1983; Schapiro *et al.*, 1984; López-Tejero *et al.*, 1986) as a consequence of chronic ethanol consumption during pregnancy. Because the normal maturation of dendritic spines on cortical neurons is characterized by the progressive appearance of mushroom-shaped and stubby spines (Marin-Padilla, 1972; Purpura, 1975), the predominance of a primitive character characterized by spines with thin, long pedicles, as observed in the present patient when compared with age-matched controls, was interpreted as the result of an abnormal development of the dendritic spine pattern on cortical pyramidal neurons. This interpretation is still more tempting given the morphological resemblance to features in brains of children with various mental deficits with a chromosomal or non-chromosomal etiology (Marin-Padilla, 1974, 1976; Purpura, 1974).

Therefore, it seems highly probable that the reported spine anomalies may be a consistent negative effect associated with chronic ethanol consumption at an early developmental stage. Abnormal dendritic spines may result in a reduced input to the dendritic arbor and modified depolarization in the 'spine-head' (Coss & Perkel, 1985; Pongrácz, 1985), thus leading to abnormal neuronal function.

This statement is further supported by the fact that similar abnormalities of the dendritic spines have been reported in a number of human diseases marked by mental retardation (Marin-Padilla, 1972; Huttenlocher, 1974; Purpura, 1974; Marin-Padilla, 1974, 1976; Suetsugu & Mehraein, 1980; Takashima *et al.*, 1981; Fábregues & Ferrer, 1983; Machado-Salas, 1984). Abnormalities of the dendritic spines, if proven to be present in the brains of other children, may be a morphological substrate for mental retardation observed in children with minor morphological abnormalities who are born to chronic alcoholic mothers.

Gliosis

Whereas the traditional neuropathological investigations of the central nervous system focused on neuronal changes such as those described above, the experimental data stressed the impairment and/or reactive changes of glial structures. After chronic exposure to ethanol an astrocytic gliosis could be demonstrated in experimental animals (Goodlett *et al.*, 1993) as well as in cell cultures (Renau-Piqueras *et al.*, 1989; Guerri *et al.*, 1993). In none of the human autopsies were glial changes reported.

Myelination

The retardation of myelination, which had been shown in cell cultures (Chiappelli *et al.*, 1991) and in rats (Phillips & Krueger, 1990; Stoltenburg-Didinger & Mayer, 1990) could be detected in children by means of magnetic resonance imaging (MRI: Knight *et al.*, 1993; Lancaster, 1994). This non-invasive procedure will probably come to replace the post-mortem investigation. Initial studies (Mattson *et al.*, 1992, 1994*a, b*) have shown a reduced thickness of the corpus callosum, indicating reduction either of myelination or of axons. In these studies the diencephalon was spared while basal ganglia and interhemispheric interconnections were reduced in size. Lesions equivalent to the linear areas of echogenicity in the thalami and basal ganglia of neonates investigated by means of sonography by another group (Hughes *et al.*, 1991) in association with FAS have not been identified by neuroimaging methods. In a Japanese study, cranial computed tomography (CCT) was performed in 3 of 26 FAS patients. There was slight cortical atrophy in the absence of more extensive structural alteration (Tanaka *et al.*, 1981).

Compared with the severity of the problem, human post-mortems are scarce. As described a survey of the international literature refers to 17 cases reported by Clarren *et al.* (1978, 4 cases), Majewski *et al.* (1976, 1 case), Peiffer *et al.* (1979, 6 cases), Wisniewski *et al.* (1983, 5 cases), and Ferrer & Galofré (1987, 1 case). In summary, a prevalence of severe malformations of the central nervous system was reported in these studies. The malformations are nonspecific. With greater awareness of the incidence of FAS more reports of random associations of FAS and other nonrelated malformations such as holoprosencephaly (Ronen & Andrews, 1991), Moebius syndrome (Hall, 1991), functional disorders such as chronic intestinal pseudo-obstruction (Vasiliauskas *et al.*, 1994), and skeletal disorders such as Klippel-Feil anomaly (Schilgen & Loeser, 1994) have been published. These rare associations do not, from the neuropathological point of view, seem to be causally related to intrauterine alcohol exposure.

The central nervous system, which is the only organ that continues to develop not only throughout pregnancy but even postnally, exhibits a special susceptibility to developmental neurotoxins such as ethanol.

Non-human primates

Due to the small number of human autopsies, it seems reasonable, even necessary, to refer to the very elegant and sophisticated neuropathological studies performed on non-human primates (Clarren *et al.*, 1990). Neuropathological and neurochemical assessments were done of 31 pigtailed macaques at 6 months of age who had been exposed weekly to ethanol throughout gestation. No structural anomalies were found in the brains by either gross inspection or light microscopy. The extent of ultrastructural alterations increased with increasing mean maternal peak plasma ethanol concentrations among the animals exposed throughout gestation. A small but statistically significant decrease in brain volume was detected in 12 animals who had received delayed exposure or exposure throughout gestation to moderate to high blood levels of ethanol. True microcephaly was noted in only one animal exposed to very high maternal blood ethanol levels administered after the fifth week of gestation. The lack of gross malformations in any brain specimen and the absence of abnormalities of cerebral cortices or nuclei, glia, or neurons (confirmed with the light microscope) suggest that there is no single pattern of structural abnormalities of the brain that accounts for the cognitive and behavioral problems associated with FAS. The study results are consistent with the clinical impression that ethanol-related behavioral teratogenesis may occur without accompanying physical anomalies. This experience is underlined by the results of masked clinical examination of MRI scans in high-functioning children with FAS (Knight *et al.*, 1993). In contrast to previous reports (Gabrielli *et al.*, 1990; Mattson *et al.*, 1992) no abnormalities could be demonstrated. This corresponds well to the majority of human neuropathological data that reveal microcephaly and minor dysplasias as being the most consistent feature of FAS (Clarren *et al.*, 1978; Peiffer *et al.*, 1979; Wisniewski *et al.*, 1983).

Ocular pathology

As part of the nervous system, the eyes are involved in FAS. Ocular abnormalities in humans exposed to alcohol during pregnancy are frequent (Strömland *et al.*, 1993; Strömland & Pinazo-Durán, 1994). The features observed are microphthalmia, microcornea, coloboma of the iris and ophthalmic nerve hypoplasia, as well as tortuosity of retinal blood vessels (Strömland, 1981).

On the basis of the clinical results of an ophthalmological study in a group of Swedish school children with FAS, in whom intraocular defects such as cataract, glaucoma, persistent hyperplastic primary vitreous, and retinal and optic nerve anomalies were observed in considerable number, a very high frequency of optic nerve hypoplasia in up to half the group was demonstrated (Strömland & Pinazo-Durán, 1994). In consequence, an experimental study was designed in rats that had been pre- and perinatally exposed to alcohol by means of a liquid diet. The optic nerve was seriously affected. The diameter of the optic nerve cross-section, glial cell nuclear area, and the total number of optic axons showed significantly lower values in the alcohol-exposed group than in the controls. In addition, the retina from the alcohol-exposed animals displayed significantly lower values of retinal thickness and ganglion cell nuclear volume compared with controls. Thus, rats exposed to alcohol *in utero* developed hypoplasia of the optic nerve – similar to the findings in children born to alcoholic mothers. Strömland & Pinazo-Durán (1994) concluded that this strongly supports the hypothesis that prenatal alcohol exposure adversely affects the development of the optic nerve.

In non-human primate infants (Clarren *et al.*, 1990) microphthalmia was noted in 3 of 26 animals exposed to ethanol. Retinal ganglion cell loss was significantly associated with intrauterine ethanol exposure. Microphthalmia and retinal ganglion cell loss were observed in animals with both delayed and full-gestational exposure. Morphometric counts of retinal ganglion cells have not been performed in humans with FAS. All the animals exposed to ethanol showed at least a mild decrease in ganglion cell numbers. This finding is in accord with observations in rats exposed to intrauterine ethanol, where mild decreases in numbers of myelinated axons were found in the optic nerve (Samorajski *et al.*, 1986; Phillips & Krueger, 1990; Phillips *et al.*, 1991; Strömland & Pinazo-Durán, 1994). FAS involves various neural-crest-derived structures, thus causing ocular malformations. Among these, anomalies of the corneal endothelium, a neural-crest-derived tissue, are frequent. Carones *et al.* (1992) described a close correlation between endothelial anomalies and auditory dysfunction in 8 children with FAS and attributed the alteration to the toxic effect of alcohol on neural crest cells destined to form both the corneal endothelium and the organ of Corti in the same embryonic period. The effects on the corneal epithelium in the patients are supported by a study that reported alterations of this tissue in embryogenic mice exposed to alcohol (Cook *et al.*, 1987).

Miller *et al.* (1984) reported alterations in the anterior segment of the eyes of children with FAS. Malformation of the anterior chamber with bilateral high intraocular pressure combined with multiple ocular anomalies was described by Martin & Rabineau (1990). All these anomalies seem to be the consequence of disturbances occurring when the three waves of mesenchymal cells migrate from the neuronal crest. Any disturbance in the induction or migration of the first wave of neuronal crest cells may result in an alteration of the final structure.

Recent data (Fox, 1995) obtained in rats demonstrate that prenatal ethanol exposure produced long-term deficits in retinal photoreceptor-mediated functions. The numbers of rods and cones were diminished. Rhodopsin content per eye was diminished. A loss of photoreceptors and possibly other cells of the distal retina contributed to these deficits. The relevance and applicability of these data to FAS and subclinical FAS have yet to be demonstrated; however, the author claims that similar retinal alterations may occur in human FAS.

In the clinical picture, strabismus convergens is frequent (Fried & Ravin, 1979). In microphthalmus and blepharophimosis, severe myopia may represent an additional visual handicap (Altmann, 1977; Strömland, 1990).

Skeletal muscle

Apart from growth deficits, muscular hypotonia – either neurogenic or myogenic – is a prominent neurological feature in FAS. One report on a constellation of unique cellular and subcellular abnormalities in the skeletal muscles of 3 infants born to alcoholic mothers is available (Adickes & Shuman, 1983). Three infants with congenital hypotonia had the same aberrations in the structure of skeletal muscles on biopsy. The hypotonia previously attributed to central nervous dysfunction is better attributed to ethanol-induced dysplasia of muscle. The hypotonicity and flaccidity of fetal alcohol myopathy are caused by disarray of the contractile proteins. The actin and myosin do not interdigitate in severely affected areas and cannot interact to produce contraction.

Placenta

A contributing factor to FAS may be the effect of ethanol on the placenta (Randall *et al.*, 1990). The evidence for alcohol-induced placental dysfunction comes mainly from studies with rats. Several studies have demonstrated impaired transport for amino acids (Henderson *et al.*, 1982), glucose (Snyder *et al.*, 1986), and folate (Lin & Lester, 1985) in pregnant rats fed liquid diets containing ethanol. However, the study of Schenker and colleagues (1989) using a human perfusion model system failed to find any effect of acute ethanol infusion on transport of amino acids or glucose. Whereas this study leaves the importance of alcohol-impaired placental transport in the etiology of fetal alcohol syndrome in doubt, it should be emphasized that the placentas used were not from alcoholic mothers and alcohol was administered acutely via perfusion. The findings from the rat studies, on the other hand, most often employed a chronic model of alcohol administration throughout pregnancy. Ethanol may adversely affect not only placental nutrient and zinc transport (Beer *et al.*, 1992) but also cAMP-dependent hormone production (Ahluwalia *et al.*, 1992; Karl & Fisher, 1993; Karl *et al.*, 1994), as shown in cultured human placental trophoblasts.

Pathogenesis of FAS

The neuropathological findings in human FAS do not provide any clues to the pathogenesis of the syndrome. Most of the case reports and even animal experiments remain purely descriptive. The key mechanisms discussed are fetal hypoxia, excessive production of certain prostaglandins and a direct effect of ethanol on developing cells, especially those of the central nervous system, altering net protein synthesis, neuronal membrane composition and/ or neuronal process formation, and production of neurotrophic factors needed for cell growth and interaction. These putative abnormalities are not, of course, mutually exclusive and, in fact, may contribute in varying degrees to alcohol-induced fetal deficits (Michaelis, 1990; Schenker *et al.*, 1990).

There is still no comprehensive understanding of the genesis of the most prominent features in FAS, i.e., the fetal growth retardation and the microcephaly. Whether the growth retardation of the brain is due to lack of trophic factors or to increased or upregulated cell death during development has not been elucidated, either in animal experiments or in the few human autopsies available. Apoptosis, i.e., genetically determined cell death, plays a major role in determining the final size of organs. Apoptosis is regulated by local growth factors. Insulin-like growth factors I and II (IGF-I, IGF-II) and IGF-binding proteins are important modulators of fetal growth. IGF-I is a key regulator of fetal growth and development (Liu *et al.*, 1993). Fetal growth retardation is a major component in FAS. Newborn mice homozygous for a targeted disruption of the IGF-I gene exhibit striking growth deficiency and attain only 60% of normal birth weight (Liu *et al.*, 1993). Null mutants for the IGF-I receptor gene die at birth and exhibit more severe growth deficiency, attaining only 45% of normal size. Null mutants of the IGF-I receptor gene also have generalized organ hypoplasia and central nervous system abnormalities (Liu *et al.*, 1993). These observations provide direct evidence that IGF-I has a continuous function throughout development and is not merely a factor that assumes a growth-promoting role in postnatal life.

Most studies on maternal alcohol exposure have revealed reduced circulating IGF-I levels in the fetus (Halmesmaki *et al.*, 1989; Sonntag & Boyd, 1989; Breese & D'Costa, 1993). In a more recent study (Singh *et al.*, 1994) the relationship between FAS and IGFs has been investigated in the offspring of ethanol-fed rats. Comparing the offspring of ethanol-fed rats with those from pair-fed and *ad libitum*-fed animals provides evidence for a specific effect of alcohol on IGF-I production in the fetus. Interestingly, IGF-I has been shown to increase alcohol dehydrogenase activity in rat hepatocyte primary culture by increasing production of this enzyme at a pretranslational level (Mezey *et al.*, 1990). Thus the alcohol-induced decrease in IGF-I levels could in turn decrease hepatic alcohol dehydrogenase activity, leading to impaired hepatic metabolism and clearance of alcohol – a vicious cycle. The findings of reduced serum concentration of IGF-I in the offspring of the alcohol-fed animals point to a direct interaction of alcohol with the growth-hormone-releasing hormone/growth hormone/insulin-like growth factor axis that is independent of indirect effects via alcohol-induced maternal malnutrition.

In contrast to these convincing findings Mauceri *et al.* (1993) did not find differences in the IGF-I levels between any of their treatment groups, using a model of feeding dams a 36% ethanol-containing liquid diet and comparing the offspring with those of dams fed isocaloric amounts of liquid diet. Fetal weight was significantly lower in the ethanol-exposed group. The data obtained suggest that circulating levels of IGF-II (but not IGF-I) and specific IGF binding proteins are altered in growth-retarded fetuses exposed to ethanol. Alterations in the expression and levels of IGFs and IGF binding proteins may contribute to the fetal growth deficiency (Mauceri *et al.*, 1993).

At the molecular level, research is now focusing on the field of mitogenic peptides, such as IGF-I and IGF-II, that exert significant effects on cell metabolism, growth, differentiation, and mitosis. The research on their role in fetal growth retardation induced by maternal alcohol ingestion seems especially rewarding and should be intensified (Krishna & Phillips, 1994).

Assuming that prenatal as well as postnatal exposure to ethanol can produce neuronal cell loss, aberrant neuronal migration, abnormalities in axonal growth and innervation, decreases in dendritic arborization and spine development as well as an overall decrease in brain weight, another common molecular event underlying these observations comes into play: the activity of intracellular calcium ions (Ca^{2+}) in the growth cone region of developing neurons. It is hypothesized that the regulation of Ca^{2+} entry into the growth cone plays an important role in neuronal process elongation. We currently do not have enough information about the systems that control Ca^{2+} in neuronal growth cones to make a clear prediction of the effects of ethanol on the function of growth cones. We do know that ethanol can affect intracellular Ca^{2+} levels in mature cells both through direct action on Ca^{2+} transport systems and channels and through receptor-regulated plasma membrane conductances, such as the NMDA receptor channels and intracellular release sites activated by inositol triphosphate (Michaelis, 1990).

Research in progress using a chick model (Pennington, 1990) indicates that pharmacologically appropriate doses of ethanol inhibit brain growth and reduce central nervous system 3',5'-cyclic adenosine monophosphate (cyclic AMP) with an associated 50% decrease in the binding of cyclic AMP by the regulatory subunit as a result of ethanol exposure. Furthermore, there is a specific loss of phosphorylation of the regulatory subunit by kinase catalytic subunit as a result of ethanol exposure. As the tissue content of cyclic AMP and the degree of regulatory subunit phosphorylation are important parameters for the regulation of protein kinase A catalytic activity, it is hypothesized that these alterations may be the biochemical transformations that underlie ethanol-induced growth suppression.

Intellectual impairment has been attributed to reduction of receptor expression in the hippocampus – the site of learning and memory in the brain of animals and humans (Savage *et al.*, 1992; Davis-Cox *et al.*, 1994). Comparable data in humans are not available. An illuminating view of the pathogenesis of FAS is still lacking.

References

Adickes, E.D. & Shuman, R.M. (1983). Fetal alcohol myopathy. *Pediatric Pathology*, **1**, 369–84.

Ahluwalia, B., Smith, D., Adeyiga, O., Akbasak, B. & Rajguru, S. (1992). Ethanol decreases progesterone synthesis in human placental cells: mechanism of ethanol effect. *Alcohol*, **9**, 395–401.

Altmann, B. (1977). Fetal alcohol syndrome. *Journal of Pediatric Ophthalmology and Strabismus*, **13**, 255.

Beer, W.H., Johnson, R.F., Guentzel, M.N., Lozano, J., Henderson, G.I. & Schenker, S. (1992). Human placental transfer of zinc: normal characteristics and role of ethanol. *Alcoholism: Clinical and Experimental Research*, **16**, 98–105.

Breese, C.R. & D'Costa, A. (1993). Long term suppression of insulin like growth factor I in rats after *in utero* ethanol exposure: relationship to somatic growth. *Journal of Pharmacological and Experimental Therapy*, **264**, 448–56.

Carones, F., Brancato, R., Venturi, E., Bianchi, S. & Magni, R. (1992). Corneal endothelial anomalies in the fetal alcohol syndrome. *Archives of Ophthalmology*, **110**, 1128–31.

Charness, M.E., Safran, R.M. & Perides, G. (1994). Ethanol inhibits neural cell–cell adhesion. *Journal of Biological Chemistry*, **269**, 9304–9.

Chiappelli, F., Tayler, A., Espinosa de los Monteros, A. & de Vellis, J. (1991). Fetal alcohol delays the developmental expression of myelin basic protein and transferrin in rat primary oligodendrocyte cultures. *International Journal of Developmental Neuroscience*, **9**, 67–76.

Clarren, S.K., Alvord, E.C., Jr & Sumi, S.M. (1978). Brain malformations related to prenatal exposure to ethanol. *Journal of Pediatrics*, **92**, 64–7.

Clarren, S.K., Astley, S.J., Bowden, D.M., Lai, H., Milam, A.H., Rudeen, K. & Shoemaker, W.J. (1990). Neuroanatomical and neurochemical abnormalities in non-human primate infants exposed to weekly doses of ethanol during gestation. *Alcoholism: Clinical and Experimental Research*, **14**, 674–83.

Committee on Substance Abuse (1993). Fetal alcohol syndrome and fetal alcohol effects. *Pediatrics*, **91**, 1004–5.

Cook, C.S., Nowotny, A.Z. & Sulik, K.K. (1987). Fetal alcohol syndrome: eye malformations in a mouse model. *Archives of Ophthalmology*, **105**, 1576–81.

Coss, R.G. & Perkel, D.H. (1985). The function of dendritic spines: a review of theoretical issues. *Behavioral Biology and Neurology*, **44**, 151–85.

Davis-Cox, M.I., Fletcher, T.L., Turner, J.N., Szarowski, D. & Shain, W. (1994). Brief ethanol exposure alters G-protein alpha-subunit expression in the developing hippocampus. Twenty-fourth annual meeting of the Society for Neuroscience, Miami Beach, Florida, USA, November 13–18, 1994. *Society for Neuroscience Abstracts*, **20**, 395.

Fábregues, I. & Ferrer, I. (1983). Abnormal perisomatic structures in non-pyramidal neurons in the cerebral cortex in Down's syndrome. *Neuropathology and Applied Neurology*, **9**, 165–70.

Ferrer, I. & Galofré, E. (1987). Dendritic spine anomalies in fetal alcohol syndrome. *Neuropediatrics*, **18**, 161–3.

Fox, D.A. (1995). Prenatal ethanol exposure alters rat retinal function, structure and biochemistry. *International Conference on Drugs of Abuse*, Funchal, Madeira, Portugal, April 29 to May 3, 1995, abstract 4.73.

Fried, R.I. & Ravin, J.G. (1979). Fetal alcohol syndrome. *Journal of Pediatric Ophthalmology and Strabismus*, **15**, 394.

Gabrielli, O., Salvolini, U., Coppa, G.V., Catassi, C., Rossi, R., Manca, A., Lanza, R. & Giorgi, B.L. (1990). Magnetic resonance imaging in the malformation syndromes with mental retardation. *Pediatric Radiology*, **21**, 16–19.

Goodlett, C.R., Leo, J.T., O'Callaghan, J.P., Mahoney, J.C. & West, R.W. (1993). Transient cortical astrogliosis induced by alcohol exposure during the neonatal brain growth spurt in rats. *Developmental Brain Research*, **72**, 85–97.

Guerri, C., Saez, R., Portoles, M. & Renau-Piqueras, J. (1993). Derangement of astrogliogenesis as a possible mechanism involved in alcohol-induced alterations of central nervous system development. *Alcohol and Alcoholism*, Suppl. **2**, 203–8.

Hall, B.D. (1991). Moebius syndrome associated with maternal alcohol abuse. *Teratology*, **43**, 437–8.

Halmesmaki, E., Valimaki, M., Karonen, S.L. & Ylikorkala, O. (1989). Low somatomedin C and high growth hormone levels in humans damaged by maternal alcohol abuse. *Obstetrics and Gynecology*, **74**, 366–70.

Hammer, R.P. & Scheibel, A.B. (1981). Morphological evidence for a delay of neuronal maturation in fetal alcohol exposure. *Experimental Neurology*, **74**, 587–96.

Hughes, P., Weinberger, E. & Shaw, D.W.W. (1991). Linear areas of echogenicity in the thalami and basal ganglia of neonates: an expanded association. *Radiology*, **179**, 103–5.

Huttenlocher, P.R. (1974). Dendritic development in neocortex of children with mental defects and infantile spasms. *Neurology*, **24**, 203–10.

Jones, K.L. (1975). Aberrant neuronal migration in the fetal alcohol syndrome. *Birth Defects: Original Article Series*, **11**, 131–2.

Jones, K.L. & Smith, D.W. (1973). Recognition of the fetal alcohol syndrome in early infancy. *Lancet*, **ii**, 999–1001.

Karl, P.I., Divald, A. & Fisher, S.E. (1994). Ethanol enhancement of ligand-stimulated cAMP production by cultured human placental trophoblasts. *Biochemical Pharmacology*, **48**, 1493–500.

Karl, P.I. & Fisher, S.E. (1993). Ethanol alters hormone production in cultured human placental trophoblasts. *Alcoholism: Clinical and Experimental Research*, **17**, 816–21.

Knight, J.E., Kodituwakku, P.W. Orrison, W.W. Jr, Lewine, J.D., Maclin, E.L., Weathersby, E.K., Cutler, S.K., McClain, C.H., Handmaker, N.S. & Handmaker, S.O. (1993). Magnetic resonance imaging in high-functioning children with fetal alcohol syndrome who exhibit specific neuropsychological deficits. *Alcoholism: Clinical and Experimental Research*, **17**, 485.

Krishna, A. & Phillips, L.S. (1994). Fetal alcohol syndrome and insulin-like growth factors. *Journal of Laboratory and Clinical Medicine*, **124**, 149–51.

Lancaster, F.E. (1994). Alcohol and white matter development: a review. *Alcoholism: Clinical and Experimental Research*, **18**, 644–7.

Lin, G.W.J. & Lester, D. (1985). Altered placental folate coenzyme distribution by ethanol consumption during pregnancy. *Nutrition Report International*, **31**, 1375–83.

Liu, J.P., Baker, J., Perkins, A.S., Robertson, E.J. & Efstratiadis, A. (1993). Mice carrying null mutations of the genes encoding insulin-like growth factor (IGF-1) and type 1 IGF receptor (IGF1r). *Cell*, **75**, 59–72.

López-Tejero, D., Ferrer, I., Dobera, M. & Herrera, E. (1986). Effects of prenatal ethanol exposure on physical growth, sensory reflex maturation and brain development in the rat. *Neuropathology and Applied Neurobiology*, **12**, 251–60.

Machado-Salas, J.P. (1984). Abnormal dendritic patterns and aberrant spine development in Bourneville's disease: a Golgi survey. *Clinical Neuropathology*, **3**, 52–8.

Majewski, F., Bierich, J.R., Löser, H., Michaelis, R., Leiber, B. & Bettecken, F. (1976). Zur Klinik und Pathogenese der Alkohol-Embryopathie. *Münchner Medizinische Wochenschrift,*, **118**, 1635–42.

Majewski, F., Fischback, H., Peiffer, J. & Bierich, J.R. (1978). Zur Frage der Interruptiones der alkoholkranken Frauen. *Deutsche Medizinische Wochenschrift*, **103**, 895–8.

Marin-Padilla, M. (1972). Structural abnormalities of the cerebral cortex in human chromosomal aberrations: a Golgi study. *Brain Research*, **38**, 1–12.

Marin-Padilla, M. (1974). Structural organization of the cerebral cortex in human chromosomal aberrations: a Golgi study. I. D1 (13–15) trisomy, Pätau syndrome. *Brain Research*, **66**, 375–91.

Marin-Padilla, M. (1976). Pyramidal cell abnormalities in the motor cortex of a child with Down's syndrome: a Golgi study. *Journal of Comparative Neurology*, **167**, 63–82.

Martin, X.D. & Rabineau, P.A. (1990). Dysgénésie de la crête neurale, de l'ectoderme, du mésoderme et syndrome alcoolique foetal. *Klinische Monatsblätter für Augenheilkunde*, **196**, 279–84.

Mattson, S.N., Jernigan, T.L. & Riley, E.P. (1994a). MRI and prenatal alcohol exposure: images provide insight into FAS. *Alcohol Health and Research World*, **18**, 49–52.

Mattson, S.N., Riley, E.P., Jernigan, T.L., Ehlers, C.L., Delis, D.C., Jones, K.L., Stern, C., Johnson, K.A., Hesselink, J.R. & Bellugi, U. (1992). Fetal alcohol syndrome: a case report of neuropsychological, MRI, and EEG assessment of two children. *Alcoholism: Clinical and Experimental Research*, **16**, 1001–3.

Mattson, S.N., Riley, E.P., Jernigan, T.L., Garcia, A., Kaneko, W.M., Ehlers, C.L. & Jones, K.L. (1994b). A decrease in the size of the basal ganglia following prenatal alcohol exposure: a preliminary report. *Neurotoxicology and Teratology*, **16**, 283–9.

Mauceri, H.J., Unterman, T., Dempsey, S., Lee, W.H. & Conway, S. (1993). Effect of ethanol exposure on circulating levels of insulin-like growth factor I and II, and insulin-like growth factor binding proteins in fetal rats. *Alcoholism: Clinical and Experimental Research*, **17**, 1201–6.

Mezey, E., Potter, J.J., Mishra, L., Sharma, S. & Janicot, M. (1990). Effect of insulin like growth factor I on rat alcoholic dehydrogenase in primary hepatic culture. *Archives of Biochemistry and Biophysics*, **280**, 390–6.

Michaelis, E.K. (1990). Fetal alcohol exposure: cellular toxicity and molecular events involved in toxicity. *Alcoholism: Clinical and Experimental Research*, **14**, 819–26.

Miller, M., Epstein, R.J., Sugar, J., Pinchoff, B.S., Sugar, A., Gammon, J.A., Mittelman, D., Dennis, R.F. & Isreal, J. (1984). Anterior segment anomalies associated with the fetal alcohol syndrome. *Journal of Pediatric Ophthalmology and Strabismus*, **21**, 8–18.

Peiffer, J., Majewski, F., Fischbach, H., Bierich, J.R. & Volk, B. (1979). Alcohol embryo- and fetopathy. *Journal of Neurological Sciences*, **41**, 125–37.

Pennington, S.N. (1990). Molecular changes associated with ethanol-induced growth suppression in the chick embryo. *Alcoholism: Clinical and Experimental Research*, **14**, 832–7.

Phillips, D.E. & Krueger, S.K. (1990). Effects of postnatal ethanol exposure on glial cell development in rat optic nerve. *Experimental Neurology*, **107**, 97–105.

Phillips, D.E., Krueger, S.K. & Rydquist, J.E. (1991). Short- and long-term effects of combined pre- and postnatal ethanol exposure three trimester equivalency on the development of myelin and axons in rat optic nerve. *International Journal of Developmental Neuroscience*, **9**, 631–47.

Pongrácz, F. (1985). The function of dendritic spines: a theoretical study. *Neuroscience*, **15**, 933–46.

Purpura, D.P. (1974). Dendritic spine dysgenesis and mental retardation. *Science*, **186**, 1126-8.

Purpura, D.P. (1975). Dendritic differentiation in human cerebral cortex: normal and aberrant developmental patterns. *Advances in Neurology*, **12**, 91–116.

Randall, C.L., Ekblad, U. & Anton, R.F. (1990). Perspectives on the pathophysiology of fetal alcohol syndrome. *Alcoholism: Clinical and Experimental Research*, **14**, 807–12.

Renau-Piqueras, J., Zaragoza, R., de Paz, P., Baguena-Cervellera, R., Megias, L. & Guerri, C. (1989). Effects of prolonged ethanol exposure on the glial fibrillary acidic protein-containing intermediate filaments of astrocytes in primary culture: a quantitative immunofluorescence and immunogold electron microscopic study. *Journal of Histochemistry and Cytochemistry*, **37**, 229-40.

Reyes, E., Rivera, J.M., Saland, L.C. & Murray, H.M. (1983). Effects of maternal administration of alcohol on fetal brain development. *Neurobehavioral Toxicology and Teratology*, **5**, 263–7.

Ronen, G.M. & Andrews, W.L. (1991). Holoprosencephaly as a possible embryonic alcohol effect. *American Journal of Medical Genetics*, **40**, 151–4.

Samorajski, T., Lancaster, F., Wiggins, R.C. (1986). Fetal alcohol exposure: a morphometric analysis of myelination in the optic nerve. *International Journal of Developmental Neuroscience*, **4**, 369–74.

Savage, D.D., Queen, S.A., Sanitez, C.F., Daxton, L.L., Mahoney, J.C., Goodlett, C.R. & West, J.R. (1992). Prenatal ethanol exposure during the last third of gestation in rat reduces hippocampal NMDA agonist binding site density in 45 day old offspring. *Alcohol*, **9**, 37–42.

Schapiro, M.B., Rosman, N.P. & Kemper, T.L. (1984). Effects of chronic exposure to alcohol on the developing brain. *Neurobehavioral Toxicology and Teratology*, **6**, 351–6.

Schenker, S., Becker, H.C., Randall, C.L., Phillips, D.K., Baskin, G.S. & Henderson, G.I. (1990). Fetal alcohol syndrome: current status of pathogenesis. *Alcoholism: Clinical and Experimental Research*, **14**, 635–47.

Schenker, S., Dicke, J.M., Johnson, R.F., Hays, S.E. & Henderson, G.I. (1989). Effect of ethanol on human placental transport of model amino acids and glucose. *Alcoholism: Clinical and Experimental Research*, **13**, 112–19.

Schilgen, M. & Loeser, H. (1994). Klippel–Feil anomaly combined with fetal alcohol syndrome. *European Spine Journal*, **3**, 289–90.

Singh, S.P., Strivenugopal, K.S., Ehmann, S., Yuan, X.H. & Snyder, A.K. (1994). Insulin-like growth factors (IGF-I and IGF–II), IGF-binding proteins, and IGF gene expression in the offspring of ethanol-fed rats. *Journal of Laboratory and Clinical Medicine*, **124**, 183–92.

Snyder, A.K., Singh, S.P. & Pullen, G.L. (1986). Ethanol-induced intrauterine growth retardation: correlation with placental glucose transfer. *Alcoholism: Clinical and Experimental Research*, **10**, 167–70.

Sonntag, W.E. & Boyd, R.L. (1989). Diminished insulin-like growth factor-I levels after chronic ethanol: relationship to pulsatile growth hormone release. *Alcoholism: Experimental Research*, **13**, 3–7.

Stoltenburg-Didinger, G. & Mayer, H. (1990). Retardation of myelination in rat spinal cord by prenatal exposure to ethanol. *X International Conference of Neuropathology*, Kyoto, 1990.

Stoltenburg-Didinger, G. & Spohr, H.L. (1983). Fetal alcohol syndrome and mental retardation: spine distribution of pyramidal cells in prenatal alcohol-exposed rat cerebral cortex: a Golgi study. *Developmental Brain Research*, **11**, 119–23.

Strömland, K. (1981). Eyeground malformation in the fetal alcohol syndrome. *Neuropediatrics*, **12**, 97–8.

Strömland, K. (1990). Contribution of ocular examination to the diagnosis of foetal alcohol syndrome in mentally retarded children. *Journal of Mental Deficiency Research*, **34**, 429–35.

Strömland, K., Hellström, A., Pinazo-Durán, M.D. & Guerri, C. (1993). Ocular abnormalities in humans and rats exposed to alcohol during pregnancy. *Teratology*, **48**, 34A.

Strömland, K. & Pinazo-Durán, M.D. (1994). Optic nerve hypoplasia: comparative effects in children and rats exposed to alcohol during pregnancy. *Teratology*, **50**, 100–11.

Suetsugu, M. & Mehraein, P. (1980). Spine distribution along the atypical dendrites of the pyramidal neurons in Down's syndrome: a quantitative Golgi study. *Acta Neuropathologica*, **50**, 207–10

Takashima, S., Becker, I.E., Armstrong, D.L. & Chan, F. (1981). Abnormal neuronal development in the visual cortex of the human fetus and infant with Down's syndrome: a quantitative and qualitative Golgi study. *Brain Research*, **225**, 1–21.

Tanaka, H., Arima, M. & Suzuki, N. (1981). The fetal alcohol syndrome in Japan. *Brain and Development*, **3**, 305–11.

Vasiliauskas, F., Piccoli, D.-A., Flores, A.F., Di Lorenzo, C. & Hyman, P.E. (1994). Chronic intestinal pseudo-obstruction in fetal alcohol syndrome. *Gastroenterology*, **106**, A637.

Wisniewski, K., Dambska, M., Sher, J.H. & Quazi, Q. (1983). A clinical neuropathological study of the fetal alcohol syndrome. *Neuropediatrics*, **14**, 197–201.

Wisniewski, K. & Lupin, R. (1979). Fetal alcohol syndrome and related CNS problems. *Neurology*, **29**, 1429–30.

Part III

Developmental issues

8

A dose–response study of the enduring effects of prenatal alcohol exposure: birth to 14 years

ANN P. STREISSGUTH, FRED L. BOOKSTEIN
AND HELEN M.BARR

Introduction

Soon after the recognition and identification of fetal alcohol syndrome (FAS) in 1968 (Lemoine *et al.*, 1968) and 1973 (Jones *et al.*, 1973; Jones & Smith, 1973), the question arose of the safety of alcohol use during pregnancy. Because the women who gave birth to children with FAS were primarily alcoholics and often not in good health or good circumstances themselves, it became imperative to sort out the effects of alcohol from other conditions associated with alcoholism and to investigate the effects of lower levels of usage. This work has progressed on two fronts: epidemiological studies of groups of women who used varying amounts of alcohol during pregnancy as part of their lifestyles, and studies of laboratory animals given alcohol during pregnancy in controlled doses.

Alcohol is now well recognized as a teratogen. Teratogens are agents that disrupt normal development of the embryo or fetus during gestation and cause various types of birth defects in the offspring (Wilson, 1977). Prenatal alcohol exposure has been demonstrated in many species to cause all four teratogenic endpoints – death, malformations, growth deficiency, and functional deficits – depending on the dose, timing, and conditions of exposure (West, 1986; Schenker *et al.*, 1990; Randall *et al.*, 1990).

Studies of experimental animals have demonstrated the direct toxic effect of alcohol on the developing embryo and fetus. In these studies, potentially confounding effects, such as nutrition, other drug exposures, and postnatal rearing conditions, can all be controlled in the study design so that it is possible to infer that alcohol itself is teratogenic.

Many experimental studies have shown that the brain is the most sensitive organ to the effects of prenatal alcohol (Riley, 1990; Goodlett & West, 1992). Effects on neurobehavioral development are often observed even in the absence of effects on growth or physical development. Several animal studies have now shown that brain defects can be produced by one or two heavy doses of alcohol at exactly the right time during early prenatal development (e.g., Sulik *et al.*, 1981). In the most recent of these studies, Dumas & Rabe (1994) demonstrated that a 'single embryonic exposure of a teratogenic dose of alcohol produced a deficit in long-term memory, but this deficit became clearly evident only as the mice aged' (p. 611). This work extends the non-human primate studies of Clarren and colleagues (1992) demonstrating that exposure to weekly binge doses of alcohol during early gestation produced a variety of neurobehavioral deficits and poorer learning in young macaque offspring free of obvious physical abnormalities.

The present paper describes the largest, most comprehensive study of the long-term effects of maternal alcohol use during pregnancy that has been carried out to date. A recent book describes the study in detail (Streissguth *et al.*, 1993).

Generally, the findings from this human population-based study are congruent with the experimental animal literature. Effects on neurobehavioral development far exceed and outlast the effects on birth weight and later size dimensions. These effects are not restricted to those subjects with physical anomalies or the facial features associated with FAS. Although some neurobehavioral deficits were observable in the first 2 days of life, they were not reliably observed on standardized developmental tests until the children were 4 years of age. Neurobehavioral deficits were even more observable at 7 years than at 4 years, and remained as strong at 14 years as at 7 years. The domains of attention, memory, speed and reliability of information processing, arithmetic functioning and phonological processing were the most affected by prenatal alcohol exposure. These neurobehavioral deficits, which are not mediated by birth weight, are highly significant statistically despite the absence of post-infancy effects of prenatal alcohol on child weight and height.

Offspring performance was not uniformly affected across all domains by prenatal alcohol exposure, and there were some age-related changes in the salience of various outcomes for prenatal alcohol. The intermittent detectability of these fetal alcohol effects does not appear to be attributable to intervening environmental conditions, but rather to our difficulty in detecting subtle teratogenic effects with standardized infant developmental tests and to our failure to incorporate more focused, individualized tests of neurobehavioral and cognitive functioning at intervening ages during infancy.

Alcohol dose was measured redundantly to express as accurately as possible the many naturally occurring variations in the pattern and timing of alcohol use by pregnant women. While our early analyses were restricted to single alcohol predictors, the lability of the associated findings from one age to another and from one outcome to another led us to experiment with multifactorial approaches to data analysis. Partial Least Squares (PLS) analytical methods (see Bookstein *et al.*, 1990, 1996; Streissguth *et al.*, 1993) have permitted us to view the saliences of each alcohol score in the context of the others in its ability to predict outcome deficits. We find that as the children reach school age, it is the binge or massed patterns of use that show the strongest relationship with offspring behavior and performance, and the scores from the earliest exposure period (prior to pregnancy recognition) that are the stronger predictors in general, compared with the midpregnancy alcohol scores.

The successful detection of prenatal alcohol effects, then, is dependent on a carefully constructed experimental design utilizing a multifactorial approach to exposure and a battery of focused and sensitive neurobehavioral tests at each age. It is crucial that the design control for competing causes of poor child outcome, including but not limited to prenatal exposure to nicotine.

Study design

The Seattle Study on Alcohol and Pregnancy was initiated in 1974 to examine the long-term effects of prenatal alcohol exposure. Our goal was to see how subtle manifestations of the characteristic deficits associated with FAS might extend to the whole range of prenatal exposure, but focusing on the moderate range of doses characteristic of 'social drinking'.

Our study was designed in keeping with the principles of teratogenic theory (Wilson, 1977). Dose, timing, and conditions of exposure were measured as precisely as possible. Three types of teratogenic outcome were examined – deficits in growth, morphology, and function – all of which were apparent in children with FAS. The functional outcomes included age-appropriate neurobehavioral and performance measures. Careful measures of dose and conditions of exposure were combined with sensitive outcome measures and assessment of many potential covariates.

The study design is prospective, longitudinal, and population-based for greater generalizability (Fig. 8.1). Data collection began with standardized maternal interviews at the fifth month of pregnancy, and the most recent data set deals with the same birth cohort of children at age 14 years. This long span, together with an unusually high follow-up rate of 82%, has permitted evaluation of the long-term effects of prenatal alcohol exposure on children's health and development.

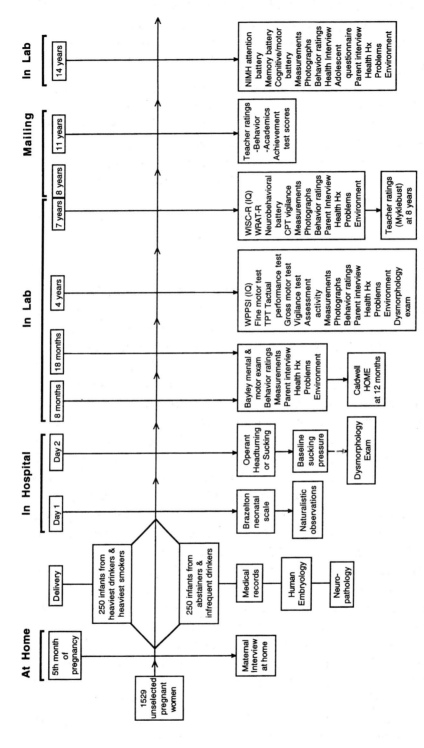

Fig. 8.1. Study design. The experimental design for the Seattle Longitudinal Prospective Study on Alcohol and Pregnancy. Sample sizes for substudies include the following: Brazelton, 469; naturalistic observation, 124; operant head-turning, 225; operant sucking, 80; baseline sucking study, 151; neonatal dysmorphology, 163; 8 month follow-up, 468; 18 month follow-up, 496; 4 year follow-up, 465; 7 year laboratory follow-up, 486; 11 year teacher rating study, 458; 14 year follow-up, 470. (Reprinted by permission of *Drug and Alcohol Dependence*.)

Table 8.1. *The Seattle Alcohol and Pregnancy Study design: 1974–94*

1529 consecutive pregnant women receiving prenatal care by the fifth month of
   pregnancy in 1974/5
'Pregnancy and Health Interview' given at home during fifth month of pregnancy
Study preceded general knowledge about not drinking during pregnancy
Follow-up cohort ≈ 500 selected at birth based on the QFV[a] interview for alcohol
Cohort oversampled for heavier drinkers and stratified for smoking
All examiners blind to exposure history and past examination performance
Follow-up rate, birth to 14 years = 82%; including 93% of those seen at 7 years
No differential loss of heavily exposed offspring

---

[a]QFV, Quantity–Frequency–Variability.

Several factors contribute to the ability of this study to detect effects where
they exist. The study began at a time when alcohol was not known to have
adverse effects on offspring, so that drinking was commonplace among pregnant women, who had less reason to minimize their reported consumption
than they would have today. Drinking and heavy drinking among Seattle
women in 1974/5 were not limited to just one end of the socioeconomic scale,
and the use of other drugs in this population was generally low.

Certain aspects of the sampling procedures precluded the serious confounding of alcohol with other risk factors such as poor prenatal care that would
have made detection of alcohol effects difficult. Selection of a cohort of
approximately 500 offspring born to the 1529 screening-study mothers enabled
us to retain all the heavier-exposed offspring within a cohort of more manage-
able size. Stratification of the follow-up sample for smoking across drinking
levels permitted separation of alcohol effects from those of smoking. The
recruitment criteria required that all women be interviewed by the fifth
month of pregnancy in order to assure that all had reasonable prenatal care,
and that alcohol use was assessed at a standard gestational age (Table 8.1).

Sample selection was biphasic. First, the screening cohort of 1529 pregnant
women was drawn consecutively from two Seattle hospitals that together
reflected the demographic characteristics of Seattle in 1974/5. The maternal
interviews were conducted in private. They covered many aspects of prenatal
life that might have contributed to the health and welfare of the offspring
(Streissguth *et al.*, 1981, 1993). The follow-up cohort of approximately 500
infants was selected at delivery on the basis of the maternal drinking and
smoking data obtained at midpregnancy in the screening study. Fig. 8.2.
shows the definitions of the Ordered Exposure Categories used to select the

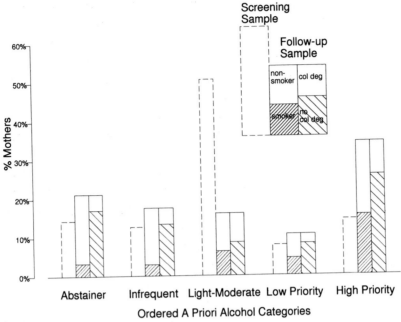

Fig. 8.2.   Alcohol exposure categories as represented in the screening sample and the follow-up sample: stratification by smoking and maternal education. The two bars at the right in each set show the proportion of smokers to nonsmokers and the proportion of mothers with college degrees to mothers without college degrees within the follow-up sample, stratified for each alcohol category. The dashed bar at the left in each set permits comparison of the follow-up sample with the screening sample according to alcohol exposure categories. The screening sample represents 1439 singleton, live-born children (from the original screening sample of 1529) who were located at delivery and alive at discharge. The follow-up sample is represented here by the 582 children seen for at least one of the follow-up examinations at day 1, 8 months, 18 months, 4 years, and/or 7 years. Definitions of alcohol exposure categories used for sample selection (ORDEXC): High Priority, AA > 1 or binge drinking of 5 or more drinks on one or more occasions with a total of at least 18 drinks per month; Low Priority, AA < 1, but 45 or more drinks per month or any reported intoxications while having no more than 4 drinks on any one occasion, or a heavy drinker according to Cahalan's (Cahalan *et al.*, 1969) score QFV = 1; Light-Moderate, AA > 0.10 and not included in either of the above two categories; Infrequent, AA < 0.10 but not an abstainer; Abstainer, no alcohol use during or in the month or so prior to recognition of pregnancy. The ORDEXC classification considered alcohol scores for both pre-pregnancy recognition and during pregnancy. For further details see Streissguth *et al.* (1981, 1993). (Reprinted by permission of the University of Michigan Press.)

follow-up cohort from the screening sample, and Streissguth *et al.* (1993) gives the selection details.

The self-reported alcohol use by these mothers was representative of the general Seattle population of pregnant women who were receiving good prenatal care by midpregnancy and who were interviewed at a time before women knew not to drink during pregnancy. Approximately 80% of women from this population reported some alcohol use during pregnancy and approximately 80% had reported some alcohol use in the month or so prior to pregnancy recognition. Fig. 8.2 shows how the sampling procedure enriched the follow-up cohort with a higher proportion of heavier drinkers, while the stratification procedure avoided an otherwise inextricable confounding of smoking with alcohol. (For further discussion of design considerations, see Streissguth *et al.*, 1994c).

The primary independent variable, alcohol, was assessed via a Quantity-Frequency-Variability (QFV) interview (Cahalan *et al.*, 1969) incorporating supplemental questions about higher levels of drinking, intoxications, and problems with drinking. Drinking during two time periods was assessed: During pregnancy (D) and Prior to pregnancy or pregnancy recognition (P) (see Streissguth *et al.*, 1993, for details). Alcohol use was quantified in several different dimensions. These are quite highly correlated, and should not be considered as independent measures of exposure. Table 8.2 lists the 12 alcohol scores usually used in the analyses, along with distribution statistics for each score from the drinking mothers in the longitudinal sample described in Streissguth *et al.* (1993) and from the mothers in the 14 year follow-up cohort. The scores include: an AA score (average ounces of absolute alcohol per day, converted in the table to approximate average number of drinks per day); a categorical QFV score incorporating volume and pattern of use; and three distinct measures of massed or binge drinking (ADOCC, average drinks per drinking occasion; MAX, maximum drinks any drinking occasion; and BINGE, a dichotomous score reflecting 5 or more drinks on any drinking occasion). These scores were all obtained for the two time periods (P and D). P or D, as the suffix to an alcohol score, identifies the score from that specific time period. Thus, AAP indicates ounces of absolute alcohol in the period prior to pregnancy recognition. A summary score was also used in the analyses: ORDEXC (ordered exposure categories), an *a priori* 'risk' score that incorporates exposure from both periods, and was used for cohort selection (ORDEXC=0 reflects abstinence during both periods; ORDEXC=4 indicates Higher Priority for cohort selection due to 'risk' drinking during at least one of the time periods).

The majority of the mothers were white, married and middle class, although the sample, representative of Seattle generally, contained a broad range of socioeconomic and racial groups. As Table 8.3 indicates, the demographic characteristics of the screening sample were very similar to those of

Table 8.2. *Alcohol use by mothers (drinkers only): screening sample versus cohort mothers*

	Screening sample		Cohort mothers	
	Mean	Median	Mean	Median
AA: drinks/day (beer, wine, liquor)				
Pre	0.8	0.4	1.6	0.8
During	0.4	0.2	0.6	0.3
MOCC: monthly occasions of drinking				
Pre	10.3	6.0	16.9	9.0
During	5.7	3.3	8.0	4.5
ADOCC: average drinks/occasion				
Pre	2.1	1.5	2.5	2.2
During	1.9	1.5	2.2	1.8
MAX: maximum drinks/occasion				
Pre	3.1	1.5	4.0	3.5
During	2.8	1.5	3.6	3.5
QFV score				
Pre	2.2	2.0	2.5	2.0
During	1.8	2.0	2.0	2.0
BINGE: % binge (5 or more drinks/ occasion)				
Pre	18.8	0	39.1	0
During	12.2	0	24.1	0

A 'drink' is calculated at 0.5 ounces or 15 g of absolute alcohol per day. Pre, before recognition of pregnancy; During, during midpregnancy. The table omits 299 mothers (20%) who abstained 'pre' and 287 (19%) who abstained 'during' in the screening study ($n = 1529$) and 124 (27%) who abstained 'pre' and 103 (22%) who abstained 'during' of the mothers of the 14 year follow-up cohort ($n = 464$). The direction order of the QFV scores has been reversed for consistency with the other drinking scales.

the follow-up cohort. Tables 8.4 and 8.5 also compare the screening sample and the follow-up cohort, showing the generally low-risk nature of the follow-up cohort even after enrichment for mothers drinking more heavily during pregnancy.

Because poor nutrition, poor maternal weight gain, and poor prenatal care are often associated with alcohol abuse, these variables were examined in relation to our alcohol use scores. There was no difference between the heavier drinkers and the rest of the sample in terms of number of sit-down meals reported per day. Maternal alcohol use was uncorrelated with total number of prenatal visits ($r = 0.04$) or weight gain during pregnancy

Table 8.3. *Maternal and household characteristics: screening sample versus follow-up cohort*

	Screening sample	Follow-up cohort
	(*n* = 1529)	(*n* = 464)
White	86%	88%
Married	87%	87%
Middle class	81%	81%
Prenatal vitamins during pregnancy	98%	98%
Prenatal care by fifth month	100%	100%
Mean educational level	13.8 years	13.7 years
Mean no. of children in household	1.0	0.9
Median annual income (14 years)	–	$45 000

All statistics except for median family income reflect maternal or household characteristics at the time of the prenatal interview in 1974/5. Number of children excludes the cohort child.

Table 8.4. *Maternal risk factors during pregnancy: screening sample versus follow-up cohort*

	Screening sample	Follow-up cohort
	(*n* = 1529)	(*n* = 464)
Alcohol use (any)	86%	80%
Cigarettes (any)	25%	31%
Marijuana (any)	12%	18%
Other illicit drugs (any)	1%	2%
Any major alcohol problems	1%	1%
No high school diploma	11%	12%
< 17 years old	2%	2%
Welfare 1975	8%	6%
Welfare (14 years) 1991	–	5%

All statistics except welfare at 14 years reflect maternal or household characteristics at the time of the prenatal interview in 1974–5.

($r = 0.00$). Maternal alcohol use was also not related to other pregnancy risk factors such as diabetes, renal disease, thyroid abnormality, or rubella (Streissguth *et al.*, 1982).

The follow-up cohort of approximately 500 subjects was examined on day 1 and day 2 of life, 8 and 18 months, and 4, 7, and 14 years, and teacher evaluations were obtained at 8 and 11 years (Fig. 8.1). All examinations were conducted blind without the examiner having knowledge about the subjects'

Table 8.5. *Rates of poor pregnancy outcome: screening sample versus follow-up cohort*

	Screening sample	Follow-up cohort
	($n = 1439$)	($n = 464$)
Prematurity (gestational age < 37 weeks)	4%	3%
Low birth weight (< 2500 g)	3%	2%
Very low birth weight (< 1500 g)	< 1%	0%

Screening study of live-born singleton infants located at delivery. Cohort infants are also only live-born singletons.

exposure history, living conditions, or previous examination scores. The sample was successfully maintained over this 15 year period by extensive tracing and outreach activity (Streissguth & Giunta, 1992). At the 14 year examination 82% of the original cohort were examined, 93% of those examined at 7 years. There has been no differential loss of heavily exposed subjects. The most frequent cause of loss to follow-up was moving out of the area.

Statistical analyses for the first 4 years primarily involved multiple regression analyses of single outcomes against single alcohol predictor variables, adjusting for co-varying conditions. These methods are discussed most fully in Streissguth *et al.* (1986, 1989*b*) Analyses from 7 years onward have involved PLS, a method of data analysis that permits the simultaneous assessment of relations among multiple alcohol predictor scores and multiple outcome scores. PLS is better suited than multiple regression or other alternatives to complex multifactorial data generated in human behavioral teratology studies such as ours. This methodology, as applied to teratology, is described in Bookstein *et al.* (1990, 1996), Sampson *et al.* (1989), and Streissguth *et al.* (1989*c*). A recent monograph on the study (Streissguth *et al.*, 1993) offers detailed descriptions of PLS analyses for cross-sectional and longitudinal designs. PLS analyses yield latent variables (LVs) for both dose (alcohol LVs) and response (outcome LVs) that demonstrate the salience of the prenatal alcohol scores for the outcomes under consideration. In particular, the Alcohol LV, which is measured as a linear combination of all the dose measures, is very stable across diverse analyses over the whole range of ages.

Data on possible confounds were obtained prospectively, at the prenatal interview and at all succeeding waves of examination. These included maternal nutrition and use of drugs and medications during pregnancy, sociodemographic and educational characteristics of the family, mother/child interactions, major life stresses in the household, childhood accidents, hospitalizations and illnesses, educational experiences of the child, and many others (Streissguth *et al.*, 1993).

All findings reported here have been evaluated in terms of many potential confounds. First, correlations between the many covariates in the database and the outcome LVs are examined. Then the covariates associated with both the Alcohol LV and the outcome LVs are examined in regression analyses to see to what extent they alter the estimated effects of alcohol dose. Scatterplots and partial residual plots are routinely examined. The results reported are not attributable to other prenatal exposures such as nicotine and illicit drugs, and are not attributable to sociodemographic variables such as parental education.

Results

Pregnancy complications, neonatal complications, and offspring growth parameters from birth to 14 years

Maternal complications of labor and delivery (including increased temperature, amnionitis, preeclampsia, and bleeding) were significantly related to 'risk level' drinking as defined by ORDEXC categories 3 and 4, as was heavy meconium in the amniotic fluid (Streissguth *et al.*, 1982). Risk level drinking, which includes infrequent binges as well as heavier average use, was also significantly related to lower Apgar scores at 1 and 5 minutes and to respiratory distress. Heart rate abnormalities were significantly related to AAP $\geq$ 1 ounce, but none of the alcohol scores were related to presentation of infant, placental and/or cord abnormalities, illness of infant prior to discharge, or length of hospitalization of the infant.

Growth parameters (height, weight, and head circumference) had a modest relationship with prenatal alcohol at birth. Although statistically significant, the alcohol effects were considerably smaller than the effects of smoking. By 8 months of age, the smoking effects were no longer statistically significant, while alcohol effects remained weakly significant (Barr *et al.*, 1984). Subsequent analyses did not reveal any further associations between prenatal alcohol and height, weight, and head circumference from 18 months through 14 years (Sampson *et al.*, 1994).

Findings during infancy, preschool, and early childhood (birth through 4 years)

Infants were examined for neurobehavioral functioning on day 1 and day 2 of life using the Brazelton Neurodevelopmental Scale (Streissguth *et al.*,

1983); naturalistic observations (Landesman-Dwyer *et al.*, 1978); operant head-turning procedures, operant sucking procedures (Martin *et al.*, 1977) and baseline sucking (Martin *et al.*, 1979; Stock *et al.*, 1985). Even after adjusting for delivery medications and other covariates, prenatal alcohol exposure was associated with poorer habituation. The more alcohol-exposed the infant, the more poorly would it habituate (show a response decrement) to a repetitive stimulus (Streissguth *et al.*, 1983). Poor habituation is generally considered to be an early manifestation of central nervous system (CNS) dysfunction. Prenatal alcohol exposure was also associated with increased 'low arousal', a cluster of behaviors involving frequent state change at the low end of the arousal continuum: for instance, frequent alternation between awake and drowsy, or difficulty in maintaining either a good alert state or a good sleep state (Streissguth *et al.*, 1983). Also, prenatal alcohol was associated with increased time with eyes open, bodily tremors, head turns to the left, hand to face activity, and decreased vigorous bodily activity in a subset of systematically observed neonates (Landesman-Dwyer *et al.*, 1978). Operant learning on day 2 (measured with both an operant head-turning paradigm and an operant sucking paradigm) was decreased by exposure to alcohol only for those infants also exposed to nicotine (Martin *et al.*, 1977). By comparison, infant sucking pressure (measured with a pressure transducer) and latency to first suck showed significant effects of prenatal alcohol exposure independent of nicotine exposure (Martin *et al.*, 1979; Stock *et al.*, 1985).

Additional analyses of newborn Brazelton and Reflex scores were carried out in conjunction with a large PLS analysis of 474 infant and early childhood outcomes measured across the first 7 years of life (Streissguth *et al.*, 1993). In these analyses, Habituation to Light (from the Brazelton scale) was the neonatal outcome most strongly correlated with prenatal alcohol exposure. Other important neonatal behaviors particularly salient for alcohol include poorer Habituation to Rattle, fewer smiles, more hand-to-mouth activity, a weaker Moro reflex, hypertonic Passive Arms reflex, hypertonic Incurvation Reflex, and a delayed Stepping Reflex threshold (Streissguth *et al.*, 1993). The neonatal findings demonstrate that subtle CNS effects of prenatal alcohol are already measurable before the infant has ever encountered a postnatal environment.

At 8 and 18 months of age, the infants were evaluated using the Bayley Scales of Infant Development (BSID) and various other checklists and rating scales. The two scales deriving from BSID are: (1) the Mental Scale, whose results are expressed in a standard score called the Mental Development Index (MDI), and (2) the Motor Scale, whose results are expressed in a standard score called the Psychomotor Development Index (PDI). At 8 months, prenatal alcohol exposure was associated with small but statistically significant decrements in MDI and PDI that could not be attributed to other risk factors such as breastfeeding, maternal separation from infant, major life changes in the household, maternal diet during pregnancy, or other prenatal exposures. Prenatal alcohol exposure was also significantly related to increased feeding problems at 8 months of age, but not to sleeping problems, colic, excess crying, or high fevers (Streissguth *et al.*, 1980). However, at 18 months there were no statistically significant relationships between prenatal alcohol and scores on the BSID. When these data were included in large PLS analyses, none of the 8 and 18 month scores were as strongly associated with the Alcohol LV as those measured at birth, 4 or 7 years (Streissguth *et al.*, 1993). This finding is probably a function of the poor sensitivity of global developmental tests at this age (see Discussion).

For the 4 year examination, a much more sensitive and comprehensive battery of neurobehavioral outcomes was assembled based on deficits observed in children with FAS (who constituted a pilot study at each examination wave). As we expected, prenatal alcohol exposure was associated with statistically significant decrements on Full Scale IQ from the Wechsler Preschool and Primary Scale of Intelligence (WPPSI). Performance Scale IQ was more strongly affected by prenatal alcohol than Verbal Scale IQ (Streissguth *et al.*, 1989*b*). Dividing the sample at 3 drinks per day, the adjusted prenatal alcohol effect was more than -4 IQ points (one-fourth of a standard deviation). Even after adjustment for other prenatal exposures and nutrition, sociodemographic characteristics, mother/child interactions, preschool attendance, and other covariates, a 3-fold relative risk of IQ below 85 is estimated for children of 'average background' in our population for exposures at or above 3 drinks per day. These CNS effects of prenatal alcohol exposure were not mediated by low birth weight.

Components of the Wisconsin Motor Steadiness Battery (WMSB) and a test of Gross Motor Performance both showed significant associations with prenatal alcohol exposure at 4 years (Barr *et al.*, 1990). On the latter test, a summary score for all balance measures was significantly associated with prenatal alcohol though measures of coordination and distance were not. These findings may relate to reports of cerebellar signs (Marcus, 1987) or frank cerebellar dysgenesis (Clarren, 1986) reported clinically in children with FAS. Performance on grip strength, finger tapping speed, and the Tactual Performance Test (TPT) were unrelated to prenatal alcohol exposure at the 4 year examination. In working on stylus-maze tasks and motor steadiness tasks, the more alcohol-exposed children showed more 'time in error'. This reflects the time it takes for a child to respond to the auditory alarm by moving the stylus away from the inner edge of the maze when an error is made (i.e., when the edge is touched) (Barr *et al.*, 1990).

Attention and reaction time at 4 years were measured with a Vigilance Test that produced an infrequently appearing target (a kitten in the window) at irregular intervals (Streissguth *et al.*, 1984*b*). The more alcohol-exposed children more often failed to press the button when the target was in sight, more often pressed the button when no target was in sight, and (particularly at the end of testing) took longer to press the button appropriately after the target appeared. Behavior ratings of the children in this setting did not reveal any associations of prenatal alcohol with gross measures of activity or failure to attend physically to the stimulus. Thus, the findings seem more pertinent to attention difficulties than to hyperactivity. Automated measures of bodily movement in the vigilance setting were unrelated to prenatal alcohol exposure (Streissguth *et al.*, 1984*b*); this may relate to the constraints upon activity in the laboratory setting.

An examiner rating of 'overall clinical impression' at the end of the 4 year neurobehavioral examination placed 19% of the children whose mothers had AA scores of at least 2.0 (4 or more drinks per day on average) in the 'suspect' or 'abnormal' categories, versus 4–5% of children of mothers with all lower levels of drinking (Streissguth *et al.*, 1984*a*).

PLS analysis by wave of measurement (Streissguth *et al.*, 1993) revealed a number of 4 year neurobehavioral effects to be among the most highly salient for the Alcohol LV. These include more 'time in error' from the WMSB, lower WPPSI IQ, lower Arithmetic and Picture Completion Subtest Scores, more frequent verbal interruptions and excessive talking during the examination, and behavior ratings (by examiner) of poorer goal directedness, poorer attention span, and more hypertonic bodily tone.

A subset of the most heavily exposed infants and hospital-matched controls ($n = 163$) was evaluated on day 1 or 2 of life for minor anomalies associated with FAS, growth deficiency, and CNS effects such as microcephaly, tremulousness, and poor suck by a dysmorphologist blind to prenatal exposures. The clinical judgment of 'fetal alcohol effects' (FAE) was associated with prenatal alcohol exposure prior to recognition of pregnancy (AAP scores) but not with exposure in midpregnancy (AAD) (Hanson *et al.*, 1978). Two infants of this subset were identified as having FAS. At the 4 year examination, another dysmorphologist conducted blind assessments of a larger group of exposed and unexposed or lightly exposed children ($n = 205$), group-matched on maternal race, age, parity, education, socioeconomic status, marital status, and smoking (Graham *et al.*, 1988). Significantly more children with possible FAE (here defined as minor anomalies characteristic of FAS, along with growth deficiency) were identified among the offspring of the heavier drinkers compared with the lightly or not exposed (20% vs 9%). The higher the exposure the greater the likelihood of the child having FAE. Eighty percent of the children identified as having FAE at birth were also identified as having FAE at 4 years, but only 50% of those identified at 4 years had been identified at birth, suggesting that only the most obviously affected neonates will be detected at birth.

The two infants clinically identified with FAS at birth by blind clinical examination by a dysmorphologist experienced in FAS diagnosis have revealed interesting growth trajectories with increasing age (Sampson *et al.*, 1994). Although they had marginally low birth weight, they were not the smallest children among the 1439 births to study mothers, nor did they show the failure to thrive that is often reported in infants with FAS. By 4 years of age they were no longer growth deficient at all and were, in fact, called only 'FAE' by the dysmorphologist conducting the blind assessments at year 4.

The mental development of these two infants revealed an uneven pattern of development during infancy: one was deviant on the 8 month Bayley scales, while the other was deviant on the Bayley MDI at 18 months. At 4 years and 7 years of age, when given the Wechsler Preschool and Preliminary Intelligence Scales and the Wechsler Intelligence Scale for Children–Revised (WISC–R), these children were both functioning in the borderline retarded range of intelligence. They have generally fallen on the low end of the many neurobehavioral and attentional tests administered between 4 years and 14 years of age, but they are not always unusually low compared with other subjects in the group of those more highly exposed to alcohol *in utero*.

Early school-age findings (7–8 years)

In the summer following their first year in school, when they averaged $7\frac{1}{2}$ years of age, the whole cohort was brought in again for a large battery of tests and measurements. Prenatal alcohol was not related to physical size at this age (Sampson *et al.*, 1994). Facial morphology, as assessed morphometrically after digitization of facial photographs that was blind to prenatal alcohol exposure, was associated with prenatal alcohol exposure in only a subgroup of the most highly exposed children (Clarren *et al.*, 1987). Neither growth nor facial morphology was as sensitive a marker of prenatal alcohol effects as the broad array of neurobehavioral outcomes.

The large battery of neurobehavioral tests administered at this $7\frac{1}{2}$ year examination and their relationship to prenatal alcohol have been described in a trilogy of papers (Streissguth *et al.*, 1989*a*, *c*; Sampson *et al.*, 1989). We observed many deficits in spatial memory and integration, verbal memory and integration, flexible problem solving, and perceptual motor function. Verbal tasks were not as strongly affected by prenatal alcohol as were visual spatial tasks. In these analyses, we exploited PLS methods for the first time, examining multifactorial alcohol predictors in relation to multiple scores from multiple tests of neurobehavioral function.

Using data from the WISC–R, a multiple regression analysis suggested an average 7 point decrement in Full Scale IQ associated with AAD ⩾ 1 (mean 1.7 oz) (Streissguth *et al.*, 1990). Decrements of 1–3 months in Arithmetic and Reading performance on the Wide Range Achievement Test–Revised (WRAT–R) were observed to be associated with a binge pattern of exposure. PLS analyses of the multiple alcohol predictors against the individual subtest scores of the WISC–R revealed that only certain subtests of this IQ test carried the alcohol effect (Arithmetic, Digit Span, and Block Design) while others showed little relationship to alcohol (Comprehension, Coding, Vocabulary, and Picture Assembly). The Alcohol LV most salient for these deficits in memory, problem solving, and speed of information processing emphasized a massed or binge drinking pattern, particularly early in gestation.

Some behavioral ratings by the psychometrist at the conclusion of testing also were associated with prenatal alcohol: distractibility, over-persistence (which can also be called rigid problem solving), reassurance-seeking, and poor organization (Streissguth *et al.*, 1989*c*).

During the school year following this examination, classroom teachers of this cohort of children were asked to fill out the Myklebust Pupil Rating Scale (MPRS) and to provide data on the children's functioning on standardized national achievement tests. Myklebust items that were the most salient for prenatal alcohol exposure included 'difficulty retaining information', 'lack of cooperation/impulsivity', and poorer 'comprehension of words', grammar, word recall, and tactfulness. Other associations suggest problems with focusing and maintaining attention and with processing and organization of information (Sampson *et al.*, 1989). Clearly, the behavioral effects of exposure noted in the one-to-one laboratory situation were still apparent 6 months later in the ratings from second-grade teachers, when the children were 7 or 8 years old.

Additional PLS analyses (Streissguth *et al.*, 1993) indicated that even after adjustment for potential confounds such as parental education and family size, the 7-year Neurobehavioral LV was as sensitive to prenatal alcohol dose as was the best neonatal performance LV. That is, these alcohol effects are not attenuating with age.

Some of the neurobehavioral tests used at this age that were the most sensitive to prenatal alcohol exposure included: written Syntax Errors and lower Mean Length of Utterance (from the Johnson Sentence Building Test), more errors of commission on the AX task of the CPT vigilance test (reflecting impulsive errors), and lower WISC–R subtest scores of Arithmetic, Digit Span and Block Designs, and lower WRAT–R Arithmetic and Spelling Achievement Scores (Streissguth *et al.*, 1993).

Across the ages from 1 day through 7 years there thus emerges a wide diversity of deficits induced by prenatal alcohol exposure. Among the most salient sequelae of exposure are neonatal habituation to light (from the Brazelton scale administered on day 1 of life); speed of information processing at age 4 (measured by the time taken to correct errors on a visual-spatial task, the Wisconsin Motor Steadiness Battery); standardized assessments of arithmetic performance following the first year in school (as measured by both the WISC–R Arithmetic subtest and the WRAT–R achievement test); and academic performance as measured by the second-grade teacher ratings. For most of these outcomes, binge drinking has more serious consequences than the same amount of steady drinking, and drinking early in pregnancy has more serious consequences than the same reported pattern of drinking in midpregnancy. There is no statistical evidence for a 'risk-free' or threshold level of prenatal drinking; and these alcohol effects cannot be 'explained away' by any of 150 covariates considered, including parents' education, maternal smoking, and nutrition during pregnancy (Streissguth *et al.*, 1993).

Late childhood and adolescent findings (11 and 14 years)

When the children were 11 years old we again mailed questionnaires to their schools. The Multigrade Inventory for Teachers (MIT) and the MPRS were found to be related to prenatal alcohol in profiles reminiscent of those for earlier teacher ratings. Behaviors that were the most salient for prenatal alcohol exposure in the cohort at 11 years included distractibility, restlessness, lack of persistence, and reluctance to meet challenges. Learning problems showing the greatest salience for prenatal alcohol exposure included those measuring information processing and reasoning problems and a lack of interest in reading. On standardized national achievement tests, arithmetic performance was the most affected by prenatal alcohol exposure, followed closely by the 'total achievement' scores (Carmichael Olson *et al.*, 1992).

The newest findings from the Seattle study involve data from assessments of the cohort at 14 years of age, when 82% of the original cohort were again evaluated (Streissguth *et al.*, 1994a, d; Sampson *et al.*, 1994). Arithmetic

Table 8.6. *Primary findings regarding prenatal alcohol exposure and attention/memory deficits at age 14 years*

1. Prenatal alcohol leads to decreased Attention/Memory in early adolescence: dose-dependent relationship
2. The strength of the relationship ($r = 0.26$) is second only to the correlation of paternal education with Attention/Memory ($r = -0.34$)
3. Alcohol effects remain significant ($p < 0.001$) after appropriate covariate adjustment
4. Attention/Memory items most salient for alcohol were impulsive errors (False Alarms) and errors of spatial orientation
5. Children identified as Neurobehavioral FAE at 7 years had Attention/Memory deficits at 14 years.

(from the WISC–R) is again highly salient for prenatal alcohol exposure, and by now a longitudinal component is clear: 91% of the heavier drinkers' children who had scored low on Arithmetic at 7 years, remained low on Arithmetic at 14 years (versus only 45% of the abstainers' children who had scored low on Arithmetic at 7 years). Findings such as these, more focal than the earlier sample-wide correlational analyses, suggest that these deficits are not a transient response to characteristics of the testing situation, but rather reflect some permanent compromise of CNS function not ameliorated by ordinary remedial programming. There are also significant effects of prenatal alcohol upon a measure of phonological processing, the Word Attack Subtest of the Woodcock Johnson Battery (Streissguth *et al.*, 1994*a*).

There are continued alcohol-related deficits in attention/memory scores, especially measures of fluctuating attentional states (observed in increased individual variability in reaction time), problems with response inhibition (assessed with increased error and 'false alarm' rates on attention tasks including the Talland Letter Cancellation Test and the Continuous Performance Test [CPT]), and spatial learning deficits (assessed with a computerized adaptation of Milner's Stepping Stone Maze [SSM]) (Streissguth *et al.*, 1994*d*). A latent variable reflecting the pattern of attention/memory deficits observed at 14 years correlated 0.67 with the composite pattern of neurobehavioral FAE at 7 years. The same binge-weighted pattern of prenatal alcohol exposure salient for neurobehavioral outcomes at 7 and 11 years was still evident in the 14 year data. (See Table 8.6 for a summary of the 14 year Attention/Memory findings.)

The most recent paper from this study (Streissguth *et al.*, 1995) examines the longitudinal components of vigilance test performance at ages 4, 7, and 14 years. Despite differences in the vigilance paradigms at each age, there are

Table 8.7. *Cross-lagged correlations: 7 year Vigilance LV with Behavior Ratings at 8, 11, and 14 years*

	r
Teacher ratings (second-grade): Attention (8 years)	−0.38
Teacher ratings (fifth/sixth-grade): Attention (11 years)	−0.36
Psychometrist ratings (14 years)	
Endurance	−0.38
Organization	−0.37
Distractibility	0.32
Persistence	−0.19
Impulsivity	0.27

From Streissguth *et al.* (1995).

Table 8.8. *Cross-lagged correlations: early parent/teacher ratings with 14 year Vigilance LV*

	r
Conners' Parent Questionnaire (7 years)	
Distractible	0.30
Impulsive/Hyperactive	0.11
Eyberg Child Behavior Inventory (ECBI) – Parent (7 years)	
Intensity	0.20
Fails to Finish Tasks	0.25
Attention	0.23
Easily Distracted	0.22
Difficulty Concentrating	0.22
Teacher ratings (second-grade): Attention (8 years)	−0.38
Teacher ratings (fifth/sixth-grade): Attention (11 years)	−0.42

From Streissguth *et al.* (1995).

clear continuities of deficit across this 10 year period of child development. Standard deviation of reaction time (SDRT), suggesting fluctuating attentional states, was the most salient for prenatal alcohol exposure at all three ages. The 19 poorest performers on the CPT at 14 years had all been poorer than average on the CPT at 7 years. Forty-seven percent of these had also been given poor ratings on attention by second-grade teachers when they were 7 or 8 years old, versus 18% of the rest of the sample. Sixty-six percent of the poor vigilance performers at 14 years had previously been given poor or below-average ratings on attention by their teachers when they were about 11 years old (versus only 26% for the rest of the sample). Tables 8.7 and 8.8

display some of the cross-lagged correlations that provide additional evidence for the longitudinal nature of these findings. Reports in progress show that prenatal alcohol also perturbs adolescent performance on cognitive tasks, particularly the speed/accuracy trade-off on a spatial visual reasoning task. Additional findings on a wide variety of school-related and adaptive behavior problems are also observed.

Discussion

The study population ($n = 1529$) reflects the demographic characteristics of Seattle, Washington, and was selected from among women who were already in prenatal care by the fifth month of pregnancy. Drinking habits of these women reflect the alcohol use patterns of women in the early 1970s before there was general knowledge about alcohol's teratogenic effects. Seven percent of the mothers reported at least 60 drinks a month before they knew they were pregnant and 2% reported this amount in midpregnancy. Seven percent reported at least 5 drinks on an occasion at least once a week and 2% reported this amount in midpregnancy.

The Seattle Longitudinal Study on Alcohol and Pregnancy has revealed marked discrepancies in the effect of prenatal alcohol on the three primary channels of teratogenic outcome: growth, morphology, and CNS dysfunction. (The fourth traditional outcome, fetal wastage, was eliminated by a design restricting measurements to liveborn.)

Alcohol effects on birth weight are generally small and unreliable, particularly in comparison with the effects of smoking, with which alcohol exposure is often linked. In our prospective study, alcohol effects were observed on three neonatal size measures – weight, length, and head circumference – and were not altered after adjustment for other factors of small size, including smoking. But the magnitude of these size effects was smaller than those of smoking. Alcohol effects on size were not detected at any follow-up after 8 months of age; and even at birth they were detectable only in the carefully stratified follow-up sample of 500 (Sampson *et al.*, 1994), *not* in the full population-based screening sample of 1529 (Streissguth *et al.*, 1994c). These paradoxical findings are congruent with many studies (including the large EUROMAC study: Forey & Taylor, 1992) showing that the prenatal effects of alcohol on birth size and subsequent child growth are variable, depending on the dose and timing of exposure measured, and on the constituency of the sample with respect to other causes of growth deficit. (Recall that the screening sample comprised mainly married, middle-class mothers at low risk for poor pregnancy outcome and all in prenatal care by midpregnancy.) Critical discussions and systematic reviews of the alcohol–birth weight relation have been published previously (Day, 1992; Kaminski, 1992; Little & Wendt, 1991; Sampson *et al.*, 1994; Streissguth *et al.*, 1994*c*; Zuckerman & Hingson, 1986). Birth weight clearly is multifactorial, and the effects of alcohol on birth weight are not as strong as the other effects of alcohol that we have detected in other domains of outcomes, particularly the neurobehavioral.

The facial dysmorphology characteristic of fetal alcohol exposure is engendered only at the very heaviest levels of prenatal alcohol exposure. Even so, in our study, it can be detected only in the infant and young child. An experienced dysmorphologist could characterize some newborns as FAE on the second day of life in blind examinations (Hanson *et al.*, 1978). Eighty percent of these were similarly classified by a different dysmorphologist, also conducting blind examinations, at 4 years of age (Graham *et al.*, 1988). Dysmorphic facial features characteristic of FAE were detected from facial photographs at 7 years only among the most highly exposed children (Clarren *et al.*, 1987). By age 14 years even this detection proved infeasible. These findings are consistent with studies of children with FAS, whose facial features are often less remarkable as they approach adolescence (Streissguth *et al.*, 1985, 1991; Spohr *et al.*, 1993). In the Seattle study, only the neurobehavioral outcomes, documented in this cohort since day 1 of life, have continued to show significant associations with prenatal alcohol up through 14 years of age (Streissguth *et al.*, 1993, 1994*a, d*).

Findings from our study are congruent with early studies such as those by Ouellette and colleagues (1977), Sander and colleagues (1977), and Scher and colleagues (1988), all of which demonstrated effects of prenatal alcohol exposure on newborn arousal. More recent research on older infants, using more sophisticated methods than ours, has replicated the small early developmental decrements we observed on the Bayley scales (Jacobson *et al.*, 1993*a*) and has expanded downward into the infancy period the finding of decrements on sensitive tasks involving speed of information processing (Jacobson *et al.*, 1993*b*).

Not all studies detect early neurobehavioral effects of prenatal alcohol (Ernhart *et al.*, 1985; Richardson *et al.*, 1989). Differences in outcome can be accounted for by differences in study design, success of follow-up, sensitivity of outcome measures, presence of other risk factors, and the like. In particular, studies that have attempted to use general scales of infant development (such as the Bayley scales) as the primary outcome for prenatal alcohol effects at later developmental ages have often met with disappointment. Like the EUROMAC study (Florey & Taylor, 1992), our Bayley examination at 18 months failed to reveal prenatal alcohol effects (Streissguth *et al.*, 1993). As we found many significant infant and child outcomes associated with prenatal alcohol both before and after 18 months of age, it may be that general developmental scales are simply not sensitive enough to capture the subtle CNS effects associated with more moderate levels of prenatal alcohol at this particular developmental age. Bayley scales at 27 months could detect prenatal alcohol effects in a much more heavily exposed group of children who were also dysmorphic (Autti-Rämö *et al.*, 1992*a*, *b*). Perhaps the variable emergence of language in 18-month-old children plays an important role in obscuring the alcohol-related deficits that seem to be measured reliably at other ages. Affirmations of the null hypothesis deriving from studies that terminate around 18 months or fail to use sensitive outcomes are certainly unwarranted. Readers wishing a fuller review of recent research in the arena of alcohol effects on human development may consult Coles (1992), Day (1992), Russell *et al.* (1991), and Streissguth *et al.* (1993).

Conclusion

At the levels of alcohol exposure reported in this longitudinal population-based study, the most reliably enduring effects of prenatal alcohol exposure are upon neurobehavioral function. These were detected at every age at which the cohort was examined (days 1 and 2, 8 months, and 4, 7, 11, and 14 years) except 18 months. Partial Least Squares (PLS) methods of data analysis have permitted consideration of multiple measures of alcohol dose and of multiple neurobehavioral outcomes. The results reported here are not attributable to such potential confounds as other teratogenic exposures, smoking, or social or demographic factors. Neurobehavioral effects of prenatal alcohol were observed from the first day of life through 14 years. These effects were dose-dependent, generally without a threshold, and, in the school-age years, more salient for binge-type drinking patterns. Self-reported drinking prior to pregnancy recognition is generally more salient for these outcomes than drinking in midpregnancy, but the two are highly correlated. Learning problems, particularly for arithmetic, were observed from 7 through 14 years, but problems with attention and speed of information processing were observable across the entire 14 year period.

To date, there is no method for directly quantifying the brain damage caused by alcohol and its relation to dysfunctional behavior in the individual affected child. (We are pursuing this direct quantification in other contexts.) The diagnostic category of 'FAS' is an insensitive guide to the extent of underlying brain pathology. People with FAS vary widely in many channels of behavior, and many other exposed offspring who fail to meet the criteria for an FAS diagnosis nevertheless show neurobehavioral deficits that may be as severe as those of FAS. Dose–response studies of these neurobehavioral profiles should lead to the development of tools for the proper identification of these children. Proper identification of the whole spectrum of alcohol-affected children should facilitate the delivery of appropriate services prior to the development of costly and debilitating secondary conditions (see Streissguth *et al.*, 1996*a*). The group of children formally diagnosed FAS is only the 'tip of the iceberg' of prenatal alcohol damage. In special programming, subtle neurobehavioral deficits, attendant psychosocial problems, lost productivity and so on, the net cost of prenatal alcohol exposure must be considerably more than the cost of FAS alone. Prevention efforts to reduce the impact of prenatal alcohol damage are clearly needed (see Streissguth *et al.*, 1996*b*).

There is no statistical evidence here of any 'risk-free' level of drinking or any 'threshold' level of prenatal alcohol exposure in the context of this dose–response analysis (see Streissguth *et al.*, 1993). Societal efforts in the United States to inform communities adequately have included: (1) a Surgeon General's warning on not drinking during pregnancy (DHSS, 1981); (2) Congressionally-mandated warning labels on containers of alcoholic beverages (United States Congress, 1988; Wagner, 1991); and (3) warning signs at point of purchase of all alcoholic beverages (stores, restaurants, and so forth) resulting from individual state and city laws and ordinances.

Acknowledgments

This research has been primarily supported by US Public Health Service grant no. AA0145501-20 from the National Institute of Alcohol Abuse and Alcoholism, with supplemental support from the University of Washington Alcoholism and Drug Abuse Institute, the University of Washington Biomedical Research Support Grant, the National Council on Alcoholism, and private contributions. The contributions of original Co-Investigators, Drs Joan C. and Donald C. Martin, and of Drs Paul D. Sampson, Ruth E. Little, Heather Carmichael Olson, Betty Darby, and Sterling K. Clarren, are gratefully acknowledged, as is the technical assistance of Pam J. Phipps, and Cara C. Ernst. We thank the children and families whose loyal support has made this study possible. This paper is an extension of earlier review papers from this study (Streissguth *et al.*, 1992; Carmichael Olson *et al.*, 1994; Streissguth *et al.*, 1994*b*).

References

Autti-Rämö, I., Gaily, E., Granström, M.-L. (1992*a*). Dysmorphic features in offspring of alcoholic mothers. *Archives of Diseases of Childhood*, **67**, 712–16.

Autti-Rämö, I., Korkman, M., Hilakivi-Clarke, L., Lehtonen, M., Halmesmäki, E. & Granström, M.L. (1992*b*). Mental development of 2-year-old children exposed to alcohol *in utero*. *Journal of Pediatrics*, **120**, 740–6.

Barr, H.M., Streissguth, A.P., Darby, B.L. & Sampson, P.D. (1990). Prenatal exposure to alcohol, caffeine, tobacco, and aspirin: effects on fine and gross motor performance in 4-year-old children. *Developmental Psychology*, **26**, 339–48.

Barr, H.M., Streissguth, A.P., Martin, D.C. & Herman, C.S. (1984). Infant size at 8 months of age: relationship to maternal use of alcohol, nicotine, and caffeine during pregnancy. *Pediatrics*, **74**, 336–41.

Bookstein, F.L., Sampson, P.D., Streissguth, A.P. & Barr, H.M. (1990). Measuring 'dose' and 'response' with multivariate data using partial least squares techniques. *Communications in Statistics*, **19**, 765–804.

Bookstein, F.L., Sampson, P., Streissguth, A.P. & Barr, H. (1996). Exploiting redundant measurement of dose and development outcome: new methods from the behavioral teratology of alcohol. *Developmental Psychology*, in press.

Cahalan, D., Cissin, I.H. & Crossley, H.M. (1969). *American Drinking Practices: A National Study of Drinking Behavior and Attitudes*. New Brunswick, NJ: Rutgers Center of Alcohol Studies Publications, Monograph no. 6.

Carmichael Olson, H., Sampson, P.D., Barr, H., Streissguth, A.P. & Bookstein, F.L. (1992). Prenatal exposure to alcohol and school problems in late childhood: a longitudinal prospective study. *Development and Psychopathology*, **4**, 341–59.

Carmichael Olson, H., Streissguth, A.P., Bookstein, F.L., Barr, H.M. & Sampson, P.D. (1994). Developmental research in behavioral teratology: effects of prenatal alcohol exposure on child development. In *Developmental Follow-up: Concepts, Domains, and Methods*, ed. S.L. Friedman & H.C. Haywood, pp. 67–112. Orlando, FL: Academic Press.

Clarren, S.K. (1986). Neuropathology in fetal alcohol syndrome. In *Alcohol and Brain Development*, ed. J.R. West, pp. 158–66. New York: Oxford University Press.

Clarren, S.K., Astley, S.J., Gunderson, V.M. & Spellman, D. (1992). Cognitive and behavioral deficits in nonhuman primates associated with very early embryonic binge exposures to ethanol. *Journal of Pediatrics*, **121**, 789–96.

Clarren, S.K., Sampson, P.D., Larsen, J., Donnell, D.J., Barr, H.M., Bookstein, F.L., Martin, D.C. & Streissguth, A.P. (1987). Facial effects of fetal alcohol exposure: assessment by photographs and morphometric analysis. *American Journal of Medical Genetics*, **26**, 651–66.

Coles, C.D. (1992). Prenatal alcohol exposure and human development. In *Development of the Central Nervous System: Effects of Alcohol and Opiates*, ed. M.W. Miller, pp. 9–36. New York: Wiley–Liss.

Day, N.L. (1992). Effects of prenatal alcohol exposure. In *Maternal Substance Abuse and the Developing Nervous System*, ed. I.S. Zagon & T.A. Slotkin, pp. 27–43. San Diego: Academic Press.

DHSS (1981). *Surgeon General's Advisory on Alcohol and Pregnancy*. FDA Drug Bulletin 11(2). Rockville, MD: Department of Health & Human Services.

Dumas, R.M. & Rabe, A. (1994). Augmented memory loss in aging mice after one embryonic exposure to alcohol. *Neurotoxicology and Teratology*, **16**, 605–12.

Ernhart, C.B., Wolf, A.W., Linn, P.L., Sokol, R.J., Kennard, M.J. & Filipovich, H.F. (1985). Alcohol-related birth defects: syndromal anomalies, intrauterine growth retardation, and neonatal behavioral assessment. *Alcoholism: Clinical and Experimental Research*, **9**, 447–53.

Florey, C.D. & Taylor, D. (project leaders) (1992). EUROMAC. A European concerted action: maternal alcohol consumption and its relation to the outcome of pregnancy and child development at 18 months. *International Journal of Epidemiology*, **21**, Suppl. **1**, S1–87.

Goodlett, C.R. & West, J.R. (1992). Fetal alcohol effects: rat model of alcohol exposure during the brain growth spurt. In *Maternal Substance Abuse and the Developing Nervous System*, ed. I.S. Zagon & T.A. Slotkin, pp. 45–75. San Diego: Academic Press.

Graham, J.M. Jr, Hanson, J.W., Darby, B.L., Barr, H.M. & Streissguth, A.P. (1988). Independent dysmorphology evaluations at birth and 4 years of age for children exposed to varying amounts of alcohol *in utero*. *Pediatrics*, **81**, 772–8.

Hanson, J.W., Streissguth, A.P. & Smith, D.W. (1978). The effects of moderate alcohol consumption during pregnancy on fetal growth and morphogenesis. *Journal of Pediatrics*, **92**, 457–60.

Jacobson, J.L., Jacobson, S.W., Sokol, R.J., Martier, S.S., Ager, J.W. & Kaplan-Estrin, M.G. (1993a). Teratogenic effects of alcohol on infant development. *Alcoholism: Clinical and Experimental Research*, **17**, 174–83.

Jacobson, S.W., Jacobson, J.L., Sokol, R.J., Martier, S.S. & Ager, J.W. (1993b). Prenatal alcohol exposure and infant information processing ability. *Child Development*, **64**, 1706–21.

Jones, K.L. & Smith, D.W. (1973). Recognition of the fetal alcohol syndrome in early infancy. *Lancet*, **ii**, 999–1001.

Jones, K.L., Smith, D.W., Streissguth, A.P. & Myrianthopoulos, N.C. (1974). Outcome in offspring of chronic alcoholic women. *Lancet*, **i**, 1076–8.

Jones, K.L., Smith, D.W., Ulleland, C.N. & Streissguth, A.P. (1973). Pattern of malformation in offspring of chronic alcoholic mothers. *Lancet*, **i**, 1267–71.

Kaminski, M. (1992). EUROMAC. A European concerted action: maternal alcohol consumption and its relation to the outcome of pregnancy and child development at 18 months. Relation of findings to other studies. *International Journal of Epidemiology*, **21** (Suppl. 1), S79–81.

Landesman-Dwyer, S., Keller, L.S. & Streissguth, A.P. (1978). Naturalistic observations of newborns: effects of maternal alcohol intake. *Alcoholism: Clinical and Experimental Research*, **2**, 171–7.

Lemoine, P., Harousseau, H., Borteyru, J.P. & Menuet, J.C. (1968). Les enfants de parents alcooliques: anomalies observées à propos de 127 cas. *Ouest Medical* (Paris), **21**, 476–82.

Little, R.E. & Wendt, J.K. (1991). The effects of maternal drinking in the reproductive period: an epidemiologic review. *Journal of Substance Abuse*, **3**, 187–204.

Marcus, J.C. (1987). Neurological findings in the fetal alcohol syndrome. *Neuropediatrics*, **18**, 158–60.

Martin, J.C., Martin, D.C., Lund, C.A. & Streissguth, A.P. (1977). Maternal alcohol ingestion and cigarette smoking and their effects on newborn conditioning. *Alcoholism: Clinical and Experimental Research*, **1**, 243–7.

Martin, D.C., Martin, J.C., Streissguth, A.P. & Lund, C.A. (1979). Sucking frequency and amplitude in newborns as a function of maternal drinking and smoking. In *Currents in Alcoholism*, vol. 5, ed. M. Galanter, pp. 359–66. New York: Grune & Stratton.

Ouellette, E.M., Rosett, H.L., Rosman, N.P. & Weiner, L. (1977). Adverse effects on offspring of maternal alcohol abuse during pregnancy. *New England Journal of Medicine*, **297**, 528–30.

Randall, C.L., Ekblad, J. & Anton, R.F. (1990). Perspectives on the pathophysiology of fetal alcohol syndrome. *Alcoholism: Clinical and Experimental Research*, **14**, 807–12.

Richardson, G.A., Day, N.L. & Taylor, P.M. (1989). The effect of prenatal alcohol, marijuana, and tobacco exposure on neonatal behavior. *Infant Behavior and Development*, **12**, 199–209.

Riley, E.P. (1990). The long-term behavioral effects of prenatal alcohol exposure in rats. *Alcoholism: Clinical and Experimental Research*, **14**, 670–3.

Russell, M. (1991). Clinical implications of recent research on the fetal alcohol syndrome. *Bulletin of the New York Academy of Medicine*, **67**, 207–22.

Russell, M., Czarnecki, D.M., Cowan, R., McPherson, E. & Mudar, P.J. (1991). Measures of maternal alcohol use as predictors of development in early childhood. *Alcoholism: Clinical and Experimental Research*, **15**, 991–1000.

Sampson, P.D., Bookstein, F.L., Barr, H.M. & Streissguth, A.P. (1994). Prenatal alcohol exposure, birthweight, and measures of child size from birth to age 14 years. *American Journal of Public Health*, **84**, 1421–8.

Sampson, P.D., Streissguth, A.P., Barr, H.M. & Bookstein, F.L. (1989). Neurobehavioral effects of prenatal alcohol. II. Partial Least Squares analysis. *Neurotoxicology and Teratology*, **11**, 477–91.

Sander, L.W., Snyder, P.A., Rosett, H.L., Lee, A., Gould, J.B. & Ouellette, E. (1977). Effects of alcohol intake during pregnancy on newborn state regulation: a progress report. *Alcoholism: Clinical and Experimental Research*, **1**, 233–41.

Schenker, S., Becker, H.C., Randall, C.L., Phillips, D.K., Baskin, G.S. & Henderson, G.I. (1990). Fetal alcohol syndrome: current status of pathogenesis. *Alcoholism: Clinical and Experimental Research*, **14**, 635–47.

Scher, M.S., Richardson, G.A., Coble, P.A., Day, N.L. & Stoffer, D.S. (1988). The effects of prenatal alcohol and marijuana exposure: disturbances in neonatal sleep cycling and arousal. *Pediatric Research*, **24**, 101–5.

Spohr, H.L., Willms, J. & Steinhausen, H.C. (1993). Prenatal alcohol exposure and long-term developmental consequences. *Lancet*, **341**, 907–10.

Stock, D.L., Streissguth, A.P. & Martin, D.C. (1985). Neonatal sucking as an outcome variable: comparison of quantitative and clinical assessments. *Early Human Development*, **10**, 273–8.

Streissguth, A.P., Aase, J.M., Clarren, S.K., Randels, S.P., LaDue, R.A. & Smith, D.F. (1991). Fetal alcohol syndrome in adolescents and adults. *JAMA*, **265**, 1961–7.

Streissguth, A.P., Barr, H.M., Carmichael Olson, H., Sampson, P.D., Bookstein, F.L. & Burgess, D.M. (1994a). Drinking during pregnancy decreases word attack and arithmetic scores on standardized tests: adolescent data from a population-based prospective study. *Alcoholism: Clinical and Experimental Research*, **18**, 248–54.

Streissguth, A.P., Barr, H.M. & Martin, D.C. (1982). Offspring effects and pregnancy complications related to self-reported maternal alcohol use. *Developmental Pharmacology and Therapeutics*, **5**, 21–32.

Streissguth, A.P., Barr, H.M. & Martin, D.C. (1983). Maternal alcohol use and neonatal habituation assessed with the Brazelton Scale. *Child Development*, **54**, 1109–18.

Streissguth, A.P., Barr, H.M. & Martin, D.C. (1984*a*). Alcohol exposure *in utero* and functional deficits in children during the first four years of life. In *Mechanisms of Alcohol Damage In Utero*, CIBA Foundation Symposium 105, pp. 176–96. London: Pitman.

Streissguth, A.P., Barr, H.M., Martin, D.C. & Herman, C.S. (1980). Effects of maternal alcohol, nicotine and caffeine use during pregnancy on infant mental and motor development at 8 months. *Alcoholism: Clinical and Experimental Research*, **4**, 152–64.

Streissguth, A.P., Barr, H.M. & Sampson, P.D. (1990). Moderate prenatal alcohol exposure: effects on child IQ and learning problems at age $7\frac{1}{2}$ years. *Alcoholism: Clinical and Experimental Research*, **14**, 662–9.

Streissguth, A.P., Barr, H.M. & Sampson, P.D. (1992). Alcohol use during pregnancy and child development: a longitudinal, prospective study of human behavioral teratology. In *Longitudinal Studies of Children at Psychological Risk: Cross-National Perspectives*, ed. C.W. Greenbaum & J.G. Auerbach, pp. 174–200. Norwood, NJ: Ablex.

Streissguth, A.P., Barr, H.M., Sampson, P.D. & Bookstein, F.L. (1994*b*). Prenatal alcohol and offspring development: the first fourteen years. *Drug and Alcohol Dependence*, **36**, 89–99.

Streissguth, A.P., Barr, H.M., Sampson, P.D., Bookstein, F.L. & Darby, B.L. (1989*a*). Neurobehavioral effects of prenatal alcohol. I. Research strategy. *Neurotoxicology and Teratology*, **11**, 461–76.

Streissguth, A.P., Barr, H.M., Sampson, P.D., Darby, B.L. & Martin, D.C. (1989*b*). IQ at age four in relation to maternal alcohol use and smoking during pregnancy. *Developmental Psychology*, **25**, 3–11.

Streissguth, A.P., Bookstein, F.L., Sampson, P.D. & Barr, H.M. (1995). Attention: prenatal alcohol and continuities of vigilance from 4 through 14 years. *Development and Psychopathology*, **7**, 419–46.

Streissguth, A.P., Bookstein, F.L., Sampson, P.D. & Barr, H.M. (1989*c*). Neurobehavioral effects of prenatal alcohol. III. PLS analyses of neuropsychologic tests. *Neurotoxicology and Teratology*, **11**, 493–507.

Streissguth, A.P., Bookstein, F.L., Sampson, P.D. & Barr, H.M. (1993). *The Enduring Effects of Prenatal Alcohol Exposure on Child Development, Birth Through 7 Years: A Partial Least Squares Solution*. Ann Arbor, MI: University of Michigan Press.

Streissguth, A.P., Clarren, S.K. & Jones, K.L. (1985). Natural history of the fetal alcohol syndrome: a ten-year follow-up of eleven patients. *Lancet*, **ii**, 85–91.

Streissguth, A.P., Grant, T.M. & Ernst, C.C. (1996*b*). Preventing fetal alcohol syndrome by working with high risk mothers and other strategies: the Seattle advocacy model. In *Proceedings of the 1994 NIAAA FAS Prevention Conference*.

Streissguth, A.P. & Giunta, C.T. (1992). Subject recruitment and retention for longitudinal research: practical considerations for a nonintervention model. In *Methodological Issues in Epidemiological, Prevention, and Treatment Research on Drug-exposed Women and Their Children*, ed. M.M. Kilbey & K. Asghar. National Institute on Drug Abuse Monograph no. 117. Rockville, MD: US Department of Health and Human Services.

Streissguth, A.P., Kopera-Frye, K. & Barr, H.M. (1996*a*). A preliminary report on primary and secondary disabilities in patients with fetal alcohol syndrome: why prevention is so needed. *Proceedings of the 1994 NIAAA FAS Prevention Conference*.

Streissguth, A.P., Martin, D.C., Barr, H.M., Sandman, B.M., Kirchner, G.L. & Darby, B.L. (1984*b*). Intrauterine alcohol and nicotine exposure: attention and reaction time in 4-year-old children. *Developmental Psychology*, **20**, 533–41.

Streissguth, A.P., Martin, D.C., Martin, J.C. & Barr, H.M. (1981). The Seattle longitudinal prospective study on alcohol and pregnancy. *Neurobehavioral Toxicology and Teratology*, **3**, 223–33.

Streissguth, A.P., Sampson, P.D., Barr, H.M., Bookstein, F.L. & Carmichael Olson, H. (1994*c*). The effects of prenatal exposure to alcohol and tobacco: contributions from the Seattle longitudinal prospective study and implications for public policy. In *Prenatal Exposure to Toxicants: Developmental Consequences*, ed. H.L. Needleman & D. Bellinger, pp. 148–83. Baltimore: Johns Hopkins University Press.

Streissguth, A.P., Sampson, P.D., Barr, H.M., Clarren, S.K. & Martin, D.C. (1986). Studying alcohol teratogenesis from the perspective of the fetal alcohol syndrome: methodological and statistical issues. *Annals of the New York Academy of Sciences*, **477**, 63–86.

Streissguth, A.P., Sampson, P.D., Carmichael Olson, H., Bookstein, F.L., Barr, H.M., Scott, M., Feldman, J. & Mirsky, A.F. (1994*d*). Maternal drinking during pregnancy: attention and short-term memory in 14-year-old offspring. A longitudinal prospective study. *Alcoholism: Clinical and Experimental Research*, **18**, 202–18.

Sulik, K.K., Johnson, M.C. & Webb, M.A. (1981). Fetal alcohol syndrome: embryogenesis in a mouse model. *Science*, **214**, 936–8.

United States Congress (1988). Public Law 100–690, 100th Cong. 2d sess. (Nov. 18, 1988). *Alcoholic Beverage Labeling Act of 1988*, 27 U.S.C. §213 et seq.

Wagner, E.N. (1991). The alcoholic beverages labeling act of 1988: a preemptive shield against fetal alcohol syndrome claims? *Journal of Legal Medicine*, **12**, 167–200.

West, J.R. (ed.) (1986). *Alcohol and Brain Development*. New York: Oxford University Press.

Wilson, J.G. (1977). Current status of teratology: general principles and mechanisms derived from animal studies. In *Handbook of Teratology*, vol. 1, ed. J.G. Wilson & F.C. Fraser, pp. 47–74. New York: Plenum Press.

Zuckerman, B.S. & Hingson, R. (1986). Alcohol consumption during pregnancy: a critical review. *Developmental Medicine and Child Neurology*, **28**, 649–54.

9

Effects of fetal alcohol exposure on early cognitive development

ILONA AUTTI-RÄMÖ AND MARJA-LIISA GRANSTRÖM

Introduction

Recognition of an association between fetal alcohol exposure and growth retardation, a particular pattern of minor and major malformations, and dysfunction of the central nervous system (CNS) (Jones *et al.*, 1973), has led to extensive clinical and animal studies. The clinically well-recognized fetal alcohol syndrome (FAS) (Rosett, 1980) has turned out to be just the tip of the iceberg. At least twice as frequently only two of the three agreed criteria for FAS (Rosett, 1980) are met, which justifies a diagnosis of fetal alcohol effects (FAE) (Clarren & Smith, 1978; Rosett, 1980). However, there seem to be many children with no diagnosis linked to fetal alcohol exposure who suffer a permanent impairment of their cognitive function despite normal growth and appearance (Autti-Rämö, 1993).

Previous chapters in this volume have discussed in detail the critical periods and doses of fetal alcohol exposure. Unlike most other organs, the CNS is sensitive to alcohol exposure throughout the prenatal period. With the CNS there seems to be a continuum of effects associated with both the duration and the degree of exposure: the longer the duration or the higher the peak concentrations, the more severe the cognitive impairment (Rosett *et al.*, 1983; Aronson *et al.*, 1984; Larsson *et al.*, 1985; Streissguth *et al.*, 1990, 1994; Olson *et al.*, 1992, Jacobson *et al.*, 1993). For any individual newborn child, however, it is still difficult to predict the degree of CNS deficiency even from objective information concerning the extent of fetal alcohol exposure. Genetic influences and other confounding factors that might interact with alcohol to affect brain development are still largely unknown.

The variety of clinical symptoms and the changing picture of impairment in psychomotor development as the CNS matures have made it difficult to define CNS symptoms specific to fetal alcohol exposure. Damage to the CNS during fetal development also leads to further abnormalities of postnatal brain maturation. Many infants exposed to alcohol prenatally have also been exposed to other factors such as prenatal maternal smoking, under-nutrition during pregnancy, or narcotics or benzodiazepines that can also adversely affect the developing CNS (Butler & Goldstein, 1973; Fogelman, 1980; Hingson *et al.*, 1982; Billing *et al.*, 1985; Fried & Watkinson, 1988; Laegreid *et al.*, 1992; Viggedal *et al.*, 1993; Griffith *et al.*, 1994). Early post-natal development can also be seriously affected by the unfavorable living conditions of such infants (Steinhausen *et al.*, 1984; Nordberg *et al.*, 1993).

There are three types of study on the association between prenatal alcohol exposure and outcome in offspring. Studies focusing on children with FAS/ FAE report clinical symptoms from just after birth to adulthood (Jones *et al.*, 1973; Hanson *et al.*, 1976; DeHaene *et al.*, 1977; Majewski, 1978; Streissguth *et al.*, 1978a, 1991a; Iosub *et al.*, 1981; Spohr & Steinhausen, 1984). Studies on children born to known alcoholics report the variety of symptoms seen in children who have been exposed to substantial amounts of alcohol (Olegård *et al.*, 1979; Kyllerman *et al.*, 1985; Aronson *et al.*, 1985). In the prospective studies the outcomes have been compared with either calculated mean amounts of alcohol consumed during pregnancy (Streissguth *et al.*, 1981, 1992) or duration of heavy alcohol exposure (Aronson *et al.*, 1984; Larsson *et al.*, 1985; Jacobson *et al.*, 1993). In this chapter we present the results of our own prospective follow-up study that was aimed at assessing the effects of the discontinuation of heavy drinking at various stages of pregnancy on the developmental outcome of the offspring.

Early cognitive development of children exposed prenatally to large quantities of alcohol for various durations

Subjects

In 1983 a special outpatient clinic for pregnant women with chronic alcohol abuse was opened at the University Central Hospital, Helsinki. During the following 3 years, 92 alcohol-abusing women were counselled at this depart-ment by the same obstetrician (Halmesmäki, 1988) at 2 to 4 week intervals. Detailed information on alcohol-induced fetal damage was given to the mothers and they were advised to abstain. In addition, special consultations by a social worker and psychiatrist were offered when needed. The alcohol consumption was calculated for each trimester separately and regarded as being moderate if it was 28–140 g per week or 110-630 g per month and as being heavy if it exceeded 140 g per week or 630 g per month. Of the 92

Table 9.1. *Social and educational level, form of the family, smoking and tranquillizer use during pregnancy, and the number of boys in the different groups*

	Group I (n = 29)	Group II (n = 27)	Group III (n = 26)
Maternal education			
1	4		2
2	1	7	1
3	5	3	6
4	18	17	17
Social class			
1	4	1	2
2	1	5	2
3	10	8	8
4	14	13	14
Single mother	15	11	8
Smoker d.p. > 10/day	14	15	12
Tranquillizer use	1	7	2
No. of boys	14	14	16

Maternal education: 1, university; 2, college; 3, vocational school; 4, elementary school.
Social class according to profession (father's when applicable): 1, leading profession; 2, senior clerical personnel, small business foreman; 3, junior, clerical personnel, skilled worker; 4, unskilled worker.
Group I, exposure to heavy alcohol during first trimester; group II, exposure to heavy alcohol during first and second trimester; group III, exposure to heavy alcohol throughout pregnancy.
d.p., during pregnancy.

newborns, 82 were reassessed at follow-up. The exposed children were divided into three groups according to the length of severe alcohol exposure: 29 of the children were exposed during the first trimester only (group I), 27 during first and second trimesters (group II), and 26 were exposed through-out pregnancy (group III).

The control groups represented low-risk, nonexposed children, and their developmental results were used when setting the acceptance limits for normal performance in Finnish children. In the original study design (Halmesmäki, 1988) the control group was not matched for the social class of the family, which limits the conclusions concerning the detrimental effects of heavy alcohol exposure during the first trimester only. The possible confounding variables of the exposed groups did not differ from each other (Table 9.1) and, thus, the main goal of our study could be achieved.

Procedures

The follow-up study consisted of five consecutive developmental assessments performed during the first 3 years. The children were examined at the mean ages of 4, 6, 12, 18 and 27 months (Fig. 9.1). The attrition rates were 68–73%.

During the first year of life, the children were examined by one of us (I.A.-R.) using a developmental assessment method based on Muenchener Funktionelle Entwicklungsdiagnostik (Hellbruegge *et al.*, 1978) that had been standardized for Finnish children. In this test the development of the child is assessed in seven or eight different areas; four of these assess motor abilities, and four cognitive abilities. Developmental age was assessed as being delayed in a particular area if the child did not pass the test items that 90% of Finnish children were able to pass at the same age (Autti-Rämö & Granström, 1991*a*). Motor development was assessed as being delayed if development was abnormal in at least two motor areas. Cognitive development was regarded as being delayed if performance in at least two cognitive areas was below that for the child's age. Psychomotor retardation was diagnosed if both motor and cognitive development were delayed.

At age 18–19 months the children were examined by one of us (I.A.-R.) using a developmental assessment test constructed and standardized for Finnish children in 1977. The test consists of fine motor, gross motor, and both objective and anamnestic language items (Autti-Rämö & Granström, 1991*b*). Fine motor and language scores were summed to determine the mental score. The test was developed for the screening of problems in early cognitive development and has a good predictive value for later IQ (Granström, 1982; Gaily *et al.*, 1990).

At the mean age of 27 months the children were examined by a psychologist and a speech therapist. The psychologist used the Bayley scales for

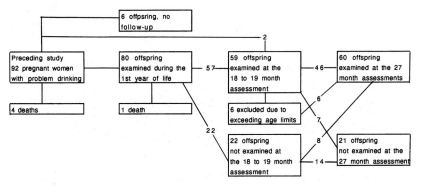

Fig. 9.1.   Participation of exposed children during various examinations.

infant development (Bayley, 1969) and the speech therapist used the Reynell verbal comprehension test (Reynell, 1977) – both widely used developmental tests. Scores of more than -2 SD below the mean for the nonexposed group's performance were considered subnormal.

Results of the longitudinal study

At the first examination at age 3–5.5 months the test was not sensitive enough to detect differences between the three groups. At the examination between 5.5 and 8 months of age the performance of the children was found to be significantly affected by increasing duration of prenatal alcohol exposure in relation to motor abilities in supine, sitting and grasping behavior (Fig. 9.2). Only by the age of 11–13 months did difficulties in comprehension and active speech become evident (Fig. 9.3).

At the age of 18–19 months the means of various developmental scores decreased as the duration of heavy alcohol exposure increased. The proportion of children falling into the abnormal range of the outcome variables was significantly larger in groups II and III. In Group I 9.5% of the children, in Group II 52.6% of the children, and in Group III 69.2% of the children had gross or fine motor difficulties. Delay in active or passive speech was observed in 23.3% of the group I children, 42.1% of the group II children and 38.5% of the group III children.

On the Bayley mental scale, at the mean age 27 months, the scores of the children in group III were significantly lower than those of the children in group I (Table 9.2) (Autti-Rämö *et al.*, 1992). Performance more than -2 SD below the mean of the nonexposed children was observed in 10% of

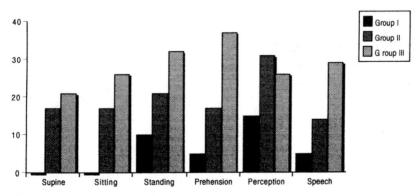

Fig. 9.2.   The percentages of 5.5- to 8-month-old children in the three exposure groups who performed poorly in various developmental areas.

Table 9.2. *Bayley mental scores transformed into SD scores relative to nonexposed children*

	Number	Mean	SEM	Range
Group I	20	−0.54	0.35	−4.9 to +2.4
Group II	20	−1.02	0.29	−4.4 to +0.7
Group III	20	−1.81	0.20	−3.4 to −0.5

ANOVA $F = 5.04$, $p = 0.0097$, I/III $p < 0.01$.

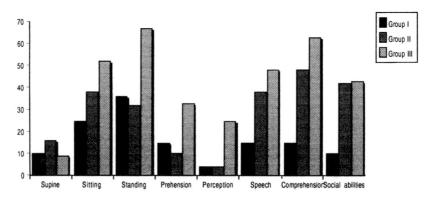

Fig. 9.3.   The percentages of 11- to 13-month-old children in the three exposure groups who performed poorly in various developmental areas.

group I children, 15% of group II children, and 45% of group III children (test for linear trend, $p = 0.0021$; chi-squared statistic, $p = 0.048$). Detailed study of the items of the Bayley test revealed that in group III visuomotor items were more difficult to overcome than language items (Korkman *et al.*, 1994). Among the children seen by a speech therapist the differences observed in the exposed children were also highly significant on the Reynell developmental language scale (Table 9.3) (Autti-Rämö *et al.*, 1992). None of the children of group I, 43.7% of the children of group II, and 52.6% of the children of group III had scores more than −2 SD below the mean scores of our nonexposed children (linear trend, $p = 0.0017$; chi-squared statistic, $p = 0.0034$).

In our study the number of children diagnosed as being delayed in development increased in all exposure groups during the first year of life (Autti-Rämö *et al.*, 1991*a*). Of all 81 infants examined during their first year of life, 23% in group I, 12% in group II, and 22% in group III were delayed in

Table 9.3. *Reynell mental scores transformed into SD scores relative to nonexposed children*

	Number	Mean	SEM	Range
Group I	15	0.67	0.27	−1.8 to +2.3
Group II	16	−1.26	0.45	−3.7 to +3.1
Group III	19	−2.28	0.42	−8.7 to −0.4

ANOVA $F=8.6$, $p=0.0007$, I/III $p<0.001$.

development at the mean age of 4 months. The corresponding figures at the age of 12 months were 40% in group I, 47% in group II, and 67% in group III. Psychomotor retardation was observed only in groups II and III. Forty percent of the children diagnosed as being normal at 12 months of age in the various groups later exhibited delay in language, fine motor, or motor development. In group I only 2 of the 6 children who exhibited motor or cognitive delay at 1 year of age showed delayed language development by the age of 27 months and 4 children performed within the normal range (Autti-Rämö, 1993). In groups II and III, however, cognitive delay at 1 year of age always predicted permanent cognitive impairment, and pure motor delay during the first year of life was followed by gross motor or fine motor difficulties, often associated with speech delay.

Altogether, 10 children were diagnosed as having FAS and 19 others as having FAE (Table 9.4). The diagnosis of FAS could be given in all cases during the first year of life and FAE in 13 of 19 cases. In 4 children the FAE diagnosis was first given at the 18 month assessment and in 2 children at the 27 month assessment. Nineteen children were diagnosed as having CNS dysfunction in the absence of growth failure or as manifesting facial features characteristic of FAS/FAE.

In group I one child was temporarily taken into custody. In group II 10 children (37%) and in group III 14 (54%) children needed intervention by child welfare authorities.

To test the effects of possible confounding variables on the Bayley scores the following background variables were forced into a model of linear regression analysis: social class at birth and at the time of assessment, maternal education, family structure, the child's having been taken into custody, smoking by the mother, gender, and duration of alcohol exposure. Only duration of alcohol exposure and social class of the family at the 27 month assessment remained in the model.

Table 9.4. *Presence of various criteria for FAS and final diagnosis by the age of 3 years*

| | No. | Criteria | | | | | Final diagnosis | | |
		Growth retardation	CNS impairment	Typical craniofacium	FAS	FAE	Pure CNS impairment	Pure growth retardation	Normal outcome
Group I	29	8	7	0	0	1	6	7	15
Group II	27	11	17	2	2	7	8	2	8
Group III	26	21	24	8	8	11	5	2	0

Discussion

Our study supports previous suggestions that fetal alcohol exposure causes a continuum of developmental defects ranging from mental retardation to slight difficulties in some areas of cognitive development. There is no typical picture of CNS dysfunction in young children who have been prenatally exposed to alcohol. During the first year of life the children were often hypotonic, exhibited abnormally high use of extensor tone, and were delayed in motor development. By the age of 1 year, early cognitive and social skills were affected. Children with mental retardation were all diagnosed by age 1 year. During the second year of life incidence of gross motor delay declined and fine motor difficulties, delay in verbal development, and other symptoms of impaired cognitive function became evident. Functional deficits vary with age as the CNS system matures, and it is difficult to find specific and sensitive tests for early childhood. Slight difficulties may easily be hidden behind the overly social behavior often observed in children who have been exposed to alcohol. The child often performs worse than expected in a test situation.

In our study with follow-up only during the first 3 years of life, no significant effect of heavy prenatal alcohol exposure restricted to the first trimester was found, with the exception of a high rate of poor articulation. Results from the Seattle prospective follow-up study (Streissguth *et al.*, 1990, 1994; Olson *et al.*, 1992) show a connection with moderate drinking and impaired performance at school age when higher cognitive abilities are tested. The preliminary results of our further follow-up also suggest that exposure only during the first trimester is connected with increased risk for later learning difficulties.

As expected from earlier studies, we saw a linear, declining relationship between the outcome scores and the duration of prenatal heavy alcohol exposure. Although the number of children performing under the acceptance limits did not differ significantly between those children exposed until the end of the second trimester and those exposed throughout pregnancy, the degree of cognitive delay was more severe if alcohol exposure was continuous. Restriction of alcohol consumption even as late as during the last trimester was of benefit to the child: every day of alcohol exposure decreases the potential of the developing fetus.

Poor social class of the family is known to be associated with poorer performance scores in older Finnish children (Gaily *et al.*, 1988, 1990; Lindahl *et al.*, 1988). In our study the social class of the family at the time of the last assessment had a significant effect on the developmental scores: at none of the assessments did the factors of social class of the family during pregnancy or maternal education have a significant effect on the outcome scores. The social class of the family had improved for 14 children by the child having been taken permanently into custody, and for 8 children by the improved employment status of their biological parents. Improved employment status may be a reflection of an increased ability to control drinking and thus better well-being of the whole family. Improving the living environment may prevent secondary impairment of developmental potential.

Although FAS is fairly easy to diagnose, FAE is not. There are no strict rules relating to how severe CNS dysfunction has to be for the CNS criterion to be fulfilled. The essential feature is that symptoms are associated with significant distress for the child and impair important areas of current or future functioning. Children with no marked somatic FAS/FAE traits but who manifest functionally disabling cognitive impairment may not be recognized as suffering from organic dysfunction caused by prenatal alcohol exposure. Developmental delay in early life may be so slight as to be considered within the range of normal, and true cognitive difficulties may go unnoticed until school age. The results of our studies clearly show that functional impairment tends to increase during childhood. Results of long-term follow-up studies on FAS children have seldom shown any significant improvement in cognitive development (Streissguth *et al.*, 1978*b*, 1985, 1991*b*; Spohr & Steinhausen, 1984; Spohr *et al.*, 1993). It is therefore very important for all children exposed prenatally to alcohol to be carefully followed up from infancy to school age. In examining young children who have been prenatally exposed to alcohol it is hazardous to rely on normal test results.

The most difficult situations we encountered during our study and in our clinical work were those in which a young child who was prenatally exposed to alcohol was taken into custody and placed in foster care or adopted. Future parents need information about the type, severity, and persistence of the cognitive problems and the rehabilitation that the child might need. Predicting the future of a very young child is, however, difficult. Results of previous studies suggest that the earlier a child is placed with a foster family the fewer the psychosocial problems that will occur (Aronson & Olegård, 1987). However, the success and permanence of early placement depends on health-care and social workers preparing foster parents adequately to face all the difficulties that prenatal exposure to alcohol may have caused.

The teratogenic effects of prenatal alcohol exposure on cognitive development are crucial to the child. The earlier they are recognized, the better can a child's future needs be assessed and attended to. In our study 58% of the children who were prenatally exposed to alcohol had signs of permanent impairment of their cognitive function before the age of 3 years. In general, mothers tend to overestimate the abilities of their children, and this is especially true in the case of mothers with drinking problems. It is important that only standardized tests with objective components are used in daily work. Only in this way can clinicians learn to recognize the wide variety of cognitive impairment in young children exposed prenatally to alcohol.

Acknowledgment

This study was supported by the Finnish Foundation for Alcohol Studies.

References

Aronson, M., Kyllerman, M., Sabel, K.-G., Sandin, B. & Olegård, R. (1985). Children of alcoholic mothers: developmental, perceptual and behavioural characteristics as compared to matched controls. *Acta Paediatrica Scandinavica*, **74**, 27–35.

Aronson, M. & Olegård, R. (1987). Children of alcoholic mothers. *Pediatrician*, **14**, 57–61.

Aronson, M., Olegård, R. & Sabel, K.-G. (1984). *Dynamics of Infant Growth and Development from Birth to 18 Months of Age in Relation to Maternal Alcohol Consumption During Pregnancy*. Reports from the Department of Applied Psychology, University of Gothenburg, vol. 9, no. 3.

Autti-Rämö, I. (1993). *The Outcome of Children Exposed to Alcohol In Utero: A prospective Follow-up Study During the First Three Years*. Thesis, University of Helsinki, Jyväskylä: Gummerus kirjapaino OY.

Autti-Rämö, I. & Granström, M.-L. (1991a). The psychomotor development during the first year of life of infants exposed to alcohol in various durations. *Neuropediatrics*, **22**, 59–64.

Autti-Rämö, I. & Granström, M.-L. (1991b). The effect of intrauterine alcohol exposition in various durations on early cognitive development. *Neuropediatrics*, **22**, 203–10.

Autti-Rämö, I., Korkman, M., Hilakivi-Clarke, L., Lehtonen, M., Halmesmäki, E. & Granström, M.-L. (1992). Mental development of 2-year-old children exposed to alcohol *in utero*. *Journal of Pediatrics*, **120**, 740–6.

Bayley, N. (1969). *Manual for the Bayley Scales of Infant Development*. New York: Psychological Corporation.

Billing, L., Eriksson, M., Steneroth, G. & Zetterström, R. (1985). Pre-school children of amphetamine-addicted mothers. *Acta Paediatrica Scandinavica*, **74**, 179–84.

Butler, N.R. & Goldstein, H. (1973). Smoking in pregnancy and subsequent child development. *British Medical Journal*, **iv**, 573–5.

Clarren, S.K. & Smith, D.W. (1978). The fetal alcohol syndrome. *New England Journal of Medicine*, **298**, 1063–7.

DeHaene, P., Samaille-Villette, C., Samaille, P.-P., Crepin, G., Walbaum, R., Deroubaix, P. & Blanc-Garin, A.P. (1977). Le syndrome d'alcoolisme fetal dans le nord de la France. *Revue de L'Alcoolisme*, **23**, 145–58.

Fogelman, K. (1980). Smoking in pregnancy and subsequent development of the child. *Child: Care, Health and Development*, **6**, 233–49.

Fried, P.A. & Watkinson, B. (1988). 12- and 24-month neurobehavioural follow-up of children prenatally exposed to marihuana, cigarettes and alcohol. *Neurotoxicology and Teratology*, **10**, 305–13.

Gaily, E., Kantola-Sorsa, E. & Granström, M.-L. (1988). Intelligence of children of epileptic mothers. *Journal of Pediatrics*, **113**, 677–84.

Gaily, E., Kantola-Sorsa, E. & Granström, M.-L. (1990). Specific cognitive dysfunction in children of epileptic mothers. *Developmental Medicine and Child Neurology*, **32**, 403–14.

Granström, M.-L. (1982). Development of the children of epileptic mothers: preliminary results from the prospective Helsinki study. In *Epilepsy, Pregnancy and the Child*, ed. D. Janz, M. Dam, A. Richens, L. Bossi & D. Schmidt. pp. 403–8. New York: Raven Press.

Griffith, D.R., Azuma, S.D. & Chasnoff, I.J. (1994). Three-year outcome of children exposed prenatally to drugs. *Journal of the American Academy of Child and Adolescent Psychiatry*, **33**, 20–7.

Halmesmäki, E. (1988). Alcohol counselling of 85 pregnant problem drinkers: effect on drinking and fetal outcome. *British Journal of Obstetrics and Gynaecology*, **95**, 243–7.

Hanson, J.W., Jones, K.L. & Smith, D.W. (1976). Fetal alcohol syndrome: experience with 41 patients. *JAMA*, **235**, 1458–60.

Hellbruegge, T., Lajosi, F., Menara, D., Schamberg, R. & Rautenstrauch, T. (eds.) (1978). *Muenchener Funktionelle Entwicklungsdiagnostik: Fortschritte der Sozialpädiatrie*. Munich: Urban and Schwarzenberg.

Hingson, A., Alpert, J.J., Day, N., Dooling, E., Kayne, H., Morelock, S., Oppenheimer, E. & Zuckerman, B. (1982). Effects of maternal drinking and marijuana use on fetal growth and development. *Pediatrics*, **70**, 539–46.

Iosub, S., Fuchs, M., Bingol, N. & Gromisch, D.S. (1981). Fetal alcohol syndrome revisited. *Pediatrics*, **68**, 475–9.

Jacobson, J.L., Jacobson, S.W., Sokol, R.J., Martier, S.S., Ager, J.W. & Kaplan-Estrin, M.G. (1993). Teratogenic effects of alcohol on infant development. *Alcoholism: Clinical and Experimental Research*, **17**, 174–83.

Jones, K.L., Smith, D.W., Ulleland, C.N. & Streissguth, A.P. (1973). Patterns of malformation in offspring of chronic alcoholic mothers. *Lancet*, **i**, 1267–71.

Korkman, M., Hilakivi-Clarke, L.A., Autti-Rämö, I., Fellman, V. & Granström, M.-L. (1994). Cognitive impairment at two years of age after prenatal alcohol exposure or perinatal asphyxia. *Neuropediatrics*, **25**, 101–5.

Kyllerman, M., Aronson, M., Sabel, K.-G., Karlberg, E., Sandin, B. & Olegård, R. (1985). Children of alcoholic mothers: growth and motor performance compared to matched controls. *Acta Paediatrica Scandinavica*, **74**, 20–6.

Laegreid, L., Hagberg, G. & Lundberg, A. (1992). Neurodevelopment in late infancy after prenatal exposure to benzodiazepines: a prospective study. *Neuropediatrics*, **23**, 60–7.

Larsson, G., Bohlin, A.-B. & Tunell, R. (1985). Prospective study of children exposed to variable amounts of alcohol *in utero*. *Archives of Disease in Childhood*, **60**, 316–21.

Lindahl, E., Michelsson, K., Helenius, M. & Parre, M. (1988). Neonatal risk factors and later neurodevelopmental disturbances. *Developmental Medicine and Child Neurology*, **30**, 571–89.

Majewski, F. (1978). Ueber Schädigende Einfluesse des Alkohols auf die Nachkommen, *Nervenarzt*, **49**, 410–16.

Nordberg, L., Rydelius, P.-A., & Zetterström, R. (1993). Children of alcoholic parents: health, growth, mental development and psychopathology until school age. *Acta Paediatrica Scandinavica Supplement*, **387**, 1–24.

Olegård, R., Sabel, K.-G., Aronson, M., Sandin, B., Johansson, P.R., Carlsson, C., Kyllerman, M., Iversen, K. & Hrbek, A. (1979). Effects on the child of alcohol abuse during pregnancy: retrospective and prospective studies. *Acta Paediatrica Scandinavica Supplement*, **275**, 112–21.

Olson, H.C., Sampson, P.D., Barr, H., Streissguth, A.P. & Bookstein, F.L. (1992). Prenatal exposure to alcohol and school problems in late childhood: a longitudinal prospective study. *Development and Psychopathology*, **4**, 341–59.

Reynell, J. (1977). *Manual for the Reynell Developmental Language Scales* (revised). Merseyside, UK: John Gardner.

Rosett, H.L. (1980). A clinical perspective of the fetal alcohol syndrome. *Alcoholism: Clinical and Experimental Research*, **4**, 119–22.

Rosett, H.L., Weiner, L., Lee, A., Zuckerman, B., Dooling, E. & Oppenheimer, E. (1983). Patterns of alcohol consumption and fetal development. *Obstetrics and Gynecology*, **61**, 539–46.

Spohr, H.-L. & Steinhausen, H.-C. (1984). Der Verlauf der Alkoholembryopathie. *Monatsschrift Kinderheilkunde*, **132**, 844–9.

Spohr, H.-L., Willms, J. & Steinhausen, H.-C. (1993). Prenatal alcohol exposure and long-term developmental consequences: a 10-year follow-up of 60 children with fetal alcohol syndrome. *Lancet*, **341**, 907–10.

Steinhausen, H.-C., Göbel, D. & Nestler, V. (1984). Psychopathology in the offspring of alcoholic parents. *Journal of the American Academy of Child and Adolescent Psychiatry*, **23**, 465–71.

Streissguth, A.P., Aase, J.M., Clarren, S.K., Randels, S.P., LaDue, R.A. & Smith, D.W. (1991*a*). Fetal alcohol syndrome in adolescents and adults. *JAMA*, **265**, 1961–7.

Streissguth, A.P., Barr, H.M., Olson, H.C., Sampson, P.D., Bookstein, F.L. & Burgess, D.M. (1994). Drinking during pregnancy decreases word attack and arithmetic scores on standardized tests: adolescent data from a population-based prospective study. *Alcoholism: Clinical and Experimental Research*, **18**, 248–54.

Streissguth, A.P., Barr, H.M. & Sampson, P.D. (1990). Moderate prenatal alcohol exposure: effects on child IQ and learning problems at age $7\frac{1}{2}$ years. *Alcoholism: Clinical and Experimental Research*, **14**, 662–9.

Streissguth, A.P., Barr, H.M. & Sampson, P.D. (1992). Alcohol use during pregnancy and child development: a longitudinal study of human behavioral teratology. In *Longitudinal Studies of Children of Psychological Risk: Cross-National Perspectives*, ed. C.W.Greenbaum & J.G. Auerbach, pp. 174–200. Norwood, NJ: Ablex.

Streissguth, A.P., Clarren, S.K. & Jones, K.L. (1985). Natural history of the fetal alcohol syndrome: a 10-year follow-up of eleven patients. *Lancet*, **ii**, 85–91.

Streissguth, A.P., Herman, C.S. & Smith, D.W. (1978*a*). Intelligence, behavior and dysmorphogenesis in the fetal alcohol syndrome: a report on 20 patients. *Journal of Pediatrics*, **92**, 363–7.

Streissguth, A.P., Herman, C.S. & Smith, D.W. (1978*b*). Stability of intelligence in the fetal alcohol syndrome: a preliminary report. *Alcoholism: Clinical and Experimental Research*, **2**, 165–70.

Streissguth, A.P., Martin, D.C., Martin, J.C. & Barr, H.M. (1981). The Seattle longitudinal prospective study on alcohol and pregnancy. *Neurobehavioural Toxicology and Teratology*, **2**, 223–33.

Streissguth, A.P., Randels, S.P. & Smith, D.F. (1991*b*). Test–retest study of intelligence in patients with fetal alcohol syndrome: implications for care. *Journal of the American Academy of Child and Adolescent Psychiatry*, **30**, 584–7.

Viggedal, G., Hagberg, B.S., Laegreid, L. & Aronson, M. (1993). Mental development in late infancy after prenatal exposure to benzodiazepines: a prospective study. *Journal of Child Psychology and Psychiatry*, **34**, 295–305.

10

The implications of attachment theory for the socioemotional development of children exposed to alcohol prenatally

MARY J. O'CONNOR

Introduction

The goal of this chapter is to describe how maternal alcohol abuse both prenatally and postnatally may contribute to the development of disturbed attachment relationships. To this end, attachment theory and research relating to individual differences in attachment security will be presented. An important aspect of this research focuses on the interaction of maternal behavior such as sensitivity and responsiveness and maternal psychopathology including depression and child maltreatment with child variables of temperament and biological risk. The relation between the early neurobehavioral sequelae of prenatal exposure and mother–infant interaction will be explored along with descriptions of the behavior of alcohol-abusing mothers and the possible impact of these behaviors on the development of attachment security. Finally, an attempt will be made to associate the characteristics seen in children of alcoholic parents with possible antecedent conditions arising from maladaptive attachment relationships.

Attachment theory

Research on infant socioemotional development in the last three decades has been directly influenced by the ethological-evolutionary theory of attachment first proposed by Bowlby ([1969] 1982, 1973, 1980). The attachment theory of Bowlby has its origins in several important trends in the behavioral sciences, including psychoanalytic theory, ethology, and neurophysiology. The major assumption of attachment theory is that attachment behaviors exhibited by the human infant are part of a species-specific behavioral system that operates to promote and maintain proximity to a primary caregiver, thus ensuring protection of the infant from danger. This behavioral system has developed through the process of evolution to ensure the survival of the species. Far from being a purely instinctual theory, Bowlby proposed that the constitutional predisposition of the infant present at birth becomes modified and elaborated through experience with the environment – particularly through social interaction with the primary caregiver. Among humans, therefore, infant–caregiver proximity depends not only on the ability of the infant to emit proximity-promoting signals but also on the complementary tendency of the caregiver to respond to these signals.

All attachment figures are not equally important in shaping personality. Bowlby proposed the term 'monotropy' to suggest the predisposition of infants to form one primary attachment relationship. This relationship, usually to the primary caregiver, develops before other attachments and remains more important. According to Bowlby, this caregiver is usually the mother but could be any primary attachment figure. Throughout this chapter, the words 'mother' and 'primary caregiver' will be used interchangeably to describe the primary attachment figure. This discussion, however, could include any primary figure such as the father, grandparent, etc.

Although it is common practice to speak of the mother's attachment to her infant, Bowlby reserves the term *attachment behavior* exclusively for the behavior of the infant toward the attachment figure. The behavior of the caregiver that is reciprocal to the attachment behavior of the infant is termed *caretaking behavior*. According to the ethological-attachment theorists, reciprocal infant and caregiver behaviors reflect evolved adaptations which form the basis for specific affective bonds between infant and caregiver on which feelings of basic trust, confidence, and security are formed.

Attachment is expressed in a system of attachment behaviors directed to the 'set goal' of maintaining optimal proximity to the attachment figure. Optimal proximity varies with the intensity of three other behavioral systems: affiliation, exploration, and fear/wariness (Bowlby, 1982). The interplay among these systems assures that the infant will seek the protection of the attachment figure when stressed and will explore the environment during periods of calm. The specific types of behaviors comprising the behavioral attachment system of the infant can be grouped into two main classes: signalling behaviors and approach behaviors. Signalling behaviors serve to attract and keep the caregiver close and include crying, smiling, babbling, calling, and gesturing. Approach behaviors bring the infant to the mother and allow for maintaining proximity. These include sucking, clinging, crawling, and walking. According to Bowlby, all the behaviors classified as part of the attachment system can serve other behavioral systems each with their own activators, terminators, predictable outcomes, and functions. It is only in certain situations, when the behaviors serve to promote and maintain proximity to the mother, that they are operating in the service of the attachment system.

In general, conditions that produce high states of arousal in the infant also activate the attachment behavioral system. Among the internal variables that may lead to activation are hunger, pain, cold, or illness. External environmental variables include the departure of an attachment figure, lack of response or rejection from such a figure, and unfamiliar situations or individuals.

It has been assumed that the nature of the child's relationship to the caregiver largely determines the attachment behavior exhibited toward her. Stress, such as that elicited by the presence of a strange adult, leads the infant to seek contact with the attachment figure. If the infant is secure with the caregiver, contact with her is comforting, and her mere presence allows the infant to explore the novel stranger, thus activating the exploration system. A child who is chronically anxious about the mother's accessibility and responsiveness will show greater fear of strangers than one who is securely attached, and will not be able to leave the mother to explore.

As Bowlby described it, attachment to the mother figure develops gradually during the first few years of life. The attachment relationship moves through four phases. In the initial or preattachment phase of development, shortly after birth, attachment behaviors are simply structured, almost reflexive in nature, and are readily elicited by stimuli provided by adult caregivers. Researchers have shown that infants are programmed to respond in specific ways to stimuli that are characteristic of human beings. For example, infants respond more strongly to sounds that are within the fundamental frequencies of the human voice (Eisenberg, 1965) and to visual stimuli that have the characteristics of the human face (Haith *et al.*, 1977).

During the first or preattachment phase, the baby is interested and responsive to all people. Infant behavior includes orientation to and gazing at people, tracking movements of the eyes, primitive grasping and reaching, smiling, and cessation of crying in response to the human voice or face. In addition, the infant can actively seek or maintain contact with the caregiver by sucking and molding when held. Bowlby suggested that these primitive behaviors become organized by a process of learning through interaction with the environment. It is during this phase that the infant begins to build expectations of how the human environment will respond. This phase terminates when the infant is capable of making discriminations among people, in particular in discriminating the mother from others, which usually occurs at around 8–12 weeks of age.

A second attachment-in-the-making phase is marked by the expansion of attachment behaviors which become more exclusively directed toward the primary attachment figure. This phase lasts about 6 months and is characterized by the infant's ability to discriminate among people. The infant begins to direct attachment behavior more toward the primary attachment figure who, in turn, is generally more successful than others in terminating attachment behavior such as crying. The baby's repertoire of attachment behaviors during this phase expands to include coordinated reaching.

The third phase, that of 'clear-cut attachment' (Ainsworth *et al.*, 1978), occurs some time during the second half of the first year of life and continues through the second and third years. Rather than relying heavily on signalling behavior to bring the primary caregiver into proximity, the toddler now actively approaches the caregiver by means of locomotion. The toddler extends the repertoire of responses to include following, greeting, and using the attachment figure as a secure base from which to explore. Other behaviors in the service of the attachment behavior system emerge, including holding on to and using language to call to the caregiver. In this phase, attachment can be viewed as a behavioral system that is normally at low intensity or activation. The system is activated when the child is separated from the caregiver or with the introduction of a stranger.

The final phase occurs during the third year of life when the caregiver is understood as an independent object who comes and goes and who is persistent in time and space. The essential feature of this phase is the lessening of egocentricity in the child. The toddler is now capable of recognizing another's point of view and is thus able to infer feelings and motives, goals, and plans to others in relation to self. Although Bowlby was specifically concerned with the attachment of a child to the primary attachment figure, the processes implicit in phase four were conceived as continuing throughout life and as being characteristic of mature attachments, which include figures other than the primary caregiver.

Basic to Bowlby's theory is that the infant's attachment is internalized as a set of enduring expectancies and self–other attributions that become a prototype for future relationships. Bowlby proposed that, during infancy, childhood, and adolescence, individuals gradually build working models or representations of the world and of themselves which then serve as the templates for interaction with others. These working models of self and world are based on the individual's experiences with attachment figures, giving the individual a sense of the accessibility and responsiveness of others and a sense of self as worthy and lovable. Attachment-relevant working models are not viewed as static but subject to revision based upon new experiences.

Nevertheless, Bowlby suggested that working models would demonstrate a degree of stability in part as a result of their being outside the realm of conscious introspection. Thus, a working model could function actually to exclude certain types of events from consciousness. Furthermore, the child's working model could also limit the child's accessibility to new opportunities for disconfirming experiences.

Main *et al.* (1985) extended Bowlby's notions to describe individual differences in attachment relationships as they related to individual differences in mental representation or working models. They defined internal models of attachment as 'a set of conscious and/or unconscious rules for the organization of information relevant to attachment and for obtaining or limiting access to . . . attachment-related experiences, feelings and ideations' (p.75). This reconceptualization of individual differences in attachment organization as individual differences in mental representation of the self allows for the investigation of attachment throughout the life span and for the study of attachment not only through overt action but through symbolic thought conveyed in language.

Main suggests that internal working models develop through generalized event representations (Main *et al.*, 1985). What is encoded by the individual is a generalized representation of events experienced, of actions, action outcomes, and associated affect. The infant–caregiver relationship will be based on the infant's actions, the infant–caregiver interactions, and the outcome of the infant's efforts to regain the caregiver in the caregiver's absence. Thus, the representation of the attachment relationship will reflect not an objective picture of the caregiver but rather a generalized event representation or history of all past interactions and intentions. The internal model of specific relationships may be formed in the first months of life, but by 1 year of age individual differences in the infant's response to separation and reunion will reflect individual differences in the infant's internal working model of the infant–caregiver relationship. These models provide rules for the direction of behavior, affective appraisal of experiences, attention and memory relevant to the attachment relationship. Although frequently unconscious, these rules are predicted to emerge in the organization of thought and language, a prediction central to the author's empirical work.

The strange situation paradigm

The empirical validation of attachment theory was made possible with the introduction of the 'strange situation', a paradigm designed to measure individual differences in the security of attachment on the basis of the infant's response to the mother during brief separations and reunions (Ainsworth *et al.*, 1978; Ainsworth & Wittig, 1969). Infants are generally tested at 12 months of age, an age when attachment behaviors are clear and easy to elicit.

The strange situation consists of eight episodes that each last approximately 3 minutes. The episodes are designed to be increasingly stressful for the infant, culminating in the most stressful episodes during which the infant is left alone. Specifically, the procedure begins with a period of direction to the mother and the introduction of the mother and infant to an unfamiliar room (episode 1). Next, the mother and infant are left alone so that the extent to which the parent is used as a secure base for exploration can be observed (episode 2). The mother and infant are then joined by a stranger (episode 3) in order to assess the infant's reaction to an unfamiliar adult and use of the parent as a haven of safety. The stranger then remains with the infant during the final separation from the mother (episode 4). Separation distress is assessed in this episode. Upon the mother's return, the stranger leaves the mother and infant alone (episode 5). During this episode, the quality of the reunion and the mother's ability to soothe the infant are observed. After the infant has recovered from the first separation, the mother again leaves the room, leaving the infant completely alone (episode 6). It is assumed that the infant will experience the most intense separation distress during this episode. In the next episode, the stranger returns (episode 7), attempts to soothe the infant, and remains with the infant until the mother enters (episode 8). The infant's reactions to the separations and, more importantly, to the reunions with the mother are thought to measure the degree to which the infant's working model of the mother provides him or her with feelings of security or trust.

Individual differences in infant responses to the situation allow for the classification of infants into one of three major attachment categories: secure (group B), insecure-avoidant (group A), or insecure-ambivalent/resistant (group C). Infants are classified as secure (group B) if they respond to the parent with a positive greeting upon reunion, if they settle easily if distressed and show little or no avoidance or resistance. Insecure-avoidant (group A) infants actively avoid the parent upon reunion and generally ignore the mother's overtures throughout the strange situation. Insecure-ambivalent/resistant (group C) infants show high levels of distress throughout the strange situation which are combined with weak-to-strong proximity seeking with mild-to-obvious resistance and an inability to be settled by the parent. This classification scheme was developed on, and has been used most extensively with, low-risk middle-class samples.

In spite of the success of the Ainsworth procedure and classification system, investigators have reported that some infants are unclassifiable – some
infants seemed insecure but could not be classified in any of the Ainsworth
categories. For other infants, the forced classification would have labelled
them secure or even very secure although independent assessments suggested
that these infants were, in fact, insecure with the parent. Furthermore, work
with maltreated infants and with other high-risk groups has resulted in difficulties in trying to force or impose the Ainsworth system of classification.
Some investigators have emphasized the qualities of apathy, disorganization,
or depression seen in these infants; others have described infants who avoid
and are ambivalent toward the parent; still others have described atypical
and even pathological behaviors such as brief 'catatonic-like' posturing
(Egeland & Sroufe, 1981; Gaensbauer & Harmon, 1982; O'Connor &
Masten, 1984; Crittenden, 1985).

After reviewing classification difficulties from other studies and viewing a
number of strange-situation videotapes of unclassifiable infants from the
Berkeley Social Development Project, Main and associates (Main &
Weston, 1982; Main *et al.*, 1985; Main & Solomon, 1986) developed a new
category of insecure attachment. Often an underlying, traditional category
remains evident, but infants representing this third category of insecurity are
characterized by their disorganized or disoriented behavior during the
reunion episodes. Under this new system, these infants are classified as
insecure-disorganized/disoriented (group D). Almost all the behavior of
these infants suggests conflict between behavioral systems and falls under
one of the following five headings: (*a*) disordering of expected temporal
sequences (i.e., greets parent brightly on reunion, then turns away);
(*b*) simultaneous display of contradictory behaviors (i.e., approaches parent,
head averted); (*c*) incomplete or undirected movements and expressions,
including stereotypic behavior; (*d*) direct indices of confusion, fearfulness,
or apprehension upon parent approach (i.e., hiding from parent, mixed or
changeable affect); and (*e*) behavioral stilling, dazed behavior, or indices of
depressed affect.

Although a forced classification may have resulted in some of these infants
being classified as secure, a review of studies of difficult-to-classify or group
D infants and of independent assessments of their attachment relationships,
suggests that these infants may be the least secure of the infants in the three
categories of insecurity. Main & Solomon (1986) also suggested that these
infants may have experienced the most extreme of family conditions, including maltreatment or depression in the mother. The majority of the infants
classified as disorganized/disoriented in the Berkeley sample had parents who

had suffered unusual trauma in their own attachment relationships and who continued to deal with their feelings of loss and rejection ineffectively.

Maternal–child characteristics and attachment

Hypotheses related to attachment theory are extremely compelling and with the provision of a paradigm to measure individual differences in infant attachment behavior, many investigators began to test the major tenets of the theory. Of particular interest was the relation between attachment and other variables of maternal personality and behavior, infant temperament and risk status, and specific transactional behaviors of the mother–infant dyad. The importance of studying early attachment derives from Bowlby's prediction that security of attachment is a source of continuity in development. For this reason, recent investigations have focused on stability of attachment classifications, behavioral sequelae associated with differences in attachment security, and working models of attachment derived from mother and child interviews.

Maternal behavior and personality

On the basis of observations that infant crying patterns were related to the mother's pattern of responsiveness to her infant, Ainsworth *et al.* (1978) predicted that the quality of infant attachment would depend upon the sensitivity of the caregiver to the infant's social signals. Implicit in this assumption was the belief that, although infant characteristics influence the mother–infant interaction, it is the mother's behavior that shapes the relationship. Mothers of secure infants were predicted to be more sensitive, more effective in soothing their infants, more positive and socially engaging in interaction, less intrusive and better able to respond to the infant's needs (Ainsworth, 1979; Ainsworth *et al.*, 1978; Main & Weston, 1982). Mothers of insecure-avoidant infants were believed to express more controlled anger and rejection of the infant, whereas mothers of insecure-ambivalent/resistant infants were described as insensitive and ineffective in their mothering.

Support for these predictions has come primarily from Ainsworth's original research group, although subsequent attempts to account for individual differences in attachment quality on the basis of global ratings of maternal sensitivity have also been successful (Ainsworth *et al.*, 1974; Egeland & Farber, 1984; Grossman *et al.*, 1985; Goldberg *et al.*, 1986; Smith & Pederson, 1988; Pederson *et al.*, 1990). The validity of the sensitivity construct has been further strengthened by the investigation of more specific maternal behavioral antecedents of attachment patterns. Mothers of secure infants have been shown to be more involved with their infants (Lyons-Ruth *et al.*, 1987); more responsive, elaborative, and appropriately stimulating in play (Blehar *et al.*, 1977; Egeland & Farber, 1984; O'Connor *et al.*, 1992); and more positive and less negative in their affective expression than mothers of insecure infants (Maslin & Bates, 1983; Lyons-Ruth *et al.*, 1987).

In contrast to the security that the child develops through sensitive maternal caregiving, maternal rejection has been investigated as playing a role in the development of insecure relationships (Main, 1981; Ainsworth, 1982). The mothers of avoidant infants have been shown to be more angry, irritable, and resentful, often opposing the infant's desires and being physically intrusive in their baby's activities. Furthermore, their verbalizations have been observed to be noncontingent and at a disproportionately high or overstimulating level (Isabella *et al.*, 1989; Isabella & Belsky, 1991).

Although less well understood, the behavior of mothers of insecure-resistant infants has been characterized as insensitive and inconsistent. These mothers have been found to be less involved with their infants, less responsive, and inconsistent in interaction (Crockenberg, 1981; Smith & Pederson, 1988; Isabella *et al.*, 1989; Isabella & Belsky, 1991). Such findings allow for the assumption that the resistant infant has developed a representational model of the mother as unavailable and unpredictable. This may lead to feelings of constant vigilance, anger, ambivalence and helplessness.

In a recent longitudinal study, Isabella (1993) focused on repeated naturalistic observations of infants at 1, 4, and 9 months of age, assessing attachment at 1 year. Results revealed that mothers of secure infants were more sensitively responsive at 1 and 4 months and less rejecting at 1 and 9 months than mothers of insecure infants. Mothers of insecure-avoidant infants were more rejecting at 9 months, whereas mothers of insecure-resistant infants were the least sensitive and most rejecting at 1 month. The mothers of resistant infants became less rejecting and the mothers of avoidant infants became more rejecting from 1 to 9 months. The author interpreted these results to mean that maternal sensitivity in the early months of life is particularly powerful in establishing later secure attachment relationships; that early experiences of rejection followed by a lessening in insensitivity might lead to incorporation in the infant's internal working model of the caregiver as unreliable (leading to insecure-resistant attachment); and that rejection experienced by the older infant would be likely to lead to conflict and avoidance as the mother's behaviors would be in more direct opposition to the infant's intentions (leading to insecure-avoidant attachment). A second important conclusion was that maternal behavior is not static but changes over time, possibly as a result of changes in the mother–infant transaction.

The effect of maternal personality in influencing infant attachment has not received much attention. In a study conducted in our laboratory (O'Connor & Sigman, 1993), we found that the mother's degree of extroversion and openness about family problems was related to infant attachment behavior. Mothers of secure infants admitted to significantly more family problems and described themselves as less introverted than mothers of insecure infants. In contrast, mothers of insecure infants evidenced more denial and increased introversion. These results are consistent with Main's (1987) speculations that mothers of insecure-avoidant infants often lack memory for childhood experiences and idealize their parents. Kobak (1987) has described these behaviors as defensive processes used by the mother in the avoidant effort to cut off negative affect. In contrast, mothers of secure infants demonstrate an ability to tolerate and integrate negative affective appraisals into organized responses. Our finding of more willingness to acknowledge family problems in mothers of secure infants may reflect less defensiveness concerning issues of rejection and dependency. This argument is particularly compelling when individual questions composing the family problems scale are reviewed. Most of the questions pertain to dimensions of acceptance–rejection and independence–overprotection, dimensions that have been shown to relate to adult attachment classifications (Kobak, 1987).

The finding that mothers of insecure infants exhibit more introversion is intriguing given that individuals scoring high on this scale are often described as conservative and self-deprecating (Dahlstrom *et al.*, 1982). Low scorers describe themselves as self-confident, independent, cheerful, adaptable, and affectionate. All these characteristics may be important for fostering security in the infant. Mothers who are comfortable and secure in their own relationships with others and who are reasonably self-confident may engender these qualities in their offspring; alternatively, mothers who are less outgoing and somewhat self-deprecating may have more trouble instilling feelings of security in their infants.

Maternal depression and child maltreatment

A continuum of parental risk exists that ranges from maternal personality problems, to deficits in judgment, to alterations in affect and impulse control. Two categories of severe parenting risk are mothers who are depressed or emotionally disturbed and mothers who neglect or maltreat their infants. There is increasing evidence that an affective disorder in the parent puts the young child at increased risk for developmental problems (Cytryn *et al.*, 1982; Sameroff & Seifer, 1983; Rolf *et al.*, 1984). In particular, insecure attachments have been shown to be more frequent in infants wth mothers suffering from severe depression or bipolar affective disorder (Radke-Yarrow *et al.*, 1985). In a study by Lyons-Ruth and associates (1986), several patterns of mother–child interaction were demonstrated and related to individual differences in chronicity, severity, and other risk factors in the mother. One pattern was characterized by flattened affect, reduced energy level, and social withdrawal. Another pattern was more overtly negative, and accompanied by hostility and interference. Yet another group of women could be characterized as labile and inconsistent. All these interactional patterns can impede the infant's sense of well-being, control, and security of attachment.

In a more recent intervention study, Lyons-Ruth *et al.* (1990) compared the infants of depressed and nondepressed mothers from low socioeconomic backgrounds. In this sample, they found that the negative effects of social risk status were significant in the untreated high-risk group as a whole, differing significantly both from the treated high-risk group and from the untreated community group. Untreated high-risk infants had a very high rate of insecure-disorganized attachment (60%) compared with the high-risk group receiving treatment (29%) and the community infants (28%). The generally favorable performance of the community infants was modified by the mother's depression status, leading to a significant difference between the treated infants of depressed mothers and all untreated infants of depressed mothers. Untreated infants of depressed mothers exhibited more than twice the rate of insecure-disorganized behavior exhibited by treated infants of depressed mothers (54% versus 22%). The positive social effect of intervention suggests that early intervention in the primary attachment relationship may modify later socioemotional adjustment in the child.

Maltreatment represents the most extreme breakdown in the parent–child relationship. In this relationship, the basic function of parenting, the protection of the child is compromised. It is logical then that maltreatment should lead to insecure attachment in the infant. There is evidence that parents who maltreat their children show deviant parental behavior and affect in many situations. Mothers who abuse their children have been shown to be extremely insensitive to them during infancy. These mothers interfere insensitively with their infants' goal-directed behavior and display more instances of covert hostility (Crittenden & Bonvillian, 1984; Lyons-Ruth *et al.*, 1987). Mothers who neglect their children often show decreased interaction, absence of affective expression, and decreased eye contact. Thus, the lives of maltreated infants are characterized by varieties of inconsistent care (Cicchetti & Rizley, 1981). As the previous discussion has shown, this type of care puts children at high risk for insecure attachment.

Confirming evidence comes from a study by Carlson and colleagues (1989) who found a preponderance of disorganized/disoriented attachments (82%) in a sample of maltreated 12-month-old infants. That maltreated infants should display such a high level of disorganized/disoriented attachment behavior may be due to the interjection of fear into the experience of caregiving. As Main & Hesse (1990) describe it, the concurrent activation of the fear/ wariness and attachment behavioral systems produces strong conflicting motivation to approach the caregiver for comfort and to retreat from her to safety. Proximity-seeking mixed with avoidance results as infants attempt to balance their conflicting approach and avoidance tendencies. Freezing, dazing, and stilling may be the result of overload causing approach and avoidance tendencies mutually to inhibit one another.

Cicchetti et al. (1990) have also suggested that the phenomenon of parent–child role reversal is another important link between child maltreatment and the insecure-disorganized/disoriented (group D) attachment pattern. A frequently observed characteristic of abused children is that they tend to be the sensitive/nurturing member of the mother–child dyad (Dean et al., 1986). This role reversal of caregiving behaviors has been observed in 6-year-olds classified as group D in the strange situation at 12 months (Main et al., 1985). The comorbidity of maltreatment and depression is only beginning to be understood and should have relevance to discussions of the parent–child relationship in alcohol-abusing mothers.

Infant temperament and biological risk status

Although attachment theory predicts that it is the mother's behavior that primarily determines the attachment relationship, a few studies have revealed that characteristics of the infant such as temperament and early biological vulnerability may also contribute (Field, 1977; Waters et al., 1980; Crockenberg, 1987; Goldsmith & Alansky, 1987; Lewis & Feiring, 1989; Wille, 1991; Ward et al., 1993). In a study of neonatal behavior, Waters and associates (1980) tested the hypothesis that some patterns of anxious attachment had antecendents in the infant's behavior and interactive abilities soon after birth. They found that, when compared with infants later classified as secure, insecure-avoidant infants scored lower on orientation, motor maturity, and state regulation at 7 days of age. These results suggested that early difficulties of the newborn may reflect problems in integrative and adaptive mechanisms which continue to influence behavior, interaction, and eventually attachment relationships, particularly if the environment is not equipped to deal sensitively with these difficulties.

Infant negative affect has also been shown to be predictive of later attachment outcome. Goldsmith & Alansky (1987), in a meta-analysis of 15 studies, demonstrated that infant proneness-to-distress predicted resistant attachment behavior. The strength of the association was low but was roughly comparable to measures of the influence of maternal behavior. In another study comparing dyads of extremely irritable infants and their mothers with dyads of nonirritable infants and mothers, van den Boom (1989) found that insecure-avoidant and insecure-resistant infants were similar in neonatal reactivity as indexed by irritability, and suggested that differences in their attachment behaviors were due to differences in maternal caretaking styles. In a recent study of distress reactivity, Calkins & Fox (1992) found that excessive crying on pacifier withdrawal at 2 days of age was related to insecure attachment at 14 months. Similarly, Crockenberg (1987) found that an increased likelihood of maternal insensitivity at 12 months was jointly determined by both negative maternal prenatal attitude and increased newborn irritability. However, infant insecurity of attachment resulted only if the mother also lacked adequate social support. Although the development of the mother–child relationship is complex, these studies suggest that it is likely that temperamental characteristics of the infant contribute to differential vulnerability to attachment disturbances.

In addition to risk associated with difficult infant temperament, biological vulnerability such as preterm birth or failure-to-thrive may predispose an infant to insecure attachments. In the early months, preterm infants tend to be less alert and responsive, show poorer motor coordination, are often irritable and drowsy, and may have an unusual cry (Field, 1977; Frodi *et al.*, 1978; Goldberg, 1978). As they mature, preterm infants are less likely to smile during interaction, and are more likely to show gaze aversion and to fuss. Although the research with regard to attachment behavior in preterm infants is equivocal, with some investigators finding detrimental effects (Wille, 1991) and others finding no effects (Goldberg *et al.*, 1986), degree of biological risk appears to be an important predictor of later attachment outcome. This conclusion extends to other biologically vulnerable infants such as those diagnosed with failure-to-thrive. In a recent study by Ward *et al.* (1993), infants with both organic and nonorganic failure-to-thrive were more likely to show anxious, disorganized attachments than normally growing controls. Furthermore, although maternal sensitivity and stressful social environments were related to infant outcome, there were no differences in patterns of attachment between organic and nonorganic groups. These results support the notion that disrupted parent–child relationships and stressful social environments are common in failure-to-thrive, regardless of the etiology of the growth failure.

Although child problems clearly interact with maternal problems to result in problems in the attachment relationship, a recent meta-analysis of 34 clinical studies on attachment found that maternal problems such as mental illness lead to more deviating attachment classification distributions than child problems (van IJzendoorn *et al.*, 1992). Results revealed that groups with a primary identification of maternal problems show attachment classification distributions highly divergent from the distributions of normal samples, whereas groups with a primary identification of child problems show distributions that are similar to normal distributions. Thus, in clinical samples, the authors concluded that the mother appears to play a more important role than the child in shaping the quality of the infant–mother attachment relationship.

Prenatal alcohol exposure and attachment

According to Coles & Platzman (1993), there are several models that can account for the effects of prenatal exposure to alcohol on the child. The *teratogenic model* explains negative consequences in terms of direct damage to the fetus during gestation. The *toxic model* assumes that the use of alcohol affects the mother physically which then leads to physical consequences to the infant. A third model, the *maternal functioning model*, attributes the outcome of the child to maternal characteristics such as personal habits, health, and caregiving competence. The *sociological model* assumes that effects result from social factors including access to prenatal care, social support, and socioeconomic status. The final or *interactive model* suggests that development results from the interaction of multiple factors including all aspects of the above models. It is this model that is most relevant to the understanding of the mother–child transaction and subsequent attachment relationship. For this reason, features of infants exposed to alcohol will be explored along with characteristics of maternal personality, social support, and child-rearing characteristics in this section.

At birth, there are signs of central nervous system (CNS) dysfunction in infants born to mothers who report consuming large quantities of alcohol during pregnancy. These include reports of jitteriness and tremulousness possibly associated with withdrawal syndrome (Coles *et al.*, 1984). Other neonatal effects include irritability, autonomic instability, increased respiratory rate, abnormal reflexes, hypotonia, less vigorous activity, slow habituation, low levels of arousal, increased levels of activity, motor immaturity, decreased sucking response, and disturbances in sleep patterns (Pierog *et al.*, 1977; Robe *et al.*, 1981; Streissguth *et al.*, 1983; Coles *et al.*, 1984, 1985). Frequently, high-pitched crying, disturbed sleep, and feeding difficulties develop following withdrawal symptoms and may persist for days or weeks (Coles & Platzman, 1993). In a study following alcohol-exposed neonates over the first few weeks of life, Coles *et al.* (1987*a*) found behavioral effects of poorer state control, motor tone, and reflexive behavior in the exposed group 28 days postpartum. Behavioral difficulties continue into the preschool period with deficits in cognitive functioning, sustained attention, emotional reactivity and independence, and an increase in activity level, rigidity, task absorption, and irritability (Landesman-Dwyer *et al.*, 1981; Steinhausen *et al.*, 1982; Morrow-Tlucuk & Ernhart, 1987).

The significance of these early neurobehavioral effects is apparent in the impact they may have on the mother–infant interaction. Investigators have shown that infant behavioral characteristics of irritability, poor state control, low responsiveness to social stimulation, poor sleep patterns, and crying all influence the mother–child relationship and may set the stage for future insecure attachment relationships (Meares *et al.*, 1982). Thus, the effects of alterations in infant behavior on infant attachment and patterns of mother–infant interaction may be the most significant result of prenatal exposure to alcohol (Hoegerman *et al.*, 1990).

In our own study of middle-class women who considered themselves social drinkers (O'Connor *et al.*, 1992), we investigated the relations between maternal alcohol use, mother–infant interaction, and infant attachment behavior using a causal modelling procedure. Our primary model was based on the research findings that maternal alcohol consumption is associated with infant irritability (Streissguth *et al.*, 1981) and that infants with difficult temperaments have been shown to have disturbances in the mother–infant relationship (Pianta *et al.*, 1989). Guided by this literature, we proposed that mothers reporting moderate to high levels of alcohol consumption during pregnancy would have infants who displayed more negative affect in interaction with their mothers. The mothers of these infants would demonstrate less optimal interaction with their infants and the mother–infant attachment patterns would appear to be less secure.

Two alternative models were also tested. The first proposed that alcohol consumption following pregnancy was directly related to the mother's interaction with the child, that the mother's interaction resulted in a negative affective response in the child, which then resulted in an insecure attachment relationship. This model put more focus on alcohol use as a moderator of interaction and less focus on the direct effects of prenatal alcohol exposure on the child's temperament. The last model tested the hypothesis that three independent and direct paths could be drawn between prenatal drinking and infant negative affect, maternal behavior, and attachment behavior, respectively. The last model was based on the possibility that alcohol consumption affected mother and infant variables independently.

The mother–child interaction and strange situation procedure were assessed when the infants were 1 year of age. The child measure was negative affect, which included whining, fussing, crying, screaming, frowning, and negative gestures such as throwing toys. Maternal behaviors were maternal elaboration of child's play and cognitive stimulation. Attachment classifications included the traditional Ainsworth categories and the insecure-disorganized/disoriented category.

Results were that this sample contained a high number of disorganized infants (32%) and that the mothers of these infants were the heaviest drinkers. Furthermore, we were able to confirm the validity of our first model as shown in Fig. 10.1. Alcohol consumption during pregnancy was positively related to infant negative affect; mothers who drank more had infants who displayed more negative affect in interaction. The mothers of negative infants were less elaborative and stimulating in interaction, and mothers who interacted less optimally with their infants had infants who displayed insecure attachment behavior. The two other models proposed in this study did not fit the data, although the concurrent drinking levels of sample mothers may

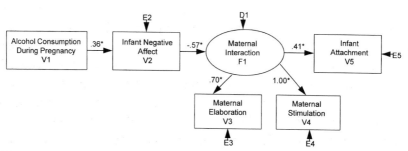

Fig. 10.1. Model for maternal alcohol use, infant affect, mother–infant interaction, and infant attachment behavior. Measured variables are V1 to V5. F1 represents the hypothesized construct of maternal interaction; E2–E5 represent errors or residuals in variables; and D1 represents disturbance or residuals in factor F1. One-way arrows are structural regression coefficients. Unidirectional arrows from E and D have fixed 1.0 values and one arrow from F1 to V4 is fixed at 1.0. $\overset{*}{p} \leqslant 0.05$, one-tailed test.

have been too low to reveal the true effects of heavy alcohol abuse on the mother–child relationship.

Studies investigating the characteristics of alcohol-abusing parents and their children are relevant for the prediction of attachment relationships and hypothesized long-term psychological effects. In a review of the interpersonal and emotional consequences of being a child of an alcoholic, Black and associates (1986) described characteristics that may be possible sequelae of early disturbances in the attachment relationship. Children of alcoholics are described as ignoring, withdrawing, and avoiding conflict. These children become self-reliant and unable to trust other people (Cork, 1979). According to Black (1979), children of alcoholics learn that other adults will not be available to them when they are in need of help. Thus, they grow up perceiving adults as uncaring and insensitive. Furthermore, parents are described as having inconsistent behavioral expectations, inconsistent physical and emotional care, inconsistent mood, as well as inconsistent responsiveness to communication and interaction (Beletisis & Brown, 1981). Problem areas cited with children of alcoholics are unresolved emotional bonds with the family, fear and denial of feelings, poor communication skills, role confusion, problems of identification, lack of trust and avoidance of intimacy, and assumption of excessive responsibility as children. Other outcomes include feelings of low self-esteem, anxiety, and depression, especially in daughters of female alcoholics (Giglio & Kaufman, 1990). Added to this list is difficulty developing close relationships, feelings of abandonment, and resistance to intervention and change (Kern, 1985). Furthermore, adult children of alcoholics report more physical and sexual abuse in the alcoholic home (Black *et al.*, 1986).

If one views attachment as a life-span task that requires continual coordination and integration as individuals adapt to their environment, one can see the importance of the mother–child relationship in negotiating this adaptation. Once an attachment develops, it continues to undergo transformations and reintegrations with each new developmental phase (Cichetti *et al.*, 1990). Research suggests possible links between insecure attachment in infancy and subsequent child behavior problems (Lewis *et al.*, 1984; Erickson *et al.*, 1985; Crowell & Feldman, 1988), thus highlighting the need to examine pathways to later maladaptation.

On the basis of the above descriptions of children of alcoholics and our current understanding of the significance of the attachment relationship, one can speculate as to how later child and adult psychopathology can begin with the early relationship between mother and child. In terms of the development of internal working models, the psychological unavailability of the mother for long periods can be seen as a powerful influence in shaping expectations that attachment figures are unavailable and that the child is unlovable. The recurrent 'loss' of the mother due to the effects of excessive drinking may be experienced by the child as recurrent separations. The psychological unavailability of the mother may lead to intense or chronic fear and feelings of insecurity. Just as the representation of sensitive mothering leads to secure attachments and subsequent feelings of trust and self-worth, the insensitive, sometimes hostile mothering of alcohol-abusing women may lead to feelings of low self-esteem, lack of trust, and depression in the offspring. Furthermore, the child's own biological vulnerability and behavioral instability often associated with prenatal alcohol exposure may further impede the development of a secure mother–infant relationship.

Recently, it has been established that women who are addicted to psychoactive drugs are likely to have a number of associated mental health and social problems (Coles & Platzman, 1993). Many women report histories of childhood physical and sexual abuse, and current abuse, and such histories are known to be associated with difficulties in parenting and an increased prevalence of abuse and neglect in offspring (Bays, 1990). Addicted women are often in situations characterized by high stress and low social support. Women who are socially isolated and addicted are likely to experience stress and depression during pregnancy and postpartum and may have a more difficult time in caring for their children. These children are at higher risk for abuse and neglect (Bays, 1990; Kelley, 1992) and for developing antisocial behavior and depression as early as the preschool period (Fitzgerald *et al.*, 1993). All these emotional and social aspects associated with maternal drinking conspire to weaken the maternal–infant bond.

Given the parallels between insensitive mothering and the behavior described in alcohol-abusing mothers, it is surprising that so few investigators have considered alcohol abuse as an important maternal variable to attachment outcome. Furthermore, given the compelling evidence that maternal affective illness and infant maltreatment relate to insecure attachment, and the high comorbidity between alcohol abuse and these maternal risk variables, it is imperative that alcohol be considered in any study on infant attachment in clinical populations.

This approach suggests fruitful directions for further research efforts in the analysis of infant behavior and environmental influences in relation to prenatal alcohol exposure. Furthermore, future research should focus on uncovering the processes and mechanisms linking insecure and secure attachment relationships to maternal substance abuse across the life span, thereby increasing our knowledge of the sequelae of alcohol abuse and the longitudinal effects of the early mother–infant bond. Through a better understanding of this rather complex developmental process, we may be better able to intervene before primary attachment relationships become disturbed. Early intervention had been found to have significant impact on the early development of infants at severe social risk due to poverty and maternal depression (Lyons-Ruth *et al.*, 1990). Similar strategies may encourage more adaptive social development in children exposed to alcohol prenatally.

References

Ainsworth, M.D.S. (1979). Attachment as related to mother–infant interaction. In *Advances in the study of Mother–Infant Interaction*, vol. 9, ed. J. Rosenblatt, R. Hinde, C. Beer & M. Bushel, pp. 1–51. New York: Academic Press.

Ainsworth, M.D.S. (1982). Attachment: retrospect and prospect. In *The Place of Attachment in Human Behavior*, ed. C.M. Parkes & J. Stevenson-Hinde, pp. 3–30. New York: Basic Books.

Ainsworth, M.D.S., Bell, S.M. & Stayton, D.J. (1974). Infant–mother attachment and social development: socialization as a product of reciprocal responsiveness to signals. In *The Integration of a Child into a Social World*, ed. M.P.M. Richards, pp. 99–135. London: Cambridge University Press.

Ainsworth, M.D.S., Blehar, M.C., Waters, E. & Wall, S. (1978). *Patterns of Attachment: A Psychological Study of the Strange Situation*. Hillsdale, NJ: Erlbaum.

Ainsworth, M.D.S. & Wittig, B.A. (1969). Attachment and exploratory behavior of one-year-olds in a strange situation. In *Determinants of Infant Behavior*, vol. 4, ed. B.M. Foss, pp. 113–36. London: Methuen.

Bays, J. (1990). Substance abuse and child abuse: the impact of addiction on the child. *Pediatric Clinics of North America*, **37**, 881–904.

Beletisis, S. & Brown, S. (1981). A developmental framework for understanding the adult children of alcoholics. *Focus on Women Journal of Addictions and Health*, **2**, 187–203.

Black, C. (1979). Children of alcoholics. *Alcohol Health and Research World*, **4**, 23–7.

Black, C., Bucky, S.F. & Wilder-Padilla, S. (1986). The interpersonal and emotional consequences of being an adult child of an alcoholic. *International Journal of the Addictions*, **21**, 213–31.

Blehar, M.C., Lieberman, A.F. & Ainsworth, M.D.S. (1977). Early face-to-face interaction and its relation to later infant–mother attachment. *Child Development*, **48**, 182–94.

Bowlby, J. (1982). *Attachment and Loss*, vol. 1, *Attachment*. New York: Basic Books (Originally published 1969).

Bowlby, J. (1973). *Attachment and Loss*, vol. 2, *Separation*. New York: Basic Books.

Bowlby, J. (1980). *Attachment and Loss*, vol. 3, *Loss, Sadness and Depression*. New York: Basic Books.

Calkins, S.D. & Fox, N.A. (1992). The relations among infant temperament, security of attachment, and behavioral inhibition at twenty-four months. *Child Development*, **63**, 1456–72.

Carlson, V., Cicchetti, D., Barnett, D. & Braunwold, K. (1989). Disorganized/disoriented attachment relationships in maltreated infants. *Developmental Psychology*, **25**, 525–31.

Cicchetti, D., Cummings, E.M., Greenberg, M.T. & Marvin, R.S. (1990). An organized perspective on attachment beyond infancy. In *Attachment in the Preschool Years: Theory, Research, and Intervention*, ed. M.T. Greenberg, D. Cicchetti & E.M. Cummings, pp. 3–49. Chicago: University of Chicago Press.

Cicchetti, D. & Rizley, R. (1981). Developmental perspectives on the etiology, intergenerational transmission, and sequelae of child maltreatment. *New Directions in Child Development*, **11**, 31–55.

Coles, C.D. & Platzman, K.A. (1993). Behavioral development in children prenatally exposed to drugs and alcohol. *International Journal of the Addictions*, **28**, 1393–433.

Coles, C.D., Smith, I.E. & Falek, A. (1987*a*). Persistence over the first month of neurobehavioral differences in infants exposed to alcohol prenatally. *Infant Behavior and Development*, **10**, 23–27.

Coles, C.D., Smith, I.E. & Falek, A. (1987*b*). Prenatal alcohol exposure and infant behavior: immediate effects and implications for later development. *Advances in Alcohol and Substance Abuse*, **6**, 87–104.

Coles, C.D., Smith, I.E., Fernhoff, P.M. & Falek, A. (1984). Neonatal alcohol withdrawal: characteristics in clinically normal, nondysmorphic infants. *Journal of Pediatrics*, **105**, 445–51.

Coles, C.D., Smith, I.E., Fernhoff, P.M. & Falek, A. (1985). Neonatal neurobehavioral characteristics as correlates of maternal alcohol use during gestation. *Alcoholism: Clinical and Experimental Research*, **9**, 454–60.

Cork, R.M. (1979). The forgotten children: a study of children with alcoholic parents. *Alcoholism: Clinical and Experimental Research*, **3**, 148–57.

Crittenden, P.M. (1985). Maltreated infants: vulnerability and resilience. *Journal of Child Psychology and Psychiatry*, **26**, 85–96.

Crittenden, P.M. & Bonvillian, J.D. (1984). The relationship between maternal risk status and maternal sensitivity. *American Journal of Orthopsychiatry*, **54**, 250–62.

Crockenberg, S.B. (1981). Infant irritability, mother responsiveness, and social support influences on the security of infant–mother attachment. *Child Development*, **52**, 857–65.

Crockenberg, S. (1987). Predictors and correlates of anger toward and punitive control of toddlers by adolescent mothers. *Child Development*, **58**, 964–75.

Crowell, J. & Feldman, S.S. (1988). Mothers' internal models of relationships and children's behavioral and developmental status: a study of mother-child interaction. *Child Development*, **59**, 1273–85.

Cytryn, L., McKnew, D.H., Bartko, J.J., Lamour, M. & Hamovitt, J. (1982). Offspring of patients with affective disorders. *Journal of the American Academy of Child Psychiatry*, **21**, 389–91.

Dahlstrom, W.G., Welsh, G.S. & Dahlstrom, L.E. (1982). *An MMPI Handbook*, vol. 1, *Clinical Interpretation*. Minneapolis, MN: University of Minnesota Press.

Dean, A.L., Malik, M.M., Richards, W. & Stringer, S.A. (1986). Effects of parental maltreatment on children's conceptions of interpersonal relationships. *Developmental Psychology*, **22**, 617–26.

Egeland, B. & Farber, E.A. (1984). Infant–mother attachment: factors related to its development and changes over time. *Child Development*, **55**, 753–71.

Egeland, B. & Sroufe, L.A. (1981). Attachment and early maltreatment. *Child Development*, **52**, 44–52.

Eisenberg, R.B. (1965). Auditory behavior in the human neonate. *Journal of Auditory Research*, **5**, 159–77.

Erickson, M.F., Sroufe, L.A. & Egeland, B. (1985). The relationship between quality of attachment and behavior problems in preschool in a high-risk sample. *Monographs of the Society for Research in Child Development*, **50**, 147–66.

Field, T.M. (1977). Effects of early separation, interactive deficits, and experimental manipulations on infant–mother face-to-face interaction. *Child Development*, **48**, 763–71.

Fitzgerald, H.E., Sullivan, L.A., Ham, H.P., Zucker, R.A., Bruckel, S., Schneider, S., Schneider, A.M. & Noll, R.B. (1993). Predictors of behavior problems in three-year-old sons of alcoholics: early evidence for the onset of risk. *Child Development*, **64**, 110–23.

Frodi, A.M., Lamb, M.E., Leavitt, L.A., Donovan, W.L., Neff, C. & Sherry, D. (1978). Fathers' and mothers' responses to the faces and cries of normal and premature infants. *Developmental Psychology*, **14**, 490–8.

Gaensbauer, T.J. & Harmon, R.J. (1982). Attachment behavior in abused/ neglected and premature infants: implications for the concept of attachment. In *The Attachment and Affiliative Systems*, ed. R.N. Emde & R.J. Harmon, pp. 245–79. New York: Plenum Press.

Giglio, J.J. & Kaufman, E. (1990). The relationship between child and adult psychopathology in children of alcoholics. *International Journal of the Addictions*, **25**, 263–90.

Goldberg, S. (1978). Prematurity: effects on parent–infant interaction. *Journal of Pediatric Psychology*, **3**, 137–44.

Goldberg, S., Perrotta, M., Minde, K. & Corter, C. (1986). Maternal behavior and attachment in low-birth-weight twins and singletons. *Child Development*, **57**, 34–46.

Goldsmith, H.H. & Alansky, J.A. (1987). Maternal and infant temperamental predictors of attachment: a meta-analytic review. *Journal of Consulting and Clinical Psychology*, **55**, 805–16.

Graham, J.M., Hanson, J.W., Darby, B.L., Barr, H.M. & Streissguth, A.P. (1988). Independent dysmorphology evaluations at birth and 4 years of age for children exposed to varying amounts of alcohol *in utero*. *Pediatrics*, **81**, 772–8.

Grossmann, K., Grossmann, K.E., Spangler, G., Suess, G. & Unzner, L. (1985). Maternal sensitivity and newborns' orientation responses as related to quality of attachment in northern Germany. *Monographs of the Society for Research in Child Development*, **50**, 233–56.

Haith, M.M., Bergman, T. & Moore, M.J. (1977). Eye contact and face scanning in early infancy. *Science*, **198**, 853–5.

Hoegerman, G., Wilson, C., Thurmond, E. & Schnoll, S. (1990). Drug-exposed neonates. *Western Journal of Medicine*, **152**, 559–64.

Isabella, R.A. (1993). Origins of attachment: maternal interactive behavior across the first year. *Child Development*, **64**, 605–21.

Isabella, R.A. & Belsky, J. (1991). Interactional synchrony and the origins of infant–mother attachment: a replication study. *Child Development*, **62**, 373–84.

Isabella, R.A., Belsky, J. & von Eye, A. (1989). The origins of infant–mother attachment: an examination of interactional synchrony during the infant's first year. *Developmental Psychology*, **25**, 12–21.

Jones, K.L. & Smith, D.W. (1973). Recognition of the fetal alcohol syndrome in early infancy. *Lancet*, **ii**, 999–1001.

Kelley, S.J. (1992). Parenting stress and child maltreatment in drug-exposed children. *Child Abuse and Neglect*, **16**, 317–28.

Kern, J.C. (1985). Management of children of alcoholics. In *Practical Approaches to Alcoholism Psychotherapy*, ed. S. Zimberg, J. Wallace & S.B. Blume. New York: Plenum Press.

Kobak, R.R. (1987). Attachment, affect regulation and defense. Paper presented at the biennial meeting of the Society for Research in Child Development, Baltimore.

Landesman-Dwyer, S., Ragozin, A.S. & Little, R. (1981). Behavioral correlates of prenatal alcohol exposure: a four-year follow-up study. *Neurobehavioral Toxicology and Teratology*, **3**, 187–93.

Lemoine, P., Harousseau, H., Borteyru, J.P. & Menuet, J.C. (1968). Les enfants de parents alcooliques: anomalies observées. *Ouest Medicale*, **25**, 476–82.

Lewis, M. & Feiring, C. (1989). Infant, mother, and mother–infant interaction behavior and subsequent attachment. *Child Development*, **60**, 831–7.

Lewis, M., Feiring, C., McGuffog, C. & Jaskir, J. (1984). Predicting psychopathology in six-year-olds from early social relations. *Child Development*, **48**, 1277–87.

Lyons-Ruth, K., Connell, D.B., Grunebaum, H.U. & Botein, S. (1990). Infants at social risk: maternal depression and family support services as mediators of infant development and security of attachment. *Child Development*, **61**, 85–98.

Lyons-Ruth, K., Connell, D.B., Zoll, D. & Stahl, J. (1987). Infants at social risk: relations among infant maltreatment, maternal behavior, and infant attachment behavior. *Developmental Psychology*, **23**, 223–32.

Lyons-Ruth, K., Zoll, D., Connell, D. & Grunebaum, H.E. (1986). The depressed mother and her one-year-old infant: environment, interaction, attachment and infant development. In *Maternal Depression and Infant Disturbance*, ed. E. Tronick & T. Field, pp. 61–82. San Francisco: Jossey-Bass.

Main, M. (1981). Avoidance in the service of attachment: a working paper. In *Behavioral Development*, ed. K. Immelman, G. Barlow, L. Petrinovich & M. Main, pp. 651–93. Cambridge: Cambridge University Press.

Main, M. (1987). Some perceptual and cognitive mechanisms acting to permit the maintenance of avoidance. Paper presented at the biennial meeting of the Society for Research in Child Development, Baltimore.

Main, M. & Hesse, E. (1990). Parents' unresolved traumatic experiences are related to infant disorganized attachment status. Is frightened and/or frightening prenatal behavior the linking mechanism? In *Attachment in the Preschool Years: Theory, Research, and Intervention*, ed. M.T. Greenberg, D. Cicchetti & E.M. Cummings, pp. 161–84. Chicago: University of Chicago Press.

Main, M., Kaplan, N. & Cassidy, J. (1985). Security in infancy, childhood and adulthood: a move to the level of representation. *Monographs of the Society for Research in Child Development*, **50**, 66–104.

Main, M. & Solomon, J. (1986). Discovery of an insecure disorganized/disoriented attachment pattern: procedures, findings and implications for the classification of behavior. In *Affective Development in Infancy*, ed. M. Yogman & T.B. Brazelton, pp. 95–124. Norwood, NJ: Ablex.

Main, M. & Weston, D.R. (1982). Avoidance of the attachment figure in infancy: descriptions and interpretations. In *The Place of Attachment in Human Behavior*, ed. C.M. Parkes & J. Stevenson-Hinde, pp. 31–59. New York: Basic Books.

Maslin, C.A. & Bates, J.E. (1983). Precursors of anxious and secure attachments: A multivariate model at age 6 months. Unpublished manuscript.

Meares, R., Penman, R., Milgrom-Friedman, J. & Baker, K. (1982). Some origins of the 'difficult' child: the Brazelton scale and the mother's view of her newborn's character. *British Journal of Medical Psychology*, **55**, 77–86.

Morrow-Tlucuk, M. & Ernhart, C.B. (1987). Maternal prenatal substance use and behavior at age 3 years. *Alcoholism: Clinical and Experimental Research*, **11**, 213A.

O'Connor, M.J. & Masten, A. (1984). Use of the strange-situation procedure in the diagnosis of attachment disorder. *Child Psychiatry and Human Development*, **15**, 64–71.

O'Connor, M.J. & Sigman, M. (1993). Maternal personality and insecure attachment. Unpublished manuscript.

O'Connor, M.J., Sigman, M. & Kasari, C. (1992). Attachment behavior of infants exposed prenatally to alcohol: mediating effects of infant affect and mother–infant interaction. *Development and Psychopathology*, **4**, 243–56.

Pederson, D.R., Moran, G., Sitko, C., Campbell, K., Ghesquire, K. & Acton, H. (1990). Maternal sensitivity and the security of infant–mother attachment: a Q-sort study. *Child Development*, **61**, 1974–83.

Pianta, R.C., Sroufe, L.A. & Egeland, B. (1989). Continuity and discontinuity in maternal sensitivity at 6, 24, and 42 months in a high risk sample. *Child Development*, **60**, 481–7.

Pierog, S., Chandavasu, O. & Wexler, I. (1977). Withdrawal symptoms in infants with fetal alcohol syndrome. *Journal of Pediatrics*, **90**, 630–3.

Radke-Yarrow, M., Cummings, E.M., Kuczynski, L. & Chapman, M. (1985). Patterns of attachment in two- and three-year-olds in normal families and families wth parental depression. *Child Development*, **56**, 591–615.

Robe, L.B., Gromisch, D.S. & Iosub, S. (1981). Symptoms of neonatal ethanol withdrawal. *Currents of Alcoholism*, **8**, 485–93.

Rolf, J.E., Crowther, J., Teri, L. & Bond, L. (1984). Contrasting developmental risks in preschool children of psychiatrically hospitalized parents. In *Children at Risk for Schizophrenia: A Longitudinal Perspective*, ed. N.F. Wyatt, E.J. Anthony, L.C. Wynne & J.E. Rolf, pp. 23–31. Cambridge: Cambridge University Press.

Sameroff, A.V. & Seifer, R. (1983). Familial risk and child competence. *Child Development*, **54**, 1254–68.

Smith, P.B. & Pederson, D.R. (1988). Maternal sensitivity and patterns of infant–mother attachment. *Child Development*, **59**, 1097–101.

Spieker, S.J. & Booth, C. (1985). Family risk typologies and patterns of insecure attachment. In 'Intervention with Infants at Risk: Patterns of Attachment', chair J.O. Osofsky. Symposium conducted at the meeting of the Society for Research in Child Development, Toronto, Ontario, Canada.

Steinhausen, H., Nestler, V. & Huth, H. (1982). Psychopathology and mental functions in the offspring of alcoholic and epileptic mothers. *Journal of the American Academy of Child Psychiatry*, **21**, 268–73.

Streissguth, A.P., Barr, H.M. & Martin, D.C. (1983). Maternal alcohol use and neonatal habituation assessed with the Brazelton scale. *Child Development*, **54**, 1109–18.

Streissguth, A.P., Martin, D.C., Martin, J. & Barr, H. (1981). The Seattle longitudinal prospective study on alcohol and pregnancy. *Neurobehavioral Toxicology and Teratology*, **3**, 223–33.

van den Boom, D. (1989). Neonatal irritability and the development of attachment. In *Temperament in Childhood*, ed. G. Kohnstamm, J. Bates & M.K. Rothbarb, pp. 299–318. New York: Wiley.

van IJzendoorn, M.H., Goldberg, S., Kroonenberg, P.M. & Frenkel, O.J. (1992). The relative effects of maternal and child problems on the quality of attachment: a meta-analysis of attachment in clinical samples. *Child Development*, **63**, 840–58.

Ward, M.J., Kessler, D.B. & Altman, S.C. (1993). Infant–mother attachment in children with failure to thrive. *Infant Mental Health Journal*, **14**, 208–20.

Waters, E., Vaughn, B. & Egeland, B. (1980). Individual differences in infant–mother attachment relationships at age one: antecedents in neonatal behavior in an economically disadvantaged sample. *Child Development*, **51**, 208–16.

Wille, D.E. (1991). Relation of preterm birth with quality of infant–mother attachment. *Infant Behavior and Development*, **14**, 227–40.

11

Fetal alcohol syndrome in adolescence: long-term perspective of children diagnosed in infancy

HANS-LUDWIG SPOHR

Introduction

Following the first European descriptions of the adverse effects on children of maternal alcohol addiction in France by Lamache (1967) and Lemoine *et al.* (1968), Jones & Smith (1973) in Seattle described fetal alcohol syndrome (FAS) as one of the most dangerous and, until then, unknown sources of developmental disorders in children born to chronic alcoholic women. The 'discovery' of the new syndrome initiated intensive research activity in all industrialized countries of the Western world, and within 20 years several thousand scientific communications dealing with FAS and other alcohol-related birth defects (ARBD) had been published, confirming that alcohol is a teratogenic drug capable of producing persisting and possibly lifelong disabilities after intrauterine exposure. Today, FAS together with trisomy 21 and spina bifida is recognized as the leading known cause of congenital mental retardation in the United States and Europe and is the only one that is 100% preventable.

A previous chapter (Streissguth, this volume) has dealt with the effects of moderate maternal alcohol consumption on child development. In contrast to the extensive research on moderate alcohol drinking during pregnancy there is still limited knowledge about the long-term developmental and adolescent outcome of children diagnosed at birth or in early childhood as having FAS. This chapter reviews the literature on FAS from a historical perspective. It starts with the first clinical reports, describes the findings of several long-term follow-up studies, and presents our own findings of the characteristic features of adolescent and young adult patients who were diagnosed with FAS in early infancy.

Early clinical reports

Jones & Smith (1973) described a distinct and visually recognizable pattern of abnormal morphogenesis and central nervous system (CNS) dysfunction in 11 children whose mothers were chronic alcoholics, for which they introduced the term 'fetal alcohol syndrome' (FAS). The syndrome is characterized by physical malformations, especially of the face (i.e., short palpebral fissures, flat midface, short nose, indistinct long philtrum, thin upper lip), stunted growth, microcephaly, delayed psychomotor maturation, and impaired intellectual development.

Although the syndrome was identified some years earlier in France, it was the first description of the syndrome in the United States in 1973 that stimulated the identification in other countries of children who were damaged *in utero* due to chronic maternal alcoholism. Only 3 years later, Hanson *et al.* (1976) had collected 41 patients with FAS, and in the same year Majewski and coworkers (1976) published a clinical report of 68 cases from southern Germany. Majewski introduced the term alcohol embryopathy (AE) into the literature, a term that is still frequently used in Germany today. The term 'embryopathy' refers to a greater extent to the teratogenic cause of alcohol damage *in utero* in contrast to the more common genetic etiology of most 'syndromes'. These first reports were supplemented by studies from France (Dehaene *et al.*, 1977; Kaminski *et al.*, 1978) as well as from Sweden (Olegard *et al.*, 1979; Kyllerman *et al.*, 1979), and the syndrome was also identified in Japan (Tanaka *et al.*, 1981). These early studies in the 1970s were focused on patients with FAS who were usually very young infants. The affected children showed great individual variations in both the extent and severity of the syndrome, but the spectrum of abnormalities in these young patients included most of the classical major and minor symptoms of FAS as described previously by Jones & Smith (1973). And because microcephaly and persistent psychomotor and developmental retardation were the major sequelae in many patients, FAS was soon recognized as one of the leading and preventable causes of congenital mental retardation with a known etiology.

Because this knowledge about the hazards of maternal alcohol abuse during pregnancy shocked the public in the United States, the issue was discussed intensively, which led to an official government warning by the Surgeon General against drinking alcoholic beverages during pregnancy (Public Health Service, 1981). In contrast to European countries or any other country of the Western world, the labelling of alcoholic beverage containers with a warning about the risks of birth defects associated with drinking alcohol during pregnancy became public law with the US Alcohol Beverage Labeling Act of 1988.

The early case reports usually described affected children with a full-blown syndrome as the most severe form of damage occurring *in utero*. Within only a few years FAS became a well-known syndrome among many pediatricians and it was quite a popular diagnosis for a while: 'peculiar looking' children who had alcohol problems in their families ran the risk of being diagnosed as having FAS at that time.

Many clinicians working with children exposed to alcohol during pregnancy appreciated the possibility of recording varying degrees of severity in the affected patients. Full-blown FAS became recognized as being located on the far end of a continuum of effects, and general agreement existed about FAS as a diagnostic entity in young infants and preadolescent children. In contrast, classification of the milder effects in alcohol-damaged children during pregnancy has been far from systematic.

Majewski *et al.* (1976) developed a clinical classification involving three levels of severity of FAS based on a weighted pediatric scoring system with quantitative cut-offs. Olegard *et al.* (1979) used the term 'partial FAS' to describe milder affected cases. Smith (1982) for the first time introduced the term 'fetal alcohol effects' (FAE) to cover the whole spectrum of recognizable effects on the offspring that are associated with maternal alcohol abuse, and Dehaene and colleagues (1977) also used a classification of 'severely to mildly affected children.' Clarren & Smith (1978) recommended using the term 'possible fetal alcohol effects' in the differential diagnosis between typical FAS and those affected children where 'the cluster of symptoms was inadequate for a definite syndrome identification'. A clear definition was lacking.

With those early reports it became evident that intrauterine alcohol damage and the impact of alcohol on the offspring are not restricted to FAS. The syndrome is only the most extreme variant of a whole spectrum of physical symptoms to be diagnosed in exposed children. The phenotype depends on, among other factors, variations in dose, timing of exposure in pregnancy, maternal metabolism, fetal susceptibility, and individual fetal resistance.

In syndromes of this kind no phenotype is ever exclusively related to a single etiology. Although children with an FAS phenotype and no history of intrauterine alcohol exposure may sometimes have been identified, the specificity of the FAS phenotype for alcohol teratogenesis is remarkably constant. Lacking other diagnostic possibilities, it was very helpful to reach an agreement on a standardized clinical definition by the Fetal Alcohol Study Group of the Research Society on Alcoholism (RSA), first published in 1980 by Rosett. As a consequence, the terms fetal alcohol syndrome (FAS) and fetal alcohol effects (FAE) as defined by Sokol & Clarren (1989) are now generally accepted.

According to this definition, a diagnosis of FAS is made when there is confirmation of a history of maternal alcohol abuse and when clinical examination reveals that a child meets the following three criteria: (1) prenatal or postnatal growth retardation, (2) CNS dysfunction, and (3) characteristic craniofacial abnormalities, including at least two of the following: (a) microcephaly, (b) short palpebral fissures, (c) poorly developed philtrum, thin upper lip, and flattening of the maxillary area. The term FAE may be used when a child shows two rather than all three of the above-listed indicators, to describe mild or abortive forms of the syndrome.

Stimulated by public interest in this issue, a number of prospective long-term follow-up and multicenter studies on moderate alcohol consumption during pregnancy as well as follow-up studies of the outcome of FAS children were initiated in the United States. Strategies of intervention and prevention programs were developed in the early 1980s that had some positive effect on pregnancy outcome. Rosett and colleagues (1980) in Boston were the first to show that reduction of alcohol consumption during late pregnancy in chronic alcoholics improved the woman's chance of having a healthier baby by preventing severe postnatal physical and developmental problems. Larsson *et al.* (1985) in Sweden clearly demonstrated in a prospective study of 40 children exposed to variable amounts of alcohol *in utero* that infants of mothers who were classified as excessive drinkers but not abusers and who reduced their alcohol consumption after the first trimester did not differ from controls with regard to the physical development or behavior of their babies; however, many infants had retarded speech development.

At the same time the notion that prenatal alcohol exposure in humans can result in long-lasting CNS dysfunction stimulated experimental animal research that addressed questions about ethanol teratogenicity impossible to study in human subjects. Animal models have enabled scientists to identify and characterize many of the harmful effects of alcohol on fetus development. These studies have provided fundamental contributions based on a variety of species and varying conditions of exposure. The increasing scientific knowledge acquired from experimental laboratory research validated the early clinical findings and corroborated the existence of FAS as a distinct syndrome (Chernoff, 1977; Diaz & Samson, 1980). Long before extended follow-up studies confirmed the early clinical suspicion that intrauterine alcohol exposure may be responsible for persistent life-long CNS disturbances, animal studies on alcohol teratogenesis demonstrated that the rapidly growing fetal brain is the most vulnerable structure of the developing child, reacting extremely sensitively to prenatal alcohol exposure with persistent structural abnormalities (West *et al.*, 1981; Stoltenburg-Didinger & Spohr, 1983; Sulik *et al.*, 1981; Clarren & Bowden, 1984).

Follow-up studies in FAS children

During the last decade clinicians who continued to diagnose and follow up children with FAS realized that there was a remarkable change in the clinical picture of the syndrome over time. On the one hand, although growth retardation and microcephaly in FAS is obvious already at birth and there is no or very little postnatal catch-up growth, irrespective of environmental and nutritional conditions, the clinical picture of FAS is not always recognized in the neonate (Little *et al.*, 1990). This is because the characteristic appearance with typical craniofacial dysmorphology, signs of neurological impairment and disturbed behavior may not become obvious before late infancy.

On the other hand, most clinicians are still very reluctant to diagnose FAS in older children or in adolescents. Whereas the recognition of the typical FAS patient in infancy and childhood is fairly well established, the adolescent phenotype is less easily recognized and, until recently, practically no adult patient has ever been diagnosed as suffering from this syndrome (Streissguth *et al.*, 1991).

The first report on older children with FAS was published by Iosub and coworkers (1981) who described longitudinal data and the developmental outcome of three siblings born to alcoholic mothers. These authors showed for the first time that two of their three patients, who had in the meantime reached maturity, were still microcephalic with some dysmorphic facial features and signs of persistent border-line to mild mental retardation. Streissguth and coworkers (1978) reported a follow-up of 20 patients and described the intelligence, behavior, and dysmorphogenesis of these children.

In 1984 a 4 year follow-up study of clinical, psychopathological, and developmental aspects in 71 children with FAS was published by our own Berlin study group (Spohr & Steinhausen, 1984). We recognized for the first time that with increasing age dysmorphic signs became less apparent in patients with FAS. Furthermore, we found a striking reduction in the severity of morphological damage, as indicated by the total number of minor craniofacial malformations. The morphometric features (i.e., head circumference, height, and weight) tended to normalize, and distinct improvements in a standardized age-adapted neurological re-examination of a subgroup of 19 children became apparent. These positive findings were supported by fewer pathological patterns in the electrocephalogram (EEG) of 45 children at follow-up as compared with their initial evaluations and with a matched control group. In contrast to these positive developmental results, the follow-up study also revealed that the persistent hyperactivity and distractability as well as the mild mental retardation seen in many of these children were responsible for failures in their social integration and school career.

The first longitudinal study was performed by the Seattle group of researchers. Streissguth *et al.* (1985) reported on the natural history of 11 children who in 1973 were the first to be diagnosed as having FAS. Ten years after the introduction of this new syndrome, 8 of the 11 original patients were reexamined. Two had died and 1 was not traceable at follow-up. The remaining patients were still dysmorphic and suffered from growth deficiency. The degree of growth deficiency and intellectual handicap were directly correlated with the extent of craniofacial abnormalities. The 4 children in this series with the most striking craniofacial dysmorphology had the most severe degree of microcephaly, the shortest stature, and the lowest level of intelligence. According to the authors, the most predictive factor in the backgrounds of the 4 severely handicapped children was the severity of maternal alcoholism.

This statement confirmed earlier findings by Majewski & Goecke (1982), who also related the severity of the clinical manifestations in affected children to the stage of maternal alcoholism. By analysing the phases in the drinking histories of 46 alcoholic mothers according to the classification by Jellinek (1946) these authors showed that the majority of children with severe forms of FAS were born to mothers in the critical and especially in the chronic stage of their alcoholism, whereas only 1 child with a mild form of the syndrome was identified from a mother in the prodromal stage of alcohol dependency. They concluded that the severity of fetal damage in a pregnant, alcohol-abusing woman is not dependent on the daily amount of alcohol consumed but on the duration of her alcoholism.

This conclusion is supported by our own observations. In our first follow-up study of 56 children with FAS, 34 patients had one or more siblings. Of a total of 75 siblings of known individual history, 27 were more than 10 years older and 19 were more than 5 years older than our index children. All were reported to be normal in terms of school career and professional education. The closer the age of the siblings was to the age of the identified FAS child the more they ran the risk of being affected by FAE themselves and taken away from their biological mothers. All younger siblings of the index-patients were diagnosed as suffering from FAS. The youngest child was very often more severely disturbed than the older siblings.

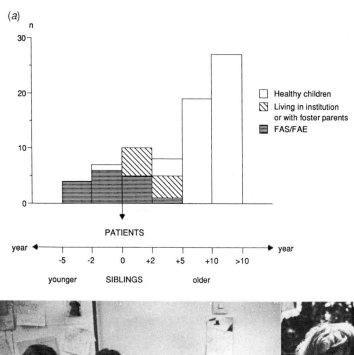

PATIENTS

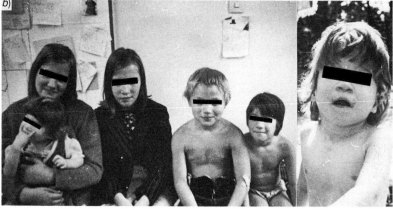

Fig. 11.1. (*a*) Age distribution and 'risk' of fetal alcohol damage in 75 siblings of 56 FAS patients. (*b*) Fetal alcohol damage in siblings of a chronic alcohol-abusing mother. The eldest two children on the picture, aged 13 and 12 years, are normally developed girls. The third child, an 8-year-old boy, is microcephalic, too small for his age, and attends a school for mentally subnormal children (diagnosis: FAE). The following 5-year-old girl is retarded and presents the typical symptoms of FAS. The youngest girl ($2\frac{1}{2}$ years), shown on the right and in the arms of the eldest sister, is the most severely affected FAS child in the family (see also the bottom row of Fig. 11.2).

There was only one exception: one of our mothers who had delivered an FAS child 2 years before had stopped drinking completely after that child was born. Two years later she gave birth to a small-for-dates but otherwise completely normal baby.

The fetal alcohol syndrome in adolescence

In recent years several long-term follow-up studies have been conducted in the United States, France, and Germany. These studies following children with FAS in adolescence and young adulthood clearly indicate that FAS can no longer be viewed as just a childhood disorder but rather as having very complex and possibly lifelong consequences for the affected patients, including a wide spectrum of physical, mental, and behavioral disabilities.

In 1991 Streissguth and co-workers presented the first data-based systematic study on the long-term consequences in 61 adolescents and adults suffering from alcohol teratogenesis. Seventy-four percent of the sample were Native Americans, 21% were Caucasian, and 5% were Afro-American blacks. Almost half the sample (47%) lived on reservations in the Southwest and Northwest United States, 14% in rural, nonreservation areas, and only 39% in urban areas. Seventy percent of the patients were diagnosed as having FAS, whereas 30% were classified as having FAE. Forty-three patients were adolescents (12–17 years old) and 18 were adults (18–40 years old).

In this study the natural history of FAS was traced into adulthood for the first time, showing that mental retardation was not necessarily predictable from the diagnosis alone and that, in particular, major psychosocial problems and life-long adjustment problems were characteristic of most of these patients. Similar to our own results (Spohr & Steinhausen, 1984), the authors stated that the facies of patients with FAS or FAE were no longer as distinctive and that facial abnormalities had become more subtle in adolescence. Obviously, the facies in FAS is highly characteristic only in small infants and children up to prepuberty. At this age one is often able to diagnose typical patients at *prima vista*. Streissguth and co-workers (1991) noted that the most discriminating facial features in childhood (i.e., short palpebral fissures, flat midface, short nose, indistinct philtrum, and thin upper lip) change over time. The authors described four characteristics of the facial phenotype in adolescence: a large nose, disappearance of the earlier midface hypoplasia, improved modelling of the philtrum and upper lip, and a large chin. However, in some adults the faces of the affected individuals had normalized so much that early childhood photographs were needed to confirm the diagnosis. In this study by the Seattle group short stature and microcephaly were the most prominent indicators of growth deficiency as the children got older. Only 25% of the adolescent and adult patients with FAS were not growth deficient for weight, only 16% were not growth deficient for height, and only 28% did not suffer from microcephaly. However, the severe developmental and cognitive handicaps persisted. The family environments were remarkably unstable, and none of the studied patients were known to be independent in terms of both housing and income.

Thirty years after FAS was first recognized in France a sample of patients very different from the Native Americans in the Seattle study was re-evaluated by Lemoine & Lemoine in Nantes, France. The authors published an important follow-up study of 105 adolescents and adults from their original sample of 127 patients whom they had described in 1968 as a 'very peculiar syndrome of children from chronic alcoholic mothers', 5 years prior to the famous first description of FAS in Seattle. Similar to the findings of the Seattle group, Lemoine & Lemoine (1992) summarized that the typical facial dysmorphism underwent changes, often with coarse features, a long face, and a bulky nose and chin, in contrast to the appearance of affected infants. The growth failure became slightly less marked but microcephaly was more pronounced. Severe physical malformations contributed to persistent disability in adolescence, although the subjects were sometimes able to function better in daily life than would have been expected. Mental retardation was seen in the many severely affected patients and disturbed behavior was present in practically all patients at follow-up. Interestingly, similar disorders were also recognized by the authors in siblings with no apparent dysmorphism, underlining the extent of the problem and, once again, demonstrating the wide range of deleterious sequelae of intrauterine alcohol exposure. In the French study a remarkably high mortality rate of 5 among 50 patients with severe FAS was found. Moreover, 2 of 28 adult patients with mild FAS had committed suicide and an additional 5 patients had attempted suicide. From this study one may learn how devastating, self-destructive, and intolerable it may be for patients to be affected with FAS and to be forced to live and to grow up with no hope and no future.

The Berlin study

In our first report on the long-term consequences of FAS (Spohr & Steinhausen 1984, 1987) we described the reduction in growth deficiency and the improvement in the dysmorphic features associated with FAS as soon as patients matured physically. On the basis of a large series of 158 children who were identified between 1977 and 1992 in Berlin as suffering from FAS/FAE, we recently completed a 10-year follow-up study of 60 adolescent patients diagnosed as having FAS during infancy and childhood. Our findings confirmed earlier assumptions of persisting sequelae due to intrauterine exposure to alcohol in a well-documented sample.

In contrast to the very selected patients in a high-risk group of Native Americans who were predominantly diagnosed during adolescence and adulthood on reservations or remote rural areas, as described by the Seattle group, we had the opportunity to follow up a large cohort of FAS children in a multidisciplinary study in West Berlin, a capital with a dense social and medical infrastructure (Spohr *et al.*, 1993; Steinhausen *et al.*, 1993). The diagnosis of these children had been known for 10–14 years, and medical therapy, advice to caretakers, and social support had been available over a long follow-up period. Despite the great differences in the selection of the patients in these two studies, the results of the long-term perspective of FAS and the developmental consequences were remarkably similar. Both studies revealed a 'growing out' of the typical FAS facies after puberty and a persistence of cognitive and psychiatric handicaps. The Berlin study findings suggested, moreover, that compensatory environmental and educational influences were less important than expected for the intellectual outcome of FAS patients at adolescence. In detail, we found that the characteristic craniofacial malformations of FAS diminish with time. This phenomenon, which was previously described in our first follow-up study, seems to be even more pronounced in adolescence and young adulthood. Ten years after the initial diagnosis, more than 70% (initially 45%) of the affected children were diagnosed as having only mild FAS, and it was difficult to diagnose FAS at all in a substantial proportion of adolescents with mild expression of the syndrome. The pediatric scoring system and the results of the initial examination and follow-up are shown in Table 11.1.

The characteristic change over time in the craniofacial dysmorphology of FAS in 44 patients who reached young adulthood is shown in Table 11.2. Although the facies in growing children with FAS loses its distinctive expression, a number of facial symptoms persist in adolescence and remain useful diagnostic features after puberty: short palpebral fissures, indistinct philtrum and, in particular, a thin upper lip, a pronounced chin or a mild form of micrognathia, and a small head circumference (which is not a facial feature *per se*, but a central nervous system characteristic). In contrast to the typical short nose with a low nasal bridge of FAS patients in infancy and childhood, a new facial feature appearing in many adolescents with FAS is a large, prominent nose with a 'distinctive' nasal bridge (see Figs. 11.2–11.4). Among the subjects in her sample of Native Americans, Streissguth recognized the same continuing growth of the nasal bridge and nasal length from root to tip, and Lemoine & Lemoine (1992) also very often described facies with typical large noses and bulky chins in their sample of adult FAS patients in France.

Table 11.1. *Pediatric scoring system and symptoms at initial examination and at 10 year follow up* (n=60)

	Item score	% of children with feature at:	
		Initial examination	Follow-up
Pediatric score items			
Postnatal growth deficiency	4	77	43
Developmental delay	4/6	90	68
Microcephaly	4	87	65
Hyperactivity	4	71	52
Hypotonia	2	75	23
Epicanthal folds	1	44	22
Short palpebral fissures	2	41	29
Ptosis	2	18	13
Short upturned nose	3	58	38
Thin upper lip	2	82	72
High arched palate	2	35	18
Cleft palate	4	7	7
Maxilla hypoplasia/flat midface	2	19	12
Abnormal palmar creases	3	58	47
Camptodactyly	2	7	2
Phalangeal anomalies (minor)	1	22	13
Limited joint movement	2	12	8
Cardiac defects	4	31	8
Hernias	2	20	3
Minor external genital anomalies	2	27	18
Coccygeal fovea	1	49	27
Renal anomalies	4	5	5
Diagnosis			
FAE	< 10	. .	15
Mild FAS	10–29	45	72
Moderate FAS	30–39	30	13
Severe FAS	> 40	25	. .

From Spohr, Willms & Steinhausen (1993).

The improvement of alcohol-induced prenatal morphological abnormalities was not restricted to the craniofacial dysmorphism; there was also a significant improvement in the internal organ malformations, skeletal abnormalities, and neurological dysfunctions, as shown in Fig. 11.5.

Despite a tendency towards catch-up growth, the morphometric parameters of adolescents suffering from FAS consistently deviated from the normal distribution, as shown in Fig. 11.6. Sixty percent of the subjects in

Table 11.2. *Craniofacial dysmorphy in FAS (n = 44)*

Symptoms	Infants (%)	Adolescents (%)
Microcephaly	81.8	61.4
Short palpebral fissures	40.9	31.8
Epicanthal folds	61.5	15.9
Low nasal bridge, short nose	54.6	29.5
Micrognathia/flat midface	65.9	45.5
Thin upper lip	81.8	65.9
Indistinct philtrum	43.2	31.8
Hypoplastic/misaligned teeth	20.5	29.5
Strabismus	38.7	29.9
Minor ear anomalies[a]	15.9	13.6
Increased growth of nose (prominent nose)	—	70.5

[a] I.e., posterior rotation and deep ear line.
From Spohr, Willms & Steinhausen (1993).

the total sample were below the population mean for head circumference and 42% below the mean for height. The pattern for weight developed differently in the two sexes. Fifty-four percent of the male subjects were 2 SD below the population mean at follow-up. In contrast, underweight persisted in only 19% of the female subjects, and quite a number of sexually mature girls manifested a significant increase in adipose tissue after puberty. This observation was not made in male subjects.

Juvenile FAS

When considering the documented developmental and physical changes in FAS from childhood to adolescence, one has to realize that a characteristic dysmorphic pattern nevertheless persists. These typical, persistent, or newly acquired symptoms are summarized in Table 11.3. Familiarity with this pattern will aid in the diagnosis of the syndrome even in patients after puberty, and may help its identification at a later age in patients who were for one reason or another not diagnosed earlier.

The cardinal signs of juvenile FAS are growth retardation and persistent microcephaly. Underweight, which is typical in infancy and only rarely amenable to therapeutic measures, is at least partially corrected, especially in adolescent female patients. The pathogenesis of this gender difference in the development of obesity in FAS patients after puberty has also been described by Streissguth (1991), Majewski (1993), and Löser (1995), and is

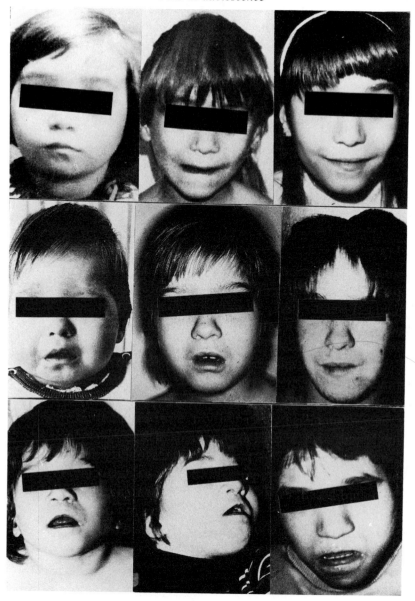

Fig. 11.2. Top line: mild female FAS child (age: 10 months, 3 years, 12 years). Middle line: moderate female FAS child (age: 8 months, 7 years, 15 years). Bottom line: severe female FAS child (age: 3 years, 5 years, 17 years).

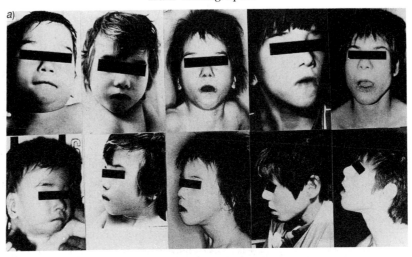

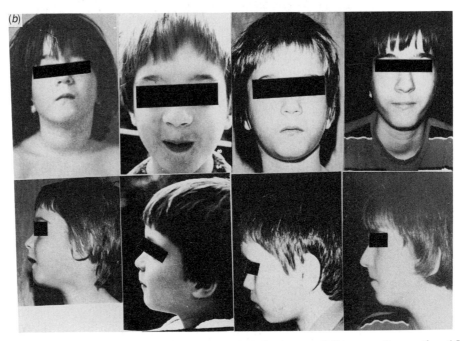

Fig. 11.3. (*a*) Child severely affected by FAS. Age at follow-up: 7 months, 15 months, 3 years, 8 years, 15 years (from left to right, in full face and in profile). (*b*) Mild FAS child. Age at follow-up: 2 years, 4 years, 7 years, 15 years (from left to right, in full face and in profile).

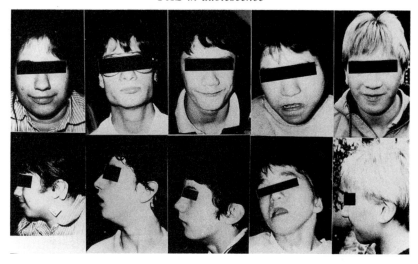

Fig. 11.4. Three female (f) and two male (m) adolescent FAS patients with different degrees of morphological damage. Upper line: 15 years (f), 16 years (m), 13 years (m), 17 years (f), 15 years (m). Lower line: same patients in profile (from left to right).

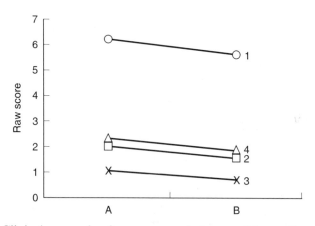

Fig. 11.5. Clinical scores for four groups of abnormalities at first assessment (A: average age 4.1 years) and follow-up (B: average age 15.1 years) in 60 children with FAS. Items are given in brackets. (1) Craniofacial dysmorphic signs (i.e. epicanthal folds, blepharophimosis, ptosis, short upturned nose, thinned upper lip, flat midface, high arched palate, cleft palate, strabismus, minor ear anomalies). (2) Skeletal dysmorphic signs (camptodactyly, clinodactyly, abnormal palm or creases, limited joint movement, coccygeal fovea, congenital hip dislocation). (3) Major malformations of internal organs (cardiac defects, renal anomalies, minor external genital anomalies, hernia, hemangioma). (4) Neurological dysfunctions (muscular hypotonia, cerebral convulsion, psychomotor developmental delay, hyperactivity, cerebral palsy, ataxia, tremor).

Table 11.3. *Juvenile FAS*

Stocky stature/growth retardation

Small head circumference/microcephaly

Craniofacial features
    Long face with mild midfacial hypoplasia
    Large nose with prominent nasal bridge
    Short palpebral fissures
Thin upper lip

Developmental and cognitive deficits

Psychiatric and behavioral problems

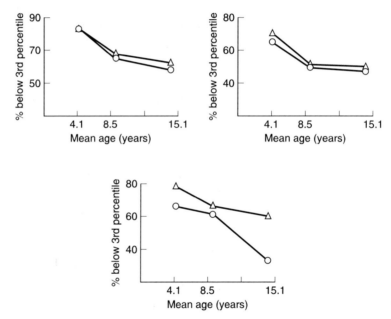

Fig. 11.6.   Physical characteristics over time of 44 adolescent patients with FAS. The proportions of patients are shown who scored below the third percentile for head circumference, height, and weight. Triangles, males; circles, females.

not clearly understood. Until now, no endocrinological disturbances have been found in a small number of female patients who were systematically studied.

    As described before in many adolescent FAS patients, the typical facies is still discernible. However, this picture changes over time, although a triad of symptoms persists: short palpebral fissures, indistinct philtrum, and a thinner upper lip. The peculiar dystrophic narrowness of the whole face, especially the midfacial hypoplasia, diminishes. The cheeks, chin, and ears appear to be better formed. The nose in particular, and less frequently the chin, also become more prominent and, in many cases, determine the character of the whole face. One could possibly speculate that the improved plastic modelling of the maturing face, especially the midface, including the sinuses, may be one of the reasons for the pronounced decrease in susceptibility to severe respiratory tract infections in older FAS children compared with those in infancy. Additional common symptoms are strabismus, myopia/hyperopia, and sometimes malformed and misaligned teeth.

Independent of growth retardation and a particular juvenile craniofacial dysmorphology, further characteristic features are essential for the typical adolescent or adult with FAS, namely persistent developmental and cognitive deficits as well as severe psychiatric and behavioral problems. These features are described in detail in the following chapter by Steinhausen.

The unfavorable developmental course caused by the teratogenic noxa alcohol was reflected even more in the school career of the adolescents. At the beginning of their schooling 30% of the children in our follow-up study went to a standard primary school, 40% to a school for pupils with learning disabilities, and 30% to a school for the mentally handicapped. However, by the end of their schooling, 55% of the sample were at a school for children with learning difficulties and another 30% at a school for the mentally handicapped. This change for the worse applied particularly to the patients with a mild degree of FAS, because the severely affected children were usually placed in an institution for severely mentally retarded children at the outset. This means that, in the course of their school career, even patients with only slight morphological abnormalities had severe learning difficulties. After initially showing age-appropriate performance, these children often developed problems in abstract reasoning and comprehension of complex relations, and they suffered from persisting deficits in central cognitive processing. Sometimes the serious intellectual shortcomings of the handicapped adolescents were masked by a lively friendliness or very effective superficial language skills.

Certainly it is difficult to assess the effects of the postnatal environment on the mental development of children with FAS. We recorded substantial changes in the children's domestic arrangements over time, as shown in Table 11.4. The numbers of children living with their biological parents or in institutions decreased and greater proportions were living with parent surrogates, foster parents, and adoptive parents. These changes had generally taken place in early childhood, and the domestic circumstances of the children

Table 11.4. *Changes in family background in FAS patients from infancy to adolescence*

	No. (%) of children ($n = 60$) at:	
	First assessment	Follow-up[a]
Both biological parents	17 (28)	4 (7)
Mother or father plus parent surrogate	6 (10)	14 (23)
Foster family	9 (15)	21 (35)
Adoptive family	4 (7)	8 (13)
Institution	24 (40)	13 (22)

From Spohr, Willms & Steinhausen (1993).
[a] After 10 years.

had been stable over many years. This stability usually started 5 to 6 years before the last follow-up assessment. Nevertheless the deleterious effects of intrauterine alcohol exposure on mental development persisted for many years, and we saw little improvement in intelligence or school achievement even when domestic circumstances changed for the better. In contrast to our original assumption of some 'biological catch-up maturation' (Spohr & Steinhausen, 1987), these findings suggest that compensatory environmental and educational influences are less important than originally expected for the developmental outcome in adolescence and young adulthood.

In summary, FAS can no longer be viewed as just a rare and peculiar childhood disorder. We have to realize that the long-term perspective of FAS in many cases implies a developmental disability beginning at birth and reaching from infancy to adulthood. The spectrum of multiple handicaps changes during different age periods and, currently, we are just beginning to identify the magnitude of physical, mental, and psychological problems that will emerge in adult FAS.

References

Abel, E.L. (1981). *Fetal Alcohol Syndrome*, vols. I–III. Boca Raton, FL: CRC Press.

Alcohol Beverage Labeling Act of 1988 (1988). *Public Law 100–690. 100th Congress 2d. Sess., November 18.*

Chernoff, G.H. (1977). The fetal alcohol syndrome in mice: an animal model. *Teratology*, **15**, 223–30.

Clarren, S.K. & Bowden, D.S. (1984). Measures of alcohol damage *in utero* in the pigtailed macaque (*Macaca nemestrina*). In *Mechanisms of Alcohol Damage In Utero*, pp. 157–72. Ciba Foundation Symposium 105. London: Pitman.

Clarren, S.K. & Smith, D.W. (1978). The fetal alcohol syndrome. Experience with 65 patients and a review of the world literature. *New England Journal of Medicine*, **298**, 1063–67.

Coles, C.D., Brown, R.T., Smith, I.E., Platzman, K.A., Erickson, S. & Falek, A. (1991). Effects of prenatal alcohol exposure at school age. I. Physical and cognitive development. *Neurotoxicology and Teratology*, **13**, 357–67.

Day, N., Richardson, G., Geva, D. & Robles, N. (1994). Alcohol, marijuana and tobacco: the effect of prenatal exposure on offspring's growth and morphology at age six. *Alcoholism: Clinical and Experimental Research*, **18**, 786–94.

Dehaene, P., Samaille-Vilette, C., Samaille, P.-P., Crépin, G., Walbaum, R., Deroubaix, P. & Blanc-Garin, A.P. (1977). Le syndrome d'alcoolisme foetal dans le nord de la France. *Revue l'Alcoölisme*, **23**, 145–58.

Diaz, J. & Sampson, H.H. (1980). Impaired brain growth in neonatal rats exposed to ethanol. *Science*, **208**, 751–60.

Hanson, J.W., Jones, K.L. & Smith, D.W. (1976). Fetal alcohol syndrome: experience with 41 patients. *JAMA*, **235**, 1458–60.

Iosub, S., Fuchs, M., Bingol, N., Stone, R.K. & Gromisch, D.S. (1981). Long-term follow-up of three siblings with fetal alcohol syndrom. *Alcoholism: Clinical and Experimental Research*, **5**, 523–7.

Jellinek, E.M. (1946). Phases in the drinking history of alcoholics: analysis of a survey conducted by the official organ AA. *Quarterly Journal of Studies on Alcohol*, **7**, 1.

Jones, K.L. & Smith, D.W. (1973). Recognition of the fetal alcohol syndrome in early infancy. *Lancet*, **ii**, 999–1001.

Kaminski, M., Rumeau, C. & Schwartz, D. (1978). Alcohol consumption in pregnant women and the outcome of pregnancy. *Alcoholism: Clinical and Experimental Research*, **2**, 155–63.

Kyllerman, M., Aronsson, A., Karlberg, E., Olegard, R., Sabel, K.-G., Sadin, J., Johansson, P.R., Carlsson, C. & Iversen, K. (1979). Epidemiologic and neuropediatric aspects of the fetal alcohol syndrome. *Neuropädiatrie, Supplement*, **104**, 435–6.

Lamache, M.A. (1967). Communications: reflections sur la descendance des alcooliques. *Bulletin de l'Academie Nationale de Medecine, Paris*, **151**, 517–21.

Larsson, G., Bohlin, A.B. & Tunell, R. (1985). Prospective study of children exposed to variable amounts of alcohol *in utero*. *Archives of Disease in Childhood*, **60**, 316–21.

Lemoine, P., Harousseau, H., Borteyru, J.P. & Menuet, J.C. (1968). Lés enfants de parents alcooliques: anomalies observées. A propos de 127 cas. *Quest-Medical*, **21**, 476–82.

Lemoine, P. & Lemoine, Ph. (1992). Avenir des enfants de meres alcooliques (étude des 105 cas retrouvés a l'âge adulte) et quelques constations d'interêt prophylactique. *Annales de pédiatrie*, **39**, 226–35.

Little, B., Little, M.A., Snell, L.M., Rosenfeld, C.R., Gilstrap, C.L. III & Gant, N.F. (1990). Failure to recognize fetal alcohol syndrome in newborn infants. *American Journal of Diseases of Children*, **144**, 1142–6.

Löser, H. (1995). *Alkoholembryopathie und Alkoholeffekte*. Stuttgart: Fiscer.

Majewski, F. (1993). Alcohol embryopathy: experience in 200 patients. *Developmental Brain Dysfunction*, **6**, 248–65.

Majewski, F., Bierich, J.R., Löser, H., Michaelis, R., Leiber, B. & Bettecken, F. (1976). Zur Klinik und Pathogenese der Alkoholembryopathie: Bericht über 68 Fälle. *Münchener Medizinische Wochenschrift*, **188**, 1635–42.

Majewski, F. & Goecke, T. (1982). Alcohol embryopathy. In *Fetal Alcohol Syndrome*, vol. 2, *Human Studies*, ed. E.L. Abel, pp. 65–88. Boca Raton, FL: CRC Press.

Olegård, R., Sabel, K.-G., Aronsson, M., Sandin, B., Johansson, P.R., Carlsson, C., Kyllerman, M., Iversen, K. & Hrbek, A. (1979). Effects on the child of alcohol abuse during pregnancy: retrospective and prospective studies. *Acta Paediatrica Scandinavica Supplement*, **275**, 112–21.

Public Health Service (1981). Surgeon General's advisory on alcohol and pregnancy. *FDA Drug Bulletin*, **11**(2), 9–10.

Rosett, H.L. (1980). A clinical perspective of the fetal alcohol syndrome. *Alcoholism: Clinical and Experimental Research*, **4**, 119–22.

Smith, D.W. (1982). *Recognizable Patterns of Human Malformation: Genetic, Embryologic and Clinical Aspects*, 3rd edn. Philadelphia: W.B. Saunders.

Sokol, R.J. & Clarren, S.K. (1989). Guidelines for use of terminology describing the impact of prenatal alcohol on the offspring. *Alcoholism*, **13**, 597–8.

Spohr, H.L. & Steinhausen, H.C. (1984). Clinical, psychopathological and developmental aspects in children with the fetal alcohol syndrome: a four year follow-up study. In *Mechanism of Alcohol Damage In Utero*, pp. 197–217. *Ciba Foundation Symposium 105*. London: Pitman.

Spohr, H.L. & Steinhausen, H.C. (1987). Follow-up studies of children with fetal alcohol syndrome. *Neuropediatrics*, **18**, 13–17.

Spohr, H.L., Willms, J. & Steinhausen, H.C. (1993). Prenatal alcohol exposure and long-term developmental consequences: a 10-year follow-up of 60 children with fetal alcohol syndrome (FAS). *Lancet*, **341**, 907–10.

Spohr, H.L., Willms, J. & Steinhausen, H.C. (1994). The fetal alcohol syndrome in adolescence. *Acta Paediatrica Scandinavica*, **404**, 19–26.

Steinhausen, H.C., Willms, J. & Spohr, H.L. (1993). Long-term psychopathological and cognitive outcome of children with fetal alcohol syndrome. *Journal of the American Academy of Child and Adolescent Psychiatry*, **32**, 990–4.

Stoltenburg-Didinger, G. & Spohr, H.L. (1983). Fetal alcohol syndrome and mental retardation: Spine distribution of pyramidal cells in prenatal alcohol-exposed rat cerebral cortex: a Golgi study. *Brain Research*, **11**, 119–23.

Streissguth, A.P. (1994). A long-term perspective of FAS. *Alcohol Health and Research World*, **18**, 74–81.

Streissguth, A.P., Aase, J.M., Clarren, S.K., Randels, S.P., LaDue, R.A. & Smith, D.F. (1991). Fetal alcohol syndrome in adolescents and adults. *JAMA*, **265**, 1961–7.

Streissguth, A.P., Clarren, S.K. & Jones, K.L. (1985). Natural history of the fetal alcohol syndrome: a ten year follow-up of eleven patients. *Lancet*, **ii**, 85–91.

Streissguth, A.P., Herman, C.S. & Smith, D.W. (1978). Intelligence, behavior and dysmorphogenesis in the fetal alcohol syndrome: a report on 20 patients. *Journal of Pediatrics*, **92**, 363–7.

Sulik, K.K., Johnston, M.C. & Webb, M.A. (1981). Fetal alcohol syndrome: embryogenesis in a mouse model. *Science*, **214**, 936–8.

Tanaka, H., Arima, N. & Suzuki, N. (1981). The fetal alcohol syndrome in Japan. *Brain Development*, **3**, 305–11.

West, J.R., Hodges, C.A. & Black, A.C. (1981). Prenatal exposure to ethanol alters the organization of hippocampal mossy fibers in rats. *Science*, **211**, 957–9.

12

Psychopathology and cognitive functioning in children with fetal alcohol syndrome

HANS-CHRISTOPH STEINHAUSEN

Introduction

Although interest in the effects of intrauterine exposure to alcohol originated only just over two decades ago when Jones & Smith (1973) gave the first Anglo-Saxon description of fetal alcohol syndrome (FAS), there is much older scientific interest in the children of alcoholics. It has been known for some time that these children may themselves develop alcoholism and further psychiatric disorders because of both genetic and environmental risk factors. The literature on the effects of these two risk factors is considerable and has recently been reviewed (Steinhausen, 1995). The present chapter will, therefore, focus exclusively on the behavioral, psychopathological, and cognitive effects of prenatal alcohol exposure in children with FAS. A preceding chapter in this volume by Streissguth deals with the effects of moderate maternal drinking and child development, so the following report will be restricted to findings in children with the characteristic features of FAS. Based both on a review of the literature and on our own research, this chapter will introduce findings on the developmental history, psychopathology and behavioral features, cognitive functioning, and follow-up status of children with FAS.

Developmental history

Most of the clinical reports dealing with FAS have noted developmental delay similar to mental retardation as a core feature of the syndrome. However, few efforts have been made to study systematically the process of development in the affected children. In our own longitudinal study we tried to overcome this deficit by retrospectively assessing the developmental history in FAS. After presenting our first analyses based on case–control studies of 68 patients and 28 healthy children (Steinhausen et al., 1982b),

Table 12.1. *Developmental history in 154 children with FAS*

Item	n	%
Prematurity	57	37.0
Neonatal complications	69	42.2
Sucking problems	82	53.1
Failure to thrive	96	62.3
Retarded motor development	104	67.5
Retarded speech development	102	66.3

we currently have data on an even larger series of FAS patients. However, it should be noted that in this series of 154 FAS patients it was not possible to obtain data on all items or on all children. This was due to the partly retrospective character of our study and the problem of obtaining reliable data from mothers who were either uncooperative or incapacitated with regard to recall of developmental data. Thus, missing data for the various items ranged from 8% to 53%.

Accordingly, the data on developmental history as presented in Table 12.1 may serve as a rather conservative estimate regarding the problems that were present in this large group of FAS children. As the data show, a large proportion of these children suffered from prematurity and neonatal complications and many had problems of adaptation to postnatal life as indicated by sucking problems and failure to thrive. In addition, the developmental milestones were typically delayed in the majority of cases. It must be added that only a minority (27%) continued to live with their biological parents, the majority living either with foster or adoptive parents (24%), in an institution (25%), or in unstable situations (20%).

It is clear from these data that there are a number of grave risks for early development of the FAS child that unfold directly at birth and lead to varying degrees of developmental delay.

Psychopathology and behavioral features

Starting with the first clinical reports on FAS in the literature, hyperactivity has been noted quite frequently (Lemoine et al., 1968; Jones & Smith, 1973; Bierich et al., 1976; Hermier et al., 1976; Dehaene et al., 1977; Streissguth et al., 1978a). However, in the majority of cases descriptions remained rather vague, and no systematic measures were taken to substantiate this impression. In fact, there are some indications that hyperactivity is the main psychopathological feature because it has been described in the majority of patients – for example, in 72% of the series of Majewski & Majewski (1988) and in 74% of the series of Iosub *et al.* (1981).

Because of the known genetic link between hyperactivity and alcoholism, it is also interesting to see hyperactivity as the main psychopathological feature in children who have been prenatally exposed to alcohol. This opens speculation regarding possible interactions of teratogenic and genetic effects – an issue that has not yet been solved. Because hyperactivity is also a component of attention deficit disorder (ADD) and hyperkinetic disorders (HD), a group of researchers have been interested in seeing whether alcoholic mothers are frequently seen among children with learning problems and hyperactivity. Shaywitz *et al.* (1980) found among 87 children of normal intelligence who had learning problems and hyperactivity, 15 who were born to mothers who were heavy drinkers. However, this study leaves open the question as to whether or not paternal alcoholism was also involved and whether or not the children's problems might have been due to poor environments or to an interaction of these factors. Furthermore, efforts to compare the 15 children born to heavy-drinking mothers with the rest of the group are lacking. Thus, the report by Shaywitz *et al.* (1980) only suggests the possibility that a high number of hyperactive children referred to clinical institutions may have been prenatally exposed to alcohol.

Other than hyperactivity, only a few behavioral features have been described in the early FAS reports. Apart from hyperactivity in the preschool period, Streissguth *et al.* (1978*a*) found no severe disorders in terms of rebellious, antisocial, excessively negativistic, or psychotic behavior. In a total of 20 cases, child abuse and neglect were noted in a few children and 2 children were withdrawn, fearful, and unresponsive when they were separated from their alcoholic mothers. School problems resulting from learning disorders and hyperactivity were frequently reported. In 3 children of normal intelligence, so-called personality problems were present. Unfortunately, this report suffers from poor documentation of data, and the reader is left with the impression that no systematic attempt to study psychopathology was undertaken.

In a study by Iosub *et al.* (1981), speech and language problems were commonly encountered. These included retarded speech development, voice dysfunctions, disorders of articulation, and fluency rate problems in from 73% to 84% of the sample.

Given this scarcity of knowledge on the psychopathology of FAS children, our own group started to assess these children more systematically. In a first attempt (Steinhausen *et al.*, 1982*a, b*) psychopathology was assessed in 49

FAS patients aged 3 years and older by using a structured interview in which each item was rated on a 3-point scale. In addition, 28 controls, matched for age, sex, and socioeconomic status were studied. These healthy children were free of prenatal, perinatal, and/or postnatal risks to central nervous system (CNS) development or other chronic diseases. The control sample included a similar percentage of foster children to control for possible deleterious effects of living away from the biological parents.

Of the 60 items in the interview, 18 gave some indication of significant differences between the two groups. In comparison with controls the FAS children had greater frequencies of outpatient therapy, eating and sleeping problems, head and body rocking, stereotyped habits (i.e., facial tics, nail biting, hair plucking), reduced vocabulary and diminished clarity of speech, stammering and/or stuttering, impaired hearing, and strabismus. Furthermore, they were more susceptible to clumsiness, hyperactivity, and attentional deficits, had more difficulties in peer relationships, tended to be more generally dependent, and had more phobias and problems with educational management. Finally, they tended to have encopresis, enuresis, and temper tantrums more frequently than the controls.

With the continuation of our studies, including a longitudinal perspective, we currently observe a far more extended series of FAS children. Table 12.2 summarizes the findings of detailed psychiatric assessments based on structured interviews at three time points during a longitudinal study. Therefore, the three subsamples partly overlap. The mean age was 63.2 months for the preschool subsample, 113.5 months for the early school subsample and 168.3 months for the late school subsample.

The figures in Table 12.2 represent a wide spectrum of disorders. During the preschool period hyperkinetic disorders were the most frequent, followed by eating disorders, speech delay, and enuresis which, by definition, was not diagnosed before the age of 5 years. However, frequencies of stereotypies, conduct disorders, anxiety disorders, and affective disorders were also far higher than in a normal population. When looking at the figures for the two school-age periods, hyperkinetic disorders are again the most common problem, followed by stereotypies, anxiety disorders, speech delay, sleep disorders, eating disorders, and conduct disorders. Obviously, the pattern of psychiatric disorders is quite complex, comprising both features of organic brain damage and disturbed adaptation to the psychosocial environment.

In our studies we repeatedly analyzed several determinants that possibly contribute to psychopathology in FAS children. Here we used an index of psychopathology comprised of the total sum of symptom scores or syndrome

Table 12.2. Psychiatric syndromes in three subsamples of FAS children during preschool, early school, and late school periods

	Preschool period (n = 49)		Early school period (n = 50)		Late school period (n = 51)	
	n	%	n	%	n	%
Eating disorders	21	42.9	14	28.0	5	9.8
Sleep disorders	7	14.3	18	36.0	17	33.3
Enuresis	15	30.6	8	16.0	4	7.8
Encopresis	2	4.1	5	10.0	1	2.0
Speech delay	15	30.6	27	54.0	18	26.5
Stereotypes	11	22.4	29	58.0	25	49.0
Hyperkinetic disorders	25	51.0	32	64.0	23	45.1
Conduct disorders	8	16.3	10	14.7	13	25.5
Anxiety disorders	6	12.2	24	48.0	30	58.8
Affective disorders	5	10.2	1	2.0	1	2.0

scores as the dependent variable. A number of predictors or independent variables were studied, namely severity of morphological damage based on a detailed pediatric assessment, milieu, gender, and IQ. Age was also considered as a determinant insofar as the analyses were performed separately for the preschool and school-age subsamples.

In our most recent analyses based on an extended cohort (Steinhausen *et al.*, 1994), we found that at preschool age, severity of morphological damage, the type of milieu, gender and IQ were significant predictors of psychopathology. In the subgroup of school-age children, some of these associations were weaker. As Fig. 12.1 shows, the children with severe morphological damage clearly had the highest psychopathology score both in the preschool ($p = 0.03$) and the school-age sample ($p = 0.01$). In addition, milieu was highly significant ($p = 0.00001$) only in the preschool sample insofar as children living in institutions had by far the highest psychopathology score, as indicated in Fig. 12.2. As is usual in child psychiatry, boys suffering from FAS had significantly higher scores than girls in both the preschool ($p = 0.02$) and the school-age sample ($p = 0.03$). Intelligence was strongly correlated with psychopathology in the preschool sample, with children with moderate or severe mental retardation having significantly higher frequencies of speech disorders, eating disorders, depression, dependency problems, and hyperkinetic disorders. In the school-age sample, these associations were restricted to speech disorders and tics.

Despite the fact that the associations between some of the predictors and psychopathology lost some power from the preschool to the school period, there is a strong overlap between severity of morphological damage, upbringing in an institution, and mental retardation. In fact, the most damaged children, both physically and mentally, were those who were raised in institutions away from their parents. This was often due to severely deprived environments characterized by both maternal and paternal alcoholism.

In summary, a detailed psychiatric assessment of FAS children revealed a broad spectrum of psychiatric disorders exceeding the common notion of the hyperkinetic disorders as the core behavioral feature of FAS. Among the various determinants of psychopathology in these children, parental alcohol consumption is the most powerful factor. In previous analyses (Steinhausen *et al.*, 1982*b*) it stood out as a predictor of psychopathology even after the milieu was controlled for. However, it cannot be ruled out that further genetic factors related to both maternal and paternal alcoholism are operating. In addition, poor environment may have contributed to the developmental and psychiatric outcome of these children.

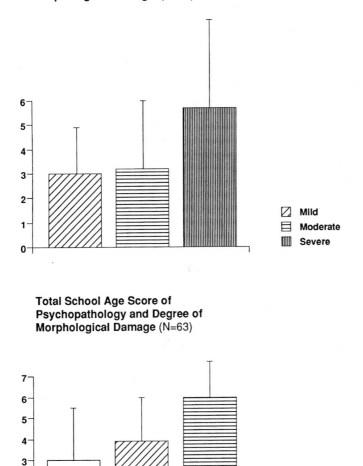

Fig. 12.1.   The relation between psychopathology and degree of morphological damage at preschool and school age.

Cognitive functioning

Mental retardation has been mentioned as one of the core features of FAS in many clinical reports covering several hundreds of patients. However, surprisingly few studies based on standardized intelligence tests and reporting the distribution of IQ are available. A compilation of the literature reporting

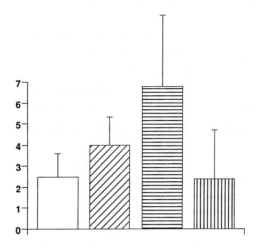

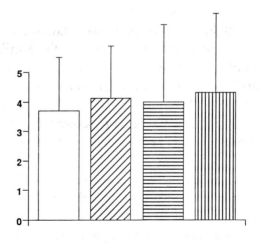

Lives with parents/surrogate
Lives with foster/adoptive parents
Lives in an institution
Changing milieu

Fig. 12.2. The relation between psychopathology and milieu at preschool and school age.

psychometric test findings is given in Table 12.3. These studies not only originate from different countries but also vary with regard to age distribution. Although the most recent series reported in the literature (Streissguth *et al.*, 1991) deals with adolescents and adults, all other series are comprised mainly of children and a few adolescents. Furthermore, a variety of tests have been used, and in some cases data from developmental tests for toddlers have been lumped together with those from intelligence tests for children, adolescents, and even adults. In addition, the issue of whether mentally retarded children may be tested with tests designed for children with normal cognitive functioning has not been addressed in these studies. Instead the dilemma has been solved covertly by using tests according to the child's functional or mental age. So, for example, a severely retarded school-age child might have been tested with a preschool measure.

Given the lack of comparability between samples and the scarcity of data reported, it is hardly surprising that the outcomes differ strikingly. In terms of proportions of mentally retarded children with FAS one may conclude from these psychometric studies only that mental retardation is overrepresented. The figures range from 19% to 60%, and it may well be that the inclusion of infants and toddlers leads to an overestimation of the proportion of mentally retarded children, given that classification may be unreliable at this age. In our own extended series of 70 children, the distribution of IQ is as follows: 24 (34.3%) of the children scored in the normal range (IQ 115–86), another 24 children (34.3%) are of borderline intelligence (IQ 85–71). Among the remaining 22 children (31.4%) with varying degrees of mental retardation, there are 8 who, in a clinical sense, are severely or moderately mentally retarded but who were not amenable to any standardized intelligence test.

Clarren & Smith (1978) claimed in their review that, of 126 patients tested with standardized instruments, 107 (85%) scored more than 2 SD below the mean. However, a more careful re-analysis of the data published at that time that had been cited by these authors reveals that psychometric data had been available for only 52 of a total of 99 FAS patients. Among these patients 33 (63%) scored below IQ 80, and it is impossible to calculate accurately the number scoring more than 2 SD below the mean. However, despite these inaccuracies and the variations in IQ found in the different studies, there is sufficient evidence from psychometric studies that there is a disproportionately high incidence of mental retardation among FAS children.

There is also considerable agreement in various studies that the severity of morphological damage in FAS is an important correlate of intelligence. Thus, seriously damaged children have lower IQs than mildly impaired children (Streissguth *et al.*, 1978*a*; Iosub *et al.*, 1981; Majewski, 1981;

Table 12.3. *IQ scores of FAS patients*

Study	Country	*n*	Age range (years)	IQ Mean	IQ Range	IQ 70–85	IQ <70
Streissguth et al. (1991)	USA	52	12–40	68	20–105		58%
Steinhausen et al. (1982)	Germany	25 (32)[a]	3–15.3	89	57–133	22%	31%[a]
Iosub et al. (1981)	USA	30	>3		50–97		46%
Majewski (1981)	Germany	18	3.7–8.8	82	47–130		
Darby et al. (1981)	USA	8	1.2–6.8	76	40–107		
Olegard et al. (1979)	Sweden	48				40%	19%
Kyllerman et al. (1979)	Sweden	16		93.8			
Streissguth et al. (1978a)	USA	20	0.9–21	65	16–105		60%[b]

[a] Seven additional patients are included who were not testable due to severe mental retardation.
[b] According to the summary, raw data indicate up to 80%.

Steinhausen *et al.*, 1982*b*). However, our recent analyses showed that this relation is not strictly linear. As Fig. 12.3 shows, among our 70 FAS patients there are children with normal or borderline intelligence who show moderate or severe degrees of morphological damage. It may be speculated that within our group of patients with varying age at first assessment, age may be a confounding factor. Because of our finding that the characteristic dysmorphic features of FAS diminish with time, but mental retardation persists (Spohr *et al.*, 1993), it is possible that a more linear relation between severity of morphological damage and intelligence is prevented by age.

Only a few studies have assessed cognitive and neuropsychological functions other than intelligence in FAS children. Kyllerman *et al.* (1979) reported that their 16 children of a prospective series had significantly poorer performance than controls with regard to tests of perception and motor development. In our first studies (Steinhausen *et al.*, 1982*a, b*) German versions of the Frostig Test of Visual Perception (FTVP) and the Illinois Test of Psycholinguistic Abilities (ITPA) were employed. In a subsample of 22 FAS children aged 4–10 years, the mean score for visual perception (37.8 on the percentile scale, SD 33.9) was significantly lower than the population norm. Even more pronounced was the pattern of psycholinguistic impairment: 24 FAS children aged 3–9 years had decreased ITPA scores in 9 of 12 subscales compared with population norms.

Two more recent studies revealed further neuropsychological deficits in FAS children. Conry (1990) compared 19 school-age children with FAS or FAE with age- and sex-matched normal controls. Using a battery of intellectual and neuropsychological tests, it was shown that FAS children differed

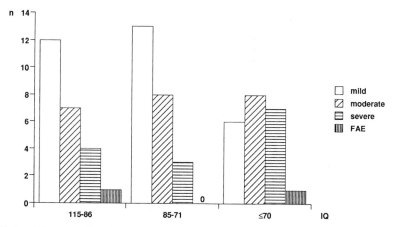

Fig. 12.3. The relation between intelligence and morphological damage at first assessment (*n* = 70).

significantly from controls. FAE children showed deficits compared with controls in only one test, whereas FAS children scored significantly lower on most measures. Nanson & Hiscock (1990) compared 20 children with FAS or FAE with 20 children with attention deficit disorder (ADD) and 20 normal controls on three experimental tasks designed to isolate four different components of attention. The study showed that, although the FAS/FAE children were significantly more impaired intellectually, their attentional problems were similar to those of ADD children. The authors speculate that the treatments known to facilitate learning in ADD children may also be beneficial to children with FAS/FAE.

Follow-up studies

Given the effects of intrauterine alcohol exposure, the question arises as to whether these effects persist over time or whether they might be mitigated through maturation or developmental factors, enriched environments, therapeutic measures, or an interaction of these factors. Furthermore, one might wonder whether all or just a proportion of children with FAS, or even only those children without dysmorphic features who had been prenatally exposed to alcohol, might improve over time. These are just some of the main questions that should be addressed by long-term follow-up studies.

The first follow-up reports were presented by the Seattle group of researchers. Streissguth *et al.* (1978b) gave follow-up IQ testing to 17 FAS patients 1–4 years after an initial evaluation. Mean IQ at the time of first testing was 66, and 67 at follow-up. The retest IQ was within 1 SD of the initial IQ scores in 77% of the sample. The 4 patients who did change did not show a consistent direction of change. There was some suggestion that apparent changes in individual IQ scores may be related to age testing. The scores of patients who were first tested at around 1 year appeared to decrease on retest, whereas the scores of patients who were first tested in the preschool years and who were retested while in primary school appeared to increase. Findings may be confounded by the fact that the different tests with different reliability and intercorrelations [i.e., the Bayley, the Stanford-Binet, the Wechsler Intelligence Scale for Children (WISC), the revised WISC (WISC-R), and the Wechsler Adult Intelligence Scale (WAIS)] form the basis of these comparisons.

Over the years, Streissguth and her associates in Seattle have continued to report on the course of FAS. In a further follow-up study they described the natural history of 11 patients who, 10 years ago, were the first to be diagnosed as having FAS (Streissguth *et al.*, 1985). At follow-up 2 former patients were dead and 1 was lost. Four of the 8 survivors were of borderline intelligence and the other 4 were severely mentally handicapped. There was a direct relation between the degree of handicap and the extent of craniofacial abnormalities in this small series.

In their study of FAS in adolescents and adults that is mentioned above, Streissguth *et al.* (1991) provide further insight into the long-term course of FAS into adulthood. The average IQ of their sample was in the range of mild retardation with extreme variation, as shown in Table 12.3, and average academic functioning was at the US second- to fourth-grade levels (ages 7–10). In terms of behavior, poor judgment, distractability, and difficulty perceiving social cues were common indicators of poor adaptation in this sample. The authors concluded that maladaptive behaviors present the greatest challenge to management in adulthood.

The stability of intelligence into mid-adolescence was assessed in the most recent report on the course of FAS by the Seattle group (Streissguth *et al.*, 1991). In 40 patients with FAS or FAE there were no significant differences in IQ scores across time. Both group means and individual IQ scores remained stable over an average test–retest interval of 8 years.

Our own group has also recently reported on the long-term outcome of a large cohort of FAS children (Steinhausen *et al.*, 1993). The study was based on a total of 158 FAS children ranging in age from 3 to 18 years. Within the entire sample only various subgroups were suitable for follow-up assessments because of changes of milieu, the scattered age pattern, and the age specificity of tests and assessments. Mean follow-up periods for the various subsamples ranged between 3 and 10 years. In this outcome study, structured psychiatric interviews for preschool and school-age children, standardized rating scales for parents and teachers, and age appropriate psychometric tests measuring intelligence were used.

The course of the psychiatric syndromes is shown in Fig. 12.4 by contrasting the findings from two of each of three assessment points. Here the findings from the first assessment are contrasted with persistent manifestations and new manifestations of psychiatric syndromes at follow-up. The top part of the figure demonstrates the course of the psychiatric syndromes from preschool into middle childhood. The following significant changes were observed. Whereas the leading diagnosis of hyperkinetic syndrome remains at about the same level, the rates increased for language disorders, sleep disorders, and tendentiously for abnormal habits and stereotypies as well as emotional disorders (anxiety and/or depression). The rates decrease for enuresis and tendentiously for eating disorders, too.

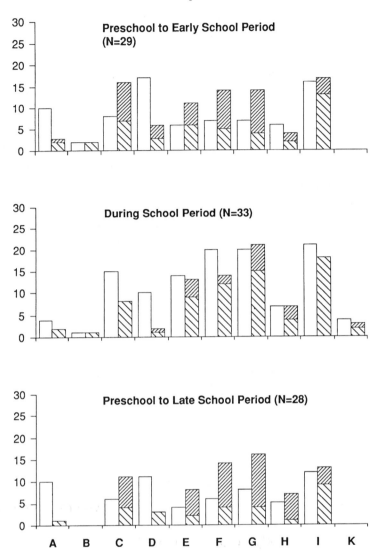

A = Enuresis
B = Enkopresis
C = Speech Disorders
D = Eating Disorders
E = Sleep Disorders

F = Habits/ Stereotypies
G = Emotional Disorders
H = Conduct Disorders
I = Hyperkinetic Disorders
K = Tics

☐ First assessment
◨ Reassessment: Persistent manifestations
▨ Reassessment: New manifestation

Fig. 12.4.   The course of psychiatric syndromes in three subsamples.

The analogous comparison of the psychiatric syndromes in the preschool period and in adolescence is presented in the middle part of Fig. 12.4. The pattern of the changes was quite comparable with those described above. There is a clear reduction of rates for enuresis and the eating disorders of early childhood, whereas there was an increase in the rate of stereotypies and a tendential increase for emotional disorders. Furthermore, it became evident that the respective manifestation of language disorders was clearly age related, especially when they were not persistent over time. Finally, the bottom part of Fig 12.4 shows the pattern of the course of psychiatric syndromes from middle childhood to adolescence. Here, too, the hyperkinetic disorders dominated, although emotional disorders as well as abnormal habits and stereotypies had similar rates of occurrence. There was, however, a clear decline in the rates for speech and language disorders and eating disorders.

In addition to the psychiatric interviews carried out with the caretakers of the children, we also asked the parents or the parent surrogates and the teachers to fill out standardized behavior checklists, i.e., the Child Behavior Check List (CBCL: Achenbach, 1978) and the Teacher Rating Form (TRF: Edelbrock & Achenbach, 1984). As evident in the long-term sample in Fig. 12.5, the profile from the parent questionnaire that was administered twice during the school-age period is characterized by peaks in the areas of attention deficit problems and social relationship problems. A decline in the scores on the scale for 'withdrawn' was the only change at follow-up. Fig. 12.5 also shows that the patterns of the follow-up profiles derived from the analogously constructed teacher questionnaire were almost identical at both follow-up assessments. There was no significant change on any of the eight scales. Here, too, both attention deficit problems and social relationship problems were most prominent.

In this longitudinal study we also obtained follow-up data on intelligence. Data on 70 FAS children at first assessment and at follow-up are compiled in Table 12.4. In 62 cases, data are based on psychometric tests. A further 8 cases were included where a clinical rating of moderate to severe and profound mental retardation was performed on the children because these patients were not amenable to intelligence testing. In this table persistent findings are represented in the diagonal, whereas improvement of mental functioning is presented in the lower triangle and deterioration of intelligence in the upper triangle. This organization of data clearly shows that the vast majority of FAS children do not change over time; their functioning remains in the same band of intelligence. There were very few children, namely 5, who improved over time, whereas 15 children deteriorated from first assessment to

CBCL

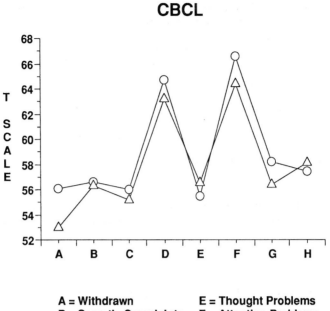

A = Withdrawn   E = Thought Problems
B = Somatic Complaints   F = Attention Problems
C = Anxious/Depressed   G = Delinquent Problems
D = Social Problems   H = Aggressive Behavior

TRF

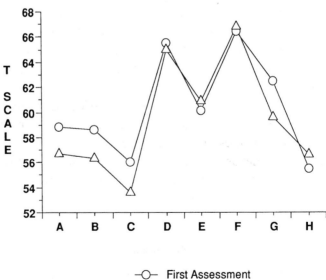

—O— First Assessment
—△— Follow-up

Fig. 12.5.   Profiles of a parent questionnaire (CBCL) and a teacher questionnaire
(TRF) at first examination and at follow-up.

Table 12.4. *Follow-up of intelligence assessment (n = 70)*

IQ	First assessment	Last assessment					
		115–86	85–71	70–51	50–36	35–21	< 20
115–86	Normal intelligence	19	4	1	—	—	—
85–71	Borderline intelligence	1	20	2	1	—	—
70–51	Mild mental retardation	—	3	6	2	—	—
50–36	Moderate mental retardation	—	—	—	2	1	—
35–21	Severe mental retardation	—	—	—	1	2	4
< 20	Profound mental retardation	—	—	—	—	—	1

follow-up. Because different tests had to be used for the various ages, changes in IQ scores may to some extent be due to problems in measurement.

In summary, our follow-up study shows that a number of psychiatric disorders persisted over time, namely hyperkinetic disorders and – especially during school age – emotional disorders, sleep disorders, and abnormal habits and stereotypies. The more age-specific disorders such as enuresis, encopresis, and eating disorders remitted over time, whereas conduct disorders had a similar frequency over time due to a mixed pattern of remissions and new manifestation. Parent and teacher questionnaires described attention deficits as the leading problems – a fact that is in good agreement with the interview findings of hyperkinetic disorders as the most prominent psychiatric syndrome. Both parents and teachers considered social relationship problems as the second most frequent deficit. There was a remarkable consistency in the rating of these two sources both at first assessment and at follow-up. Finally, the devastating effects of intrauterine exposure to alcohol were shown both by the high proportion of mentally handicapped children and by the stability of intelligence over time.

Conclusions

This chapter summarizes current knowledge on the mental development, psychopathology and behavior, cognitive functioning and long-term developmental outcome of FAS children. The summary was based on studies performed in various countries including our own longitudinal project, which followed a considerable number of FAS children. It has been shown that the affected children are subject to varying degrees of developmental handicaps. Intrauterine exposure to alcohol due to maternal alcoholism not only results in a specific dysmorphic syndrome but, perhaps even more importantly, in behavioral symptoms and cognitive impairment that have a limiting effect on successful life adaptation.

These limitations are obvious from the beginning of life. Immediately after birth a chain of developmental hazards starts to unfold. The most obvious signs are various medical complications and developmental delays. A considerable number of FAS children start to develop psychiatric symptoms at an early age. Both during preschool and school age, a great variety of disorders can be observed. Although hyperactivity and attention deficit are common problems, psychopathology is not restricted to these core symptoms. The pattern is more widespread and age dependent. In the preschool period, eating disorders, enuresis, speech delay, and stereotypies play an additional role. Later, during early school age, some of these problems such as speech delay and stereotypies are even more common. New problems such as a high prevalence of anxiety or sleep disorders emerge now. In addition, the enormous variety of symptoms and the high prevalence for any psychopathology is impressive: in our own extended sample 63% of the FAS children were psychiatrically abnormal. This means that these children were suffering from either a single or (more commonly) more than one psychiatric disorder.

However, there is a considerable variation both in behavior or psychopathology and in cognitive functioning. Sadly, there is sufficient evidence from various studies that severity of morphological damage, psychopathology, and mental retardation tend to coincide in a subgroup of severely affected FAS children who often come from extremely deprived backgrounds that include chronic maternal alcoholism and very often also paternal alcoholism. Currently, no study has tried to disentangle the effects of the teratogenic and the environmental risk factors on the child's development. Whereas this may prove to be extremely difficult for scientific analyses, there are some hints from the longitudinal studies that even a stimulating environment with sensitive adoptive or foster parents or a good institution may not be sufficient to compensate for the deleterious effects of prenatal damage due to alcohol exposure.

Although mental retardation and cognitive deficits are extremely overrepresented among FAS children it should not be overlooked that there is a wide variation of mental functioning. A considerable proportion of these children function normally and obtain age-appropriate grade levels at school. Interestingly, our own recent analyses, in contrast to other reports, no longer show a linear relation between degree of morphological damage and intelligence. As speculated above, this relation may level off with increasing age or reflect the fact that dysmorphic features may be a relatively crude measure of morphological damage, especially of the brain. More sensitive measures based, for example, on neuro-imaging techniques, may better serve this purpose and reveal new insights in the future.

Finally, extended follow-up studies show that many FAS children, due to persisting mental impairment and psychiatric disorder, continue to be problematic during adolescence and even young adulthood. The chain of developmental impairments starting early in life progresses into later life and causes serious problems for management and life adaptation. A considerable proportion of these patients remain dependent on support from a caring environment, that is, at home, in the school, and in the society at large. Other chapters in this volume deal with these important tasks of environmental interventions and rehabilitation of FAS patients.

References

Achenbach, T.M. (1978). The Child Behavior Profile. I. Boys aged 6–11. *Journal of Consulting and Clinical Psychology*, **46**, 478–88.

Bierich, J.R., Majewski, F., Michaelis, R. & Tilner, I. (1976). Das embryofetale Alkoholsyndrom. *European Journal of Pediatrics*, **121**, 155–77.

Clarren, S.K. & Smith, D.W. (1978). The fetal alcohol syndrome: experience with 65 patients and a review of the world literature. *New England Journal of Medicine*, **298**, 1063–7.

Conry, J. (1990). Neuropsychological deficits in fetal alcohol syndrome and fetal alcohol effects. *Alcoholism: Clinical and Experimental Research*, **14**, 650–5.

Darby, B.L., Streissguth, A.P. & Smith, D.W. (1981). A preliminary follow-up of 8 children diagnosed fetal alcohol syndrome in infancy. *Neurobehavioral Toxicology and Teratology*, **3**, 157–259.

Dehaene, P., Titran, M., Samaille-Vilette, C., Samaille, P.P., Crépin, G., Delahousse, G., Walbaum, R. & Fasquelle, P. (1977). Frèquence du syndrome d'alcoolisme foetal. *Nouvelle Press Médicale*, **6**, 1763–8.

Edelbrock, C. & Achenbach, T.M. (1984). The teacher version of the Child Behavior Profile. I. Boys aged 6–12. *Journal of Consulting and Clinical Psychology*, **52**, 207–17.

Hermier, M., Leclercq, F., Duc, H., David, L. & Francois, R. (1976). Le nanisme intrautérin avec débilité mentale et malformations dans le cadre de l'embryofoetopathie alcoolique: à propos de quatre cas. *Pediatrie*, **31**,749–62.

Iosub, S., Fuchs, M., Bingol, N. & Gromisch, D.S. (1981). Fetal alcohol syndrome revisited. *Pediatrics*, **68**, 475–9.

Jones, K.L. & Smith, D.W. (1973). Recognition of the fetal alcohol syndrome in early infancy. *Lancet*, **ii**, 999–1001.

Kyllerman, M., Aronsson, A., Karlberg, E., Olegard, R., Sabel, K.-G., Sandin, J., Johansson, P.R., Carlsson, C. & Iversen, K. (1979). Epidemiologic and neuropediatric aspects of the fetal alcohol syndrome. *Neuropädiatrie*, Supplement *10*, 435–6.

Lemoine, P., Harousseau, H., Boteyru, J.P. & Menuet, J.C. (1968). Les enfant des parents alcooliques: anomalies observées à propos de 127 cas. *Quest Médicale*, **25**, 476–82.

Majewski, F. (1981). Alcohol embryopathy: some facts and speculations about pathogenesis. *Neurobehavioral Toxicology and Teratology*, **3**, 129–44.

Majewski, F. & Majewski, B. (1988). Alcohol embryopathy: symptoms, auxological data, frequency among the offspring and pathogenesis. In , pp. 837–44. Amsterdam: Excerpta Medica.

Nanson, J.L. & Hiscock, M. (1990). Attention deficits in children exposed to alcohol prenatally. *Alcoholism: Clinical and Experimental Research*, **14**, 656–61.

Olegard, R., Sabel, K.-G., Aronsson, M., Sandin, B., Johansson, P.R., Carlsson, C., Kyllerman, M., Iversen, K. & Hrbek, A. (1979). Effects on the child of alcohol abuse during pregnancy. *Acta Psychiatrica Scandinavica Supplement*, **275**, 112–21.

Shaywitz, S.E., Cohen, D.J. & Shaywitz, B.A. (1980). Behavior and learning difficulties in children of normal intelligence born to alcoholic mothers. *Journal of Pediatrics*, **96**, 978–82.

Spohr, H.-L., Willms, J. & Steinhausen, H.-C. (1993). Prenatal alcohol exposure and long-term developmental consequences: a 10-year follow-up of 60 children with fetal alcohol syndrome (FAS). *Lancet*, **341**, 907–10.

Steinhausen, H.-C. (1995). Children of alcoholic parents. *European Child and Adolescent Psychiatry*, **4**, 143–52.

Steinhausen, H.-C., Nestler, V. & Huth, H. (1982a). Psychopathology and mental functions in the offspring of alcoholic and epileptic mothers. *Journal of the American Academy of Child and Adolescent Psychiatry*, **21**, 268–73.

Steinhausen, H.-C., Nestler, V. & Spohr, H.-L. (1982b). Development and psychopathology of children with the fetal alcohol syndrome. *Journal of Developmental and Behavioral Pediatrics*, **3**, 49–53.

Steinhausen, H.-C., Willms, J. & Spohr, H.-L. (1993). Long-term psychopathological and cognitive outcome of children with fetal alcohol syndrome. *Journal of the American Academy of Child and Adolescent Psychiatry*, **32**, 990–4.

Steinhausen, H.-C., Willms, J. & Spohr, H.-L. (1994). Correlates of psychopathology and intelligence in children with fetal alcohol syndrome. *Journal of Child Psychology and Psychiatry and Allied Disciplines*, **35**, 323–31.

Streissguth, A.P., Aase, J.M., Clarren, S.K., Randels, S.P., La Due, R.A. & Smith, D.F. (1991). Fetal alcohol syndrome in adolescents and adults. *JAMA*, **265**, 1961–67.

Streissguth, A.P., Clarren, S.K. & Jones, K.L. (1985). Natural history of the fetal alcohol syndrome: a 10-year follow-up of eleven patients. *Lancet*, **ii**, 85–92.

Streissguth, A.P., Herman, C.S. & Smith, D.W. (1978a). Intelligence, behavior and dysmorphogenesis in the fetal alcohol syndrome: a report on 20 patients. *Journal of Pediatrics*, **92**, 363–7.

Streissguth, A.P., Herman, C.S. & Smith, D.W. (1978b). Stability of intelligence in the fetal alcohol syndrome: a preliminary report. *Alcoholism: Clinical and Experimental Research*, **2**, 165–70.

Streissguth, A.P., Randels, S.P. & Smith, D.F. (1991). A test–retest study of intelligence in patients with fetal alcohol syndrome: implications for care. *Journal of the American Academy of Child and Adolescent Psychiatry*, **30**, 584–7.

Part IV

Intervention

13

Rehabilitation approaches for fetal alcohol syndrome

BARBARA A. MORSE AND LYN WEINER

Introduction

Alcohol's capacity adversely to affect pregnancy outcome is well documented. Several thousand clinical and experimental studies have reported somatic and neurological problems in children of women who drank heavily during pregnancy. Yet, beyond the recognized clinical and diagnostic features, little has been reported on the development of children with fetal alcohol syndrome (FAS) or fetal alcohol effects (FAE). Few studies have reported intervention strategies and no specific therapeutic protocols have been systematically investigated among children with FAS. This lack of information frustrates caregivers and parents and impedes provision of appropriate treatment. Clinical issues have become increasingly important to the community at large, although most research has addressed mechanisms of damage. While experimental studies should ultimately benefit clinicians, the immediate needs of families with FAS and FAE demand a comprehensive look at systematic intervention and treatment. Development of strategies for intervention begins with an understanding of the unique needs of affected children.

Central nervous system deficits in FAS

For children, families, and educators struggling with FAS/FAE, abnormalities of the brain and central nervous system (CNS) pose the greatest challenge. FAS/FAE manifests itself in a broad range of effects with a considerable amount of variability in the behavioral, psychological and cognitive deficits (Rosett & Weiner, 1984). Epidemiological studies and case reports demonstrate that CNS problems can include hyperactivity, diminished intelligence, learning disabilities, inappropriate or unusual social behaviors, delays in speech and language, poor eating and sleeping patterns, impaired hearing, longer reaction time and delayed developmental milestones (Rosett & Weiner, 1984; Streissguth, 1986; Nanson & Hiscock, 1990). Many of these problems are evident even in children with FAS who have normal intelligence.

Lemoine *et al.* described these behaviors in 1968, and they have been noted repeatedly in subsequent reports. Observations by individual clinicians suggest additional behavioral concerns, including failure to learn from mistakes, lack of judgment, lack of remorse for misbehavior, lying, immature behaviors, persistent sleeplessness, extreme mood changes, unusual aggressiveness or physical strength and wide variation in learning abilities at different times.

The aberrant behaviors of these children give an illusion of 'purposefulness'. For example, they may remember the alphabet one day but have forgotten it the next. Parents report frequent lying, but done in such a way that the lie is transparent. This leads to the impression that children with FAS are naughty, devious, lazy, willfully disobedient, or otherwise intractable.

Some children have subtle problems; others are so severely affected that they cannot function in the community. The average IQ is reported to be 70, with a range from 45 to 110. According to estimates from the Centers for Disease Control, more than 45% of children with FAS have IQs greater than 85. Yet the literature has consistently reported on only the most severely affected children and outcomes predicted for all children with FAS have been based on these extreme cases. Obstacles to intervention include the lack of an adequate description of children with mild and moderate FAS and an assumption that children with the diagnosis of FAS are beyond help. Affected children are often described as lacking conscience and prone to criminal activity. Such dire predictions have failed to consider the enormous heterogeneity of the population or the possible benefits of targeted intervention strategies.

Outcomes among children with FAS

No intervention

The earliest reports described outcomes over time among children with FAS who were not offered systematic interventions. Most were case studies of children who had been referred to research centers having received a diagnosis of FAS from their primary providers. The age at which the children were evaluated varied from infancy to adolescence. Few of these studies employed a control population. Nonetheless, they provided a preliminary understanding of the development of children with FAS.

In a group of 20 children with FAS ranging in age from 9 months to 21 years, Streissguth and colleagues (1978) found that intelligence scores remained stable 1–4 years after the first testing. Mean IQs were similar; 77% of the patients scored within 1 SD of their initial IQ. There were, however, 4 children who showed considerable change on retest. There was no consistent direction of change; 2 manifested a decrease greater than 1 SD, and 2 had an increase. Neither original IQ scores nor home environment explained the change.

Spohr & Steinhausen (1984) evaluted children with FAS at two points in time. The severity of morphological damage and the total number of malformations were less apparent over time. There was a catch-up growth (head size, weight, and height) as well as improvement in electroencephalogram recordings. Four years after diagnosis, fewer children were receiving care for a number of symptoms including eating problems, clumsiness, impaired concentration, negative mood and phobias. Improvement observed in some of the children was associated with a positive home environment. However, children were not normal in all psychiatric areas. Hyperactivity and distractibility remained major handicaps to academic achievement. An increase in IQ score was seen in children who initially scored between 70 and 115. The most severely dysmorphic children had lasting retardation which did not respond to rehabilitative measures.

A later follow-up of 158 children ranging in age from newborn to 11.5 years showed a high rate of psychiatric disorders, with almost two-thirds of the children having at least one problem (Steinhausen *et al.*, 1993, 1994). Most common psychiatric disorders which persisted included hyperkinetic disorders, emotional disturbances, sleep disorders, abnormal habits, and stereotypies. Age-specific disorders, such as enuresis and encopresies, remitted over time. Parents and teachers reported attention deficit disorders and problems with social relationships. The severity of the psychopathology was related to morphological damage and was predicted by the amount of alcohol exposure *in utero*. Children who were most severely damaged were living in institutions and had the highest total psychopathology score.

Aronson & Olegard (1987) observed uneven developmental profiles in children exposed to alcohol *in utero*. Hand and eye coordination, form perception and concept formation were impaired. Severely disturbed visual and/ or auditory perception was found in the majority of children. Difficulties in interpreting sensory input resulted in insecurity and low self-confidence. Learning was further complicated by hyperactivity. There was also a high

frequency of attention deficit and perseveration. A stable environment did
not eliminate mental and perceptual problems but did seem to improve the
outcome, especially in interpersonal skills and social development.

These early, descriptive studies laid the foundation for future investigations. However, as they provided no interventions, these reports fuelled the
belief that FAS was an irremediable condition for which there was little hope.
Improvement was viewed as random, and targeted intervention seemed unlikely to provide significant benefit.

Interventions not specific to FAS

Interventions to help maximize the potential of children with FAS have been
reported in a few early pilot programs. Bierich (1978) observed that learning
ability and other mental functions were inhibited by restlessness, an inability
to concentrate and a lack of initiative. Long-term occupational therapy
reduced hyperexcitability among moderately affected children and enabled
them to advance. External structure and concrete cues were necessary to
compensate for the lack of internal control. Koranyi & Csiky (1978) reported
that medical and educational intervention alleviated some symptoms among
5 children with FAS (age 2–13 years) although normalcy was not reached.
Interventions developed for other handicapped children were helpful to children with FAS. They concluded that symptomatology can be altered by
socioeconomic conditions, maternal–infant interactions, and medical care.

W.A. Zaleski (personal communication 1984) conducted an early intervention program in which one group of 14 preschool children born to alcoholic
women was provided with intensive early intervention while another group
received support but no specific program. On retesting after 6 months, the
children in the intensive program showed significant gains in intelligence as
compared with the controls, although IQ levels were not reported. One focus
of the program was teaching parents techniques to stimulate their children at
home.

In Massachusetts, children with FAS were compared with other children
enrolled in the Massachusetts early intervention programs between 1985 and
1987 (Weiner & Morse, 1988). These statewide programs provide therapeutic
services to children aged from birth to 3 years who have, or are at risk for,
developmental delay. Among the 6831 children served in this time period,
there were 34 with a diagnosis of FAS (0.5%). Analysis compared the occurrence of specific medical problems and the prevalence of functional and
family problems for which treatment was provided.

At admission to the early intervention program, children with FAS were significantly more likely to have three or more physiological problems than were other developmentally delayed children (46% vs 9%). They also exhibited more problems in gross and fine motor ability, expressive language, and social skills. Families with an FAS child differed significantly from other families with at-risk children on the following demographic variables: annual income below $10 000, unemployed parents, protective services, foster family, four or more children, substance abuse, and ethnicity (black/non-black). Children with FAS lived in families with five or more of these characteristics significantly more often than other at-risk children.

At discharge from the program, the total number of reported functional, familial, and diagnosed problems for children with FAS was significantly greater than for other at-risk children. Program staff reported that they perceived children with FAS to have unique problems compared with other children in the population which they served and that many of these problems did not respond to general intervention strategies.

From these studies it is clear that early intervention can benefit some children with FAS, consistent with our understanding of neural plasticity and developmental improvement. However, in the absence of knowledge about the CNS deficits which are specific to FAS, development of targeted intervention strategies could not progress beyond this point.

Interventions specific to FAS

Identification of CNS impairments

Recent studies suggest specific impairments in children with FAS/FAE. Brown *et al.* (1991) reported that 25 school-age children exposed to alcohol throughout gestation showed deficits in their ability to sustain attention and had more behavioral problems as assessed by teacher and parent versions of the Child Behavior Checklist. There were, moreover, distinctions between children with FAS and those with classic attention deficit, hyperactivity disorder (ADHD), most notably in a low level of impulsivity. In addition, the pattern of errors on the vigilance task was not typical of hyperactive children. The alcohol-exposed children had a higher number of errors due to omissions rather than commissions. This finding is characteristic of children with mild neurological impairments. Outcomes related to internalizing behaviors (depression and withdrawal) were related more strongly to current maternal alcohol use than to prenatal exposure.

Kodituwakku *et al.* (1992) reported that children with FAS (mean age 13 years) had significant deficits in flexible problem solving, regulating behavior, and planning and utilizing feedback. These researchers also reported a pattern of deficits in mental manipulation of information in working memory in 10 non-mentally-retarded children with FAS (Kodituwakku *et al.*, 1994). Don *et al.* (1993) found that a group of young adults with FAS (mean age 19 years) and IQs greater than 86 showed a lower than average slope of learning but a good rate of retention. Tasks requiring mental control and efficient processing were difficult. Traditional academic and intellectual testing did not fully reflect these cognitive disabilities.

Sensory processing has also been identified as a specific deficit for FAS (Morse & Cermak, 1994). Children with FAS/FAE demonstrated significantly greater problems with touch, movement, visual and auditory stimuli and taste/smell when compared with a control group. The behavioral manifestations of poor sensory processing (activity levels, organization, social skills, feeding and sleep) were also greater.

Experimental research suggests mechanisms that underlie some of the behavioral problems. Behaviors and specific sites of damage have been correlated – for example, learning and memory deficits with the hippocampus, and motor control with the cerebellum (Riley, 1990; West *et al.*, 1990). In pilot studies, Mattson & Riley (1994) linked decreased volume of basal ganglia in children exposed to large doses of alcohol during gestation with impaired implicit memory in procedural learning. (For a lengthy discussion on this topic see Bond & West, this volume).

Clinical and experimental studies as well as observations of clinicians, parents and teachers have established a commonality and uniqueness to the problems seen in FAS. It is important to note that children with FAS are not all alike. The range of severity varies widely; no one child will have all the problems which have been reported. However, as a group, children with FAS display unique developmental and behavioral problems. Specific interventions, targeted to identified needs, should be the most effective strategies (Weiner & Morse, 1991, 1994). Early intervention has been successful in improving developmental outcome among children with other disorders such as Down syndrome (Hayden & Haring, 1976; Bricker, 1978). However, to date there have been no systematic investigations of effective interventions for FAS. Parent reports (from hot-line calls, newsletters, support groups) and a recently published book by Kleinfeld & Westcott (1993) on experiences educating children with FAS are currently the best source of effective techniques for addressing many of the problems associated with FAS. These strategies, developed independently by parents and teachers, are consistent with the research findings and reflect many of the basic under-standings of the problems encountered by these children (Morse & Weiner, 1993). They acknowledge the centrality of the dysfunctional CNS in children with FAS. Those parents and teachers who have used these intervention techniques were able to see growth and improvement in children previously considered unlikely to improve (Kleinfeld & Westcott, 1993).

For optimal development, early educational intervention with individual instruction in a consistent and supportive environment is required. While severely affected children may experience only slight improvement, the majority will benefit from targeted strategies utilizing existing knowledge about learning disabilities and other developmental disorders.

Strategies

The environment

The intervention technique most commonly recommended by professionals and parents is to structure the environment to facilitate a child's functional behavior. This principle is crucial to the classroom environment, although it can be used in other settings as well. Tanner-Halverson (1993) suggests orga-nizing the environment, defining work and play areas. Work spaces should be kept clear and free of distraction; materials not currently being used should be out of sight. Visual and pictorial cues in the immediate view of the child should not be simply decorative, but used as reminders about classroom activities only.

Hinde (1993) also encourages parents to structure the home environment. In her experience, parents are the most important factors for success in working with children birth to 3 years. Parents must alter their lifestyles and make changes as children with FAS are often unable to make adapta-tions themselves. Parents also need to provide a positive atmosphere, identi-fying skill strengths in their child and building on those skills. Hinde suggests task analysis (breaking down each desired behavior into small steps, and teaching/rewarding each step) as a successful teaching method.

Children with FAS respond well to a highly consistent routine, including the behavior and responses of people in the child's world. For example, the same activities should occur at the same time each day. Children benefit from having assigned seats in school which do not change during the year. When changes in schedule or set-up need to occur, advance preparation eases the transition. Following experiences of her son in four different educational programs, Caldwell (1993) delineated his need for consistency. The goal of successful programs was to teach and problem solve, but not to punish. In programs where the activities varied widely from day to day, her son misbehaved and achieved little. He was also reluctant to attend these programs. In the classrooms that were consistent, her son thrived and behaved appropriately. She identified the keys to his success as:

1. Teachers who were explicit, consistent and used preventive discipline.
2. Visual aids and class arrangement which reinforced class rules and activities.
3. Program routine which varied little from day to day.
4. Techniques designed to empower, not intimidate, children.

> Getting dressing in the wrong clothes was a constant source of friction between John and his mother. The difference between school clothes and play clothes was so clear to her. It wasn't until she recognized that John couldn't see this difference that she came up with a solution. She put all of John's playclothes in the dresser and his school clothes in the closet. She provided a further visual reminder by putting a picture of play activities on the dresser drawers and a picture of school activities on the closet door. John learned the new system quickly and the problem was solved.

Sleep patterns

Sleep disturbances, which occur commonly, have been reported to have a physiological component. Infants born to women who drank heavily throughout pregnancy experienced more interruptions in quiet sleep and were less apt to develop night/day sleep cycles (Sander *et al.*, 1977). Techniques to regulate and calm infants and help them go back to sleep on their own included swaddling and dark and quiet rest areas. The sleep disturbances are believed to persist well into childhood, and may be helped through consistent bedtime routines, the use of white noise in a bedroom, snug bedclothes, and sensory integration therapy.

> Henry is a 9-year-old adopted child who was diagnosed with FAS at birth. His sleep patterns have been consistently poor, and include difficulty falling asleep, easy wakenings, wandering around the house at night and waking parents. His parents tried multiple strategies without success, from punishment to allowing him to sleep on their bedroom floor. Improvement was seen when traditional sheets and blankets were replaced with a mummy-type sleeping bag which enveloped him tightly. In addition, his parents placed a fan in the room to mask general household noises. They gave Henry a headset and a tape of relaxing sounds (i.e., ocean waves) to help him get to sleep. These combined efforts improved both Henry's sleep and his general functioning during the day.

Eating problems

Infants with FAS may present feeding problems due to neuromuscular delays or anatomical abnormalities. Failure to thrive is a common concern. Older children may eat little and gain weight slowly. Hypersensitivity to the feeling of food or utensils in their mouths can cause children to play with food in their fingers or to chew over and over without swallowing. Success can be achieved by allowing ample time to eat, having reasonable expectations on portion size, and carefully controlling temperature and texture of foods. Reducing distractions (particularly for infants) may also improve intake.

> Sally, a 4-year-old with FAS, had severe eating problems. She weighed only 10 kg. Some days she refused food altogether. At other times, she put food in her mouth but did not swallow it. Sally's pediatrician revised weight gain estimates for her to a more realistic goal of 1 kg per year. This enabled her parents to relax more about her eating and be less concerned about Sally's position on growth charts. Sally received sensory integration therapy focusing on the oral cavity to improve her tolerance for foods of varying textures and temperature. Her parents lengthened meal times and offered frequent, small portions. At Sally's preschool program, they gave her half her lunch at morning snack and the remainder at lunch time. The combination of these strategies have led to an overall improvement in her eating and a resulting weight gain of 1.2 kg in 1 year.

Sensory processing

Children with FAS often demonstrate exaggerated responses to sensory input, another example of the disorganized CNS. The brain's inability to control and sort sensory information can easily overwhelm the child with FAS. This disorder contributes to feeding, sleeping, activity, learning, and behavioral problems. Children may be misperceived as aggressive when they strike back after being accidentally bumped. In some cases it may contribute to an inappropriate diagnosis of psychosis in children who seek sensory stimulation through body rocking, touching others, or tearing bits of paper into tiny shreds. It may also contribute to difficulty in achieving bladder and bowel control as sensations remain unrecognized.

Children have several common behavioral responses to sensory overload. They may perseverate (repeating words, actions and thoughts), shut down, throw temper tantrums or become frustrated. Interventions to minimize sensory processing problems include reducing all stimulation for a period of time and using calming techniques. Modifying the environment to reduce intrusive sensations includes loose clothing to lessen the pressure at waists, wrists and ankles, sunglasses to reduce glare of lights, and avoiding crowds and jostling.

Sitting in a bean bag chair, rocker, or hammock, taking a warm bath or shower, or listening to quiet music over headphones can help a child refocus.

Sensory integration therapy which focuses on helping the brain adapt to tactile, auditory, visual and kinesthetic stimuli is helpful for long-term therapy and should be initiated as soon after birth as possible. For the older child, Murphy (1993) recommends planning teaching activities to prevent mental or physical overstimulation, such as ensuring that reading occurs in a quiet room.

> John is a 13-year-old child with FAS whose behaviors at home and school are becoming increasingly disruptive. He often changes clothing several times, complaining that the 'pants give me a stomach ache' or 'the sock hurts my foot.' He refuses to comb his hair or brush his teeth. He is negligent about using toilet paper. He is considered aggressive at school, hitting other children who may touch or bump him. He often complains that things are 'too loud' or that the 'lights are too bright'. Physical guidance from the teacher (such as a hand on the shoulder) is met with anger, yet he may ask to sit on the teacher's lap or stroke her clothing.
>
> John was identified as having multiple sensory processing problems affecting his behavior and his ability to learn. Through therapy and work with a sensory integration specialist, several strategies were employed. His mother removed all stiff, scratchy, tight clothing from his wardrobe and replaced it with soft, knit fabrics, including socks without seams in the toe. Substituting commercial baby diaper wipes for toilet paper resolved this problem. To reduce his aggressive responses in the classroom, the teacher seated him in an area where other children would not bump him. His parents provided a bean-bag chair for the classroom, giving John a comforting space to go when he needed to calm down. When the lights bother him, he may wear sunglasses. If the teacher is going to touch him, she tells him first, to allow him to prepare. She also gives him advance preparation for any changes in the schedule. To meet his need for tactile stimulation, John keeps two very smooth rocks in his pocket. These strategies have greatly reduced John's behavior problems and improved his ability to learn.

Learning problems

Difficulties with learning may be associated with organizational and processing deficits in the areas of input, integration, memory and output. Memory and retrieval difficulties contribute to the perception that children are willful or lazy. In addition, learning often occurs in 'spurts,' with apparently easy periods followed by difficult ones. This contributes to the notion that children are able to choose when they want to learn and when they do not.

Many of the techniques for learning and using information which underlie traditional teaching are unavailable to children with FAS. Thus even the most basic skills (e.g., distinguishing friends from strangers) must be carefully taught. Winick (1993) has demonstrated that role-playing can be effective in teaching children with FAS how to understand consequences and appropriate behavior. By allowing children to act out various parts in a situation, appropriate responses may become internalized in a way they cannot with simple instruction or observation. Phillpot & Harrison (1993) modify this technique and emphasize that children should be encouraged to find strategies of their own to improve memory and learning. When the child is able to suggest a strategy, she may be able to use it better than one which is imposed on her.

As our understanding of the disabilities of FAS improves, the approach to teaching also changes. Rather than relying on standard teaching methods which emphasize visual and auditory learning, context-specific learning environments, visual and kinesthetic activity-based methods and creative, flexible strategies become more important. Children with FAS often have difficulty generalizing information from the situation in which they learned it to another one. Cues, which help most people identify appropriate context, are often missed. Utilizing all the senses for learning, rather than just the visual and auditory systems, increases the likelihood of successful input. Visual information (picture, charts) should back up all spoken information. Facilitated communication (microphone on the teacher, headphones on the child) may improve focus and concentration. Compensatory plans can be developed to remove or diminish learning barriers – for example, providing a typewriter or computer for the child whose fine motor skills impede his progress.

Mark's IQ score was 103, but his academic achievement was poor. He had difficulty retaining what he had learned. Assignments and tests never were completed.

Working as a team, Mark's parents and teachers determined that he learned best if he could hear the material repeated many times. They placed a small tape recorder on his desk so that he could replay the day's lessons and assignments. They also created a pictorial chart for his schoolwork so Mark could check-off for himself when he competed his work. When possible, the teacher would ask Mark to answer test questions orally, because it is difficult for him to write, even if he knows the answer. The teacher has also learned to be more patient with Mark, understanding that he is trying hard, but that some days are more difficult for him than others.

Social skills

Children with FAS often appear socially inappropriate, unable to consider the consequences of their actions and unresponsive to subtle non-verbal cues (gestures, facial expressions, tone of voice). Distinctions between public and private behavior may be blurred. While perceived as behavior problems, these reflect a learning disability. Social skills may be improved through careful, repetitive and concrete teaching of appropriate behavior. Clear, consistent, and immediate rewards help reinforce positive behaviors. Rewards and punishments should be clearly linked to the desired behaviors, e.g., children who throw food should help clean the spill rather than be deprived of favorite activities. Changes in routine and transitions should be explained well in advance, with role playing or practice sessions used to ease the adjustment. Some parents have found that video-taping appropriate and inappropriate behavior is a useful way to teach social skills.

> Eight-year-old Jill's inability to make and keep friends left her feeling lonely and depressed. After one or two visits, other children refused to come back or teased her. Several times she told her mother that she wished she could die. To help her daughter, Jill's mother started by including one other child in a brief excursion to get an ice cream cone or do an errand. She gradually lengthened the excursion and had the other child come home with Jill for an hour of play. These trips were planned for weekend afternoons, when Jill was less likely to be overtired or over-stimulated from school. Jill's mother stayed nearby to monitor the play   at first, but moved away as Jill's social skills improved. She also volunteered to be a Girl Scout troop leader, providing Jill with a controlled, small group experience.

Steps towards improving treatment

In the field of developmental psychology, there is a general understanding that early intervention and a facilitating environment can help to maximize every child's potential, no matter what the problem. Providing intervention early in life capitalizes on the brain's plasticity and capacity for adaptation. Early intervention also increases the likelihood that delays will be identified before they become major problems, and therefore remediation can be more effective. The ability to provide early intervention is predicated on at least two premises: (1) that diagnosis is made efficiently and accurately; and (2) that the nature of the disability is well enough understood that targeted, effective interventions can be designed. These are two weak areas within the field of study for FAS. To date, most of the intervention strategies are based on anecdotal clinical reports or small pilot studies.

While systematic evaluation is conducted to determine which strategies are effective, several steps can improve intervention and treatment now.

Pediatrician's role

Diagnosis of FAS is the important first step in linking children with appropriate intervention strategies. But the diagnosis remains elusive and rate of diagnosis varies with the individual physician and within some populations. As there are no biochemical tests to confirm FAS, diagnosis is based on the clinical judgment of the examiner (Morse & Weiner, 1995). Assessment is difficult in the newborn period when CNS anomalies cannot be documented and facial dysmorphology may not yet be obvious. Difficulty in making the diagnosis is further exacerbated by the lack of a single uniform response to alcohol exposure. Variability of effects will also be seen due to individual differences in children. It is important to remember that all the reported problems may not be the result of alcohol exposure but may be associated with other risk factors, genetics and maternal illnesses. As the child grows, environmental factors may also influence development.

A survey of pediatricians in Massachusetts demonstrated that while knowledge of FAS is high, clinicians feel unprepared to deal with the issues (Morse *et al.*, 1992). More had suspected FAS/FAE than had made the diagnosis. In some settings, physicians are reluctant to give a diagnosis which is seen as little more than a pejorative label with few perceived benefits. Physicians express a reluctance to make a diagnosis unless there is an established treatment protocol. In the absence of specific therapeutic modalities, FAS is treated as a generalized CNS disorder. This often means children do not benefit as fully as they might from early intervention strategies. An additional impediment to the diagnosis is the poor description of problems which children with FAS manifest. With a few exceptions, the literature has been content to reiterate the problems which were identified initially. There has also been an emphasis on the most severely affected children (who represent only 10–20% of those affected) and a neglect of the more subtle problems of the majority. When a physician is suspicious about the diagnosis of FAS in a patient, he or she often has only this literature as a reference. If the child does not fit the severity represented, the diagnosis of FAS may be inappropriately discarded. Conversely, an incomplete understanding of FAS can lead to the diagnosis being over-used. In some clinics, as many as two-thirds of the children referred for a confirmation of FAS were found to have other, non-alcohol-related developmental problems (J.L. Nanson, personal communication 1993).

When children are undiagnosed or inaccurately diagnosed, or when there is a misunderstanding of FAS, inappropriate school placement often results. Children with FAS have been incorrectly labelled as emotionally disturbed, or placed in special education classes when they could function in regular classrooms. Others need special services and are denied them. Their inconsistent responses and behavioral problems mask their educational needs, making it difficult to assess whether they require special classes. Many school systems base service eligibility on IQ scores, eliminating children with IQs above 69. Children with FAS often have IQ scores above 69 but have severe CNS disorders which render them unable to use their intelligence effectively. Neurobehavioral disorders are misidentified as bad or malicious behavior, compromising appropriate intervention. In addition, teachers lack guidance and protocols to address the unique problems of FAS. There also remains a stigma to the diagnosis of FAS, further compromising effective intervention.

Accurate identification of children who have FAS will lead to more efficient linkage to intervention services. Early diagnosis will make services available to the family in the child's most formative years. Planning which begins in early childhood can facilitate the development of coordinated services for as long as they are required.

Physicians who understand FAS can form effective partnerships with parents (Olsen *et al.*, 1992). Together, realistic expectations will be developed for the child's growth and development. In addition, physicians who are working closely with the biological parents of children with FAS have an opportunity to identify current substance abuse and to make referrals for treatment.

Engaging parents

Families are integral to maintaining the consistent supportive environment which is critical for affected children. However, the very circumstances which result in FAS/FAE may necessitate alternative family placements. Children are often placed within the foster or adoptive care systems or are living with relatives other than their biological parents. In a study of 61 adolescents and adults with FAS, Streissguth & Randels (1988) found that 77% were not living with a biological parent. The average age at which the children had left their biological homes was 46 months.

The needs of children with FAS demand energy, resourcefulness and flexibility. If parents are to meet the demands of raising a child with FAS, they need access to the best possible information and services. Yet parents often report inadequate information, difficulty in obtaining a diagnosis, and a lack of supportive services. This is equally true for biological, foster and adoptive families. When they express concern over their children's behaviors, skills or development, their observations are dismissed or invalidated. Instead of being acknowledged as the best source of information about their child, parents are often left out of the planning process.

Parental involvement is critical to the success of any treatment strategy. It has been identified as one of the most consistent factors leading to an improved outcome for a child and sustained interest in a child's development and education (Bronfenbrenner, 1975; Horton, 1976; Bricker, 1978). Parents who have participated in early intervention report an increased sense of control over their own lives, higher general life satisfaction, and increased self-confidence (Hubell, 1983).

A gap in information and services has multiple consequences. Parents become frustrated and feel inadequate, blaming themselves for their child's problems. Social service agencies in Massachusetts have reported that the average length foster placement for a child with FAS is 6 months, considerably briefer than for other special needs children. Agencies attribute these frequent moves both to the infant's difficult and unpredictable behavior, and to a lack of information available to caregivers. Placing or assigning custody of children is further hampered when their behaviors are misunderstood and no clear treatment protocols exist. Families who assume temporary custody become frustrated with their lack of knowledge and support and terminate their responsibility for the child.

Partnerships between families and the medical and educational communities facilitate development of the optimal environment. The expertise of each party should be acknowledged and combined. Sharing all available information builds trust and increases the knowledge base.

Support groups

Parents helping parents represents a cost-effective and efficient way to facilitate optimal development of children with alcohol-related birth defects. Other families with similar children offer a pragmatic means by which information can be shared. Sharing techniques and tips facilitates coping with daily activities. Parents can benefit from the advice and experience of other parents in coming to terms with their child's handicaps. Acknowledgement of the difficulty of raising children with FAS helps to relieve frustration and releases energy to more productive parenting roles. When parents help one another understand the constitutional bases of the behavioral and learning problems seen in FAS, they develop more appropriate expectations. They are better able to distinguish between what their child cannot do and what he or she will not do. Until the professional community acquires more experience with FAS, parents may be the best source of information on available resources, such as ancillary services, summer programs, and respite care. Support groups are a source of encouragement to advocate for the child at school, in the extended family, and in the community.

Support groups for those raising children with FAS have become active throughout the United States, Canada, Germany and other countries. In many cases they simply provide a comfortable forum in which to discuss the issues common to foster, adoptive and biological parents. In other circumstances, groups have become proactive, planning and sponsoring conferences, writing and distributing newsletters, and contributing to educational materials for other parents. Some groups connect parents by telephone for support. Others have become active in legislative issues. Alliances have also developed between some support groups and the scientists doing clinical research in FAS/FAE. This vital link helps to assure the relevance of new research while allowing families to feel they are contributing to improved understanding of FAS.

Support groups can also provide a forum for expression of guilt and anger over the child's problems. Biological, adoptive and foster parents need to come to the understanding that both mother and child were victims of the disease of alcoholism. Excessive drinking was not malicious nor done willfully with the intent to harm the baby. They must recognize that the mother's options were limited by her disease. Moralistic views need to be replaced with therapeutic plans. Anger and remorse need to be channelled to a focus on the child's positive traits and to planning remedial strategies.

Need for sobriety

Several researchers have noted the potential problems of growing up in a home rendered chaotic by continuing alcohol abuse (Aronson & Olegard, 1985; Streissguth & La Due, 1987; Zuckerman & Bresnahan, 1991). The disabilities of FAS make a child more vulnerable to the adverse effects of an environment which is unstable or inconsistent. The complex interrelationships of environmental stress, inadequate parenting, lack of enrichment, and poor nutrition all contribute to poor development. These problems are often present in homes where alcohol abuse continues. Sobriety by both parents is essential to the optimal development of the child. Therefore, intervention strategies must include the provision of treatment for parents and training for professionals to ensure identification and referral.

Future directions for research and intervention

Pilot research suggests that children with FAS differ in the nature of their disabilities from children with developmental delays associated with factors other than alcohol, including exposure to illicit drugs. Researchers, clinicians, parents, and teachers have observed that the difficulties encountered by affected children have a number of common characteristics. While the research is far from complete, these findings provide invaluable information to caregivers and point to areas for future research. There is a need to further evaluate the specificity of alcohol's effects to increase our understanding of the differences and similarities in comparison with other CNS disorders. As the understanding of the characteristics of FAS and their etiology increases, more effective interventions for children at home, school, and in the community will be developed, drawing on our existing knowledge of developmental and learning disabilities. Medical, social services, and educational professionals will be better equipped to address the complex problems which children and their families now face. The outcome for all individuals with FAS and FAE will improve.

References

Aronson, M. & Olegard, R. (1985). Fetal alcohol effects in pediatrics and child psychology. In *Alcohol and the Developing Brain*, ed. U. Ryberg, C. Alling & J. Engel. New York: Raven Press.

Aronson, M. & Olegard, R. (1987). Children of alcoholic mothers. *Pediatrician*, **14**, 57–61.

Bierich, J.R. (1978). Pränatale Schadigungen durch Alkohol. (Prenatal damage from alcohol.) *Der Internist*, **19**, 131–9.

Bricker, D. (1978). Early intervention: the criteria for success. In 'Early Intervention with Infants and Young Children'. *Allied Health and Behavioral Science Journal*, **1**, 567–82.

Bronfenbrenner, U. (1975). Is early intervention effective? In *Handbook of Evaluation Research*, vol. 2, ed. E.L. Strevnning & M. Guttentag. Beverly Hills: Sage Publications.

Brown, R.T., Coles, C.D., Smith, I.E., Platzman, K.A., Silverstein, J., Erickson, S. & Falek, A. (1991). Effects of prenatal alcohol exposure at school age. II. Attention and behavior. *Neurotoxicology and Teratology*, **13**, 369–76.

Caldwell, S. (1993). Nurturing the delicate rose. In *Fantastic Antone Succeeds!*, ed. J. Kleinfeld & S. Westcott, pp. 97–130. Fairbanks, AK: University of Alaska Press.

Don, A., Kerns, K., Mateer, C.A. & Streissguth, A.P. (1993). Cognitive deficits in normal IQ and borderline IQ adults with fetal alcohol syndrome. *Alcoholism: Clinical and Experimental Research*, **17**, 458.

Hayden, A.H. & Haring, N.G. (1976). Early intervention for high risk infants and children: programs for Down syndrome children. In *Intervention Strategies for High Risk Infants and Children*, ed. T.D. Tjossem. Baltimore: University Park Press.

Hinde, J. (1993). Early intervention for alcohol affected children. In *Fantastic Antone Succeeds!*, ed. J. Kleinfeld & S. Westcott, pp. 131–48. Fairbanks, AK: University of Alaska Press.

Horton, K.B. (1976). Early intervention for hearing impaired infants and young children. In *Intervention Strategies for High Risk Infants and Young Children*, ed. T.D. Tjossem. Baltimore: University Park Press.

Hubell, R. (1983). *A Review of Head Start Research Since 1970*. Washington: CSR, Inc.

Kleinfeld, J. & Westcott, S. (eds.) (1993). *Fantastic Antone Succeeds!* Fairbanks, AK: University of Alaska Press.

Kodituwakku, P.W., Handmaker, N.S., Cutler, S.K., Weathersby, E.K., Handmaker, S.D. & Aase, J.M. (1992). Specific impairments of self regulation in FAS/FAE: a pilot study (abstract). *Alcoholism: Clinical and Experimental Research*, **16**, 381.

Kodituwakku, P.W., Handmaker, N.S., Cutler, S.K., Weathersby, E.K., Cutler, S.K. & Handmaker, S.D. (1994). Impaired goal management in working memory in FAS/FAE. *Alcoholism: Clinical and Experimental Research*, **18**, 502.

Koranyi, G. & Csiky, E. (1978). Az embryopathia alcoholica gyermekkorban eszleheto tuneteirol. (Signs of alcohol embryopathy apparent in childhood.) *Orvosi Hetilap*, **119**, 2923–9.

Lemoine, P., Harousseau, H., Borteyru, J.-P. & Menuet, J.-C. (1968). Les enfants de parents alcooliques: anomalies observées. A propos de 127 cas. (Children of alcoholic parents: observed anomalies in 127 cases.) *Ouest Médicale*, **21**, 476–82.

Mattson, S.N. & Riley, E.P. (1994). Implicit memory in children with fetal alcohol syndrome. I. Procedural learning. *Alcoholism: Clinical and Experimental Research*, **18**, 502.

Morse, B.A. (1993). Information processing: a conceptual approach to understanding the behavioral disorders of fetal alcohol syndrome. In *Fantastic Antone Succeeds!*, ed. J. Kleinfeld & S. Westcott, pp. 23–36. Fairbanks, AK: University of Alaska Press.

Morse, B.A. & Cermak, S. (1994). Sensory processing in children with FAS. *Alcoholism: Clinical and Experimental Research*, **18**, 503.

Morse, B.A., Idelson, R.K., Sachs, W.H., Weiner, L. & Kaplan, L.C. (1992). Pediatricians' perspectives on fetal alcohol syndrome. *Journal of Substance Abuse*, **4**, 187–95.

Morse, B.A. & Weiner, L. (1993). *FAS: Parent and Child*. Brookline, MA: Fetal Alcohol Education Program, Boston University School of Medicine.

Morse, B.A. & Weiner, L. (1995). Fetal alcohol syndrome. In *Behavioral and Development Pediatrics: A Handbook for Primary Care*, ed. B. Zuckerman & S. Parker, pp. 149–52. Boston: Little, Brown.

Murphy, M. (1993). Shut up and talk to me. In *Fantastic Antone Succeeds!*, ed. J. Kleinfeld & S. Westcott, pp. 189–200. Fairbanks, AK: University of Alaska Press.

Nanson, J.L. & Hiscock, M. (1990). Attention deficits in children exposed to alcohol prenatally. *Alcoholism: Clinical and Experimental Research*, **14**, 656–61.

Olsen, H.C., Burgess, D.M. & Streissguth, A.P. (1992). Fetal alcohol syndrome (FAS) and fetal alcohol effects (FAE): a lifespan view, with implications for early intervention. *Zero to Three*, **13**, 24–9.

Phillpot, B. & Harrison, N. (1993). A one-room schoolhouse for children with FAS/FAE. In *Fantastic Antone Succeeds!*, ed. J. Kleinfeld & S. Westcott, pp. 233–52. Fairbanks, AK: University of Alaska Press.

Riley, E.P. (1990). The long term behavioural effects of prenatal alcohol exposure in rats. *Alcoholism: Clinical and Experimental Research*, **14**, 670–3.

Rosett, H.L. & Weiner, L. (1984). *Alcohol and the Fetus: A Clinical Perspective*. New York: Oxford University Press.

Sander, L.W., Snyder, P.A., Rosett, H.L., Lee, A., Gould, J.B. & Ouellette, E.M. (1977). Effects of alcohol intake during pregnancy in newborn state regulation. *Alcoholism: Clinical and Experimental Research*, **1**, 233–41.

Spohr, H.-L. & Steinhausen, H.-C. (1984). Clinical, psychopathological and developmental aspects in children with the fetal alcohol syndrome: a four-year follow-up study. In *Mechanisms of Alcohol Damage In Utero*, pp. 197–217. Ciba Foundation Symposium 105. London: Pitman.

Steinhausen, H.-C., Willms, J. & Spohr, H.-L. (1993). Long-term psychopathological and cognitive outcome of children with fetal alcohol syndrome. *Journal of the American Academy of Child and Adolescent Psychiatry*, **32**, 990–4.

Steinhausen, H.-C., Willms, J. & Spohr, H.-L. (1994). Correlates of psychopathology and intelligence in children with fetal alcohol syndrome. *Journal of Child Psychology and Psychiatry*, **35**, 323–31.

Streissguth, A.P. (1986). The behavioral teratology of alcohol: performance, behavioral and intellectual deficits in prenatally exposed children. In *Alcohol and Brain Development*, ed. J.R. West, pp. 3-44. New York: Oxford University Press.

Streissguth, A.P., Herman, C.S. & Smith, D.W. (1978). Stability of intelligence in the fetal alcohol syndrome: a preliminary report. *Alcoholism: Clinical and Experimental Research*, **2**, 165–70.

Streissguth, A.P. & LaDue, R.A. (1987). Fetal alcohol: teratogenic causes of developmental disabilities. In *Toxic Substances and Mental Retardation*, ed. S. Schroeder. Washington, DC: American Association for Mental Deficiency Monograph 8.

Streissguth, A.P. & Randels, S. (1988). Long term effects of fetal alcohol syndrome. In *Alcohol and Child/Family Health*, ed. G.C. Robinson & R.W. Armstrong. Vancouver: BC FAS Resource Group.

Tanner-Halverson, P. (1993). Snagging the kite string. In *Fantastic Antone Succeeds!*, ed. J. Kleinfeld & S. Westcott, pp. 201–22. Fairbanks, AK: University of Alaska Press.

Weiner, L. & Morse, B.A. (1988). Behavioral manifestations of FAS: implications for care. *American Public Health Association Meetings*, Boston, Massachusetts.

Weiner, L. & Morse, B.A. (1991). Facilitating development for children with fetal alcohol syndrome. *Brown University Child and Adolescent Behavior and Development Letter: Special Supplement*, Nov.

Weiner, L. & Morse, B.A. (1994). Intervention and the child with FAS. *Alcohol, Health and Research World*, **18**, 67–72.

West, J.R., Goodlett, C.R. & Brandt, J.P. (1990). New approaches to research on the long-term consequences of prenatal exposure to alcohol. *Alcoholism: Clinical and Experimental Research*, **14**, 674–89.

Winick, P. (1993). Mainstreaming children with FAS in a small rural school. In *Fantastic Antone Succeeds!*, ed. J. Kleinfeld & S. Westcott, pp. 223–32. Fairbanks, AK: University of Alaska Press.

Zuckerman, B. & Bresnahan, K. (1991). Developmental and behavioral consequences of prenatal drug and alcohol exposure. *Pediatric Clinics of North America*, **38**, 1387.

14

Fetal alcohol syndrome: a framework for successful prevention

LYN WEINER AND BARBARA A. MORSE

Introduction

The cost of fetal alcohol syndrome (FAS) is staggering – an enormous toll is extracted from the patient, the family, and the community. The intellectual and behavioral problems which the child and adult with FAS must face have been well documented in clinical and experimental findings (Rosett & Weiner, 1984; Streissguth *et al.*, 1994). The families are challenged and often frustrated in their attempts to provide the optimal developmental environment (Kleinfeld & Westcott, 1993). The economic costs to the community are high (Bloss, 1994). In three studies, estimates of the annual costs in the United States ranged from $321 million to $3236 million. All estimates included the cost of care for low birth weight babies, surgical correction of birth defects, and the care of people with moderate or severe mental retardation until age 21 years. The higher estimates also included the value of productivity lost as well as the cost of treatment and residential care for patients of all ages with FAS. The lifetime cost for a single case of FAS has been estimated at $596 000. Monies saved in the prevention of one case of FAS would finance prevention programs which reduce the emotional and physical pain of the patients and their families.

Prevention programs

Numerous prevention strategies have been employed in the United States since the recognition of FAS in 1974 and were energized in 1981 when the Surgeon General advised all women to abstain from alcohol consumption during pregnancy (Public Health Service, 1981). There are several potential audiences for prevention programs and each requires a distinct approach. The general population needs information on alcohol's potential to affect pregnancy outcome. This allows people to be knowledgeable and to make appropriate choices about their use of alcohol. The woman who is drinking heavily requires motivation to seek treatment for her addiction and prenatal care when pregnant. She needs reassurance that help is available and effective. The parents of children with birth defects need an understanding of alcohol's actions and the role they may or may not have played in their child's problems. If FAS is the problem, diagnosis and treatment should follow. If it is not, parents need guidance to understand the true etiology of their child's problems.

Educational campaigns

To date, prevention programs have focused on increasing information about alcohol's effects on pregnancy among the general population. These programs have been successful. Among adults age 18–44 years, there was a significant increase in knowledge between 1985 and 1990 (Dufour *et al.*, 1994). In 1990, the vast majority (89–92%) responded that heavy drinking during pregnancy increases the chance of some adverse pregnancy outcome: miscarriage, mental retardation, low birth weight, and birth defects. This belief was significantly higher than the 87–88% reported in 1985. Awareness of the term 'FAS' also increased, from 25% to 39%, in the 5 year period. Men reported lower levels of knowledge than women, although their understanding had also increased since 1985.

Analysis of the female population by demographic characteristics revealed lower levels of knowledge or beliefs among women who were black, Hispanic, had fewer than 12 years of education, had a family income less than $20 000, were unemployed, and were divorced or separated. The authors suggest the need to seek additional prevention strategies for this subgroup of women who are already at risk for poor pregnancy outcome. This suggestion is underscored by findings of the Behavioral Risk Factor Surveillance System which reported that frequency of alcohol use among pregnant women declined from 32% to 20% between 1985 and 1988 (Serdula *et al.*, 1991). However, there were no differences in the amount consumed among those who continued to drink.

These findings have been reinforced by a study on the warning labels which have been placed on all alcoholic beverage containers sold or distributed in the United States since 1989. The warning states, 'According to the Surgeon General, women should not drink alcoholic beverages during pregnancy because of the risk of birth defects.' The goal of this measure was to advise all consumers about the risks of drinking. The effectiveness of the warning labels has been evaluated among 3572 inner-city women at Hutzel Hospital Prenatal Clinic in Detroit (Hankin *et al.*, 1993). Two questions were explored: (1) whether women were more aware of the risks of alcohol and (2) whether drinking behavior changed. Two years following implementation of the warning label requirement, 57% of this group reported seeing the warning on alcoholic beverages. Drinking decreased among the non-risk women. The decrease was small – about 1.42 grams absolute alcohol per week or 28.4 g of beer. There was no change among the risk drinkers. Parity was significantly different among drinking groups, with more risk drinkers being multiparous. The authors suggest that the mothers' belief that their earlier pregnancies had successful outcomes outweighed the message on the warning label. Women who have this sense of personal invulnerability may remain impervious to public service announcements as well as to warning labels.

A recent Canadian study of the effectiveness of public service announcements about FAS also showed increased knowledge (Casiro *et al.*, 1994). After a 10 week public service announcement campaign more women correctly answered questions about alcohol's effects during pregnancy. However, this study did not assess behavioral change and did not compare knowledge levels among risk and non-risk women. The authors concluded that methods such as public service announcements were valuable as part of a multifaceted strategy.

Campaigns which disseminate information and increase knowledge have not been found to change behavior (LaPierre, 1967). An evaluation of women's attitudes and behavior following delivery revealed that 20% of the women consumed alcohol during pregnancy at levels they themselves defined as 'risk' (Minor & Van Dort, 1982). Participants in focus groups demonstrated familiarity with general guidelines for prenatal health; however, the majority indicated that they did not comply with most of the recommended health practices (DHSS, 1986).

Clinical prevention

There is a need for strategies which focus directly on changing the behavior of the at-risk population. An opportunity exists when the health care provider, in a primary care setting, assesses alcohol use routinely, provides education to all, and identifies and treats (or refers for treatment) women at risk. Ideally, this would occur before conception to ensure that no stage of fetal development is compromised by exposure to alcohol. More typically, however, concerns about alcohol use during pregnancy are raised when a woman enters prenatal care. Even at this time primary care intervention can have significant impact.

Theoretical basis for clinical intervention

The strategy of intervention with heavy drinkers in the prenatal period is based on an understanding of mediating factors in ethanol's actions on fetal development, particularly the role of dose, timing of exposure, pattern of consumption and parity. The role of mediating factors is underscored by the observation that not all children exposed to high levels of alcohol *in utero* suffer from alcohol-related birth defects (Rosett & Weiner, 1984). Prospective studies suggest 2–10% have FAS, 40% have fetal alcohol effects (FAE), and 50% show neither on examination. The expression of FAS itself varies, with a broad range of adverse outcomes from subtle to severe.

Dose

While the precise dose of alcohol which causes adverse outcomes has not been established, it is clear that alcohol's effects are dose related. The association between alcohol consumption and low birth weight, which serves as a marker for morbidity and mortality, has been investigated in many sites. In early prospective studies, neonatal growth retardation was observed only among babies born to the 2–11% of women who reported drinking most heavily (although definitions of drinking categories have differed) (Seidenberg & Majewski, 1978; Sokol *et al.*, 1980; Silva *et al.*, 1981; Plant, 1985; Du Ve Florey, 1988). Lower birth weights, but not growth retardation, were reported in association with moderate levels of consumption in two studies (Little, 1977; Mills *et al.*, 1984). Researchers at four additional sites found no effect of alcohol on birth weight (Tennes & Blackard, 1980; Hingson *et al.*, 1982; Marbury *et al.*, 1983; Gibson *et al.*, 1983).

Prospective follow-up studies of children exposed to a range of alcohol *in utero* also demonstrate a dose-response. Detailed psychological and morphological examination of 4-year-old children found a higher incidence of abnormal children when maternal alcohol consumption was greater than 4 drinks a day (19% vs 4%) (Streissguth *et al.*, 1984*a*). Another study from this same group found deficits in attention span at low levels of alcohol (Streissguth *et al.*, 1984*b*). However, in a later analysis, massed drinking (5 or more drinks per occasion) was reported to be the most consistent predictor of neurobehavioral deficits in school-age children (Streissguth *et al.*, 1989, 1994). Other researchers observed that the deficits in weight and head circumference among 6-year-olds were in direct proportion to the amount of alcohol exposure *in utero* (Day *et al.*, 1994). In another study, there were no adverse effects on attention or cognitive ability among 4-year-olds at any level of exposure in the absence of FAS (Boyd *et al.*, 1991). Yet another study found no relationship between prenatal alcohol exposure and neurobehavioral development at 48 months (Freid & Watkinson, 1990).

Evaluation of infant processing revealed a threshold at the level between 7 and 28 drinks per week for most neurobehavioral deficits (Jacobson *et al.*, 1993). Although some reductions in neurobehavioral scores occurred at lower levels, the authors note that there is little functional significance to these effects. Moreover, the authors are careful to note that this 'average' consumption does not reflect actual consumption patterns. For example, an average score of 7 drinks per week does not represent 1 drink on each day, but typically represents relatively heavy intake on one drinking day. In this sample, mothers who averaged more than 7 drinks per week exposed their infants to an average of 6 drinks per day (range 1.2–24.8 per day) on an average of 2.6 days per week (0.6–7.0 days). These data suggest that blood alcohol concentrations (BAC) are an important factor in the expression of alcohol-related disorders.

The animal model, in which precise doses are administered and BACs are monitored, demonstrates a direct association between BACs and adverse fetal development. Congenital abnormalities and growth retardation occur in the animal model in association with BACs in excess of 100 mg% (Abel & Greizerstein, 1979; Randall, 1982). Peak BAC rather than alcohol dose has been demonstrated to be the critical factor in reducing brain growth in the rat (West *et al.*, 1990; Bonthius & West, 1990).

Among humans, risk increases not only with consumption level, but also with chronicity of alcoholism. High morbidity and mortality rates have been reported among mothers of children with FAS. It has been estimated that 75% of the mothers are dead or missing from alcohol-related problems within 5 years of the birth of their baby (Clarren, 1981).

Timing of exposure

Another important variable in the occurrence of alcohol-related damage is timing of exposure. Alcohol has the capacity to interfere with every stage of fetal development (Rosett *et al.*, 1981). Vulnerability of particular organ systems is greatest at the time of their most rapid cell division. In the first trimester, when organs are developing, high concentrations of alcohol can modify cell membranes and cell migration, and can disturb embryonic organization of tissue, causing morphological anomalies. Severe damage at this stage may result in spontaneous abortions or miscarriages. Throughout pregnancy, disturbances in the metabolism of carbohydrates, lipids and proteins can retard cell growth and division. In the third trimester, the human brain has a period of rapid growth. High blood alcohol concentrations at this time may impair central nervous system growth and development and limit future intellectual and behavioral capacities. FAS is the result of the cumulative actions of high BACs throughout the pregnancy.

An understanding of the mediating factors suggests that intervention with heavy drinkers has the potential to lessen alcohol-related birth defects. When dose and timing of exposure are reduced, then risk is also reduced.

Clinical models of intervention

Neonatal period

At Boston City Hospital, between 1974 and 1979, in one of the first prospective studies in the United States, we investigated the impact of a range of drinking patterns on fetal development (Rosett *et al.*, 1983*a,b*). Women interviewed at the time of registration for prenatal care were asked a series of questions about their lifestyles, including drinking, smoking and eating patterns. Women who reported consumption of at least 45 drinks a month with 5 or more on some occasions were classified as heavy drinkers. Moderate drinkers drank more than once a month but did not meet criteria for heavy drinking. Rare drinkers either abstained or drank less than once a month.

Among the 1711 women who participated, 9% were heavy drinkers, 37% were moderate, and 53% were rare. As in other studies of drinking patterns, the reported daily mean consumption of absolute alcohol by the heavy drinkers was significantly higher than that reported by the moderate drinkers; the heavily drinking women reported daily absolute alcohol consumption 15 times higher (131.4 g vs 8.6 g).

Women were provided with education about the risks of alcohol consumption during pregnancy. Heavily drinking women were encouraged to join counselling sessions or to enter treatment focused on cessation of alcohol use. A supportive approach was emphasized. Women were advised that they had a better chance of having a healthy baby if they stopped drinking heavily. Treatment approaches were individualized to a woman's needs; some required detoxification and intensive treatment, others met weekly with a counsellor. No woman refused participation. A positive hopeful message of the benefits of reduction and an attempt to build self-esteem in the women were emphasized in counselling. An alcohol history was taken at each coun-selling session, including quantity, frequency and circumstances of use. Women were informed that equal risk existed from all alcoholic beverages. Myths about the weakness or strength of various beverage types were dis-pelled. While abstinence was the goal, both reduction in use and achievement of abstinence were praised. Women who continued drinking or relapsed, were reminded of the benefits of abstinence. Criticism and provocation of guilt were avoided.

In addition to reduction of alcohol use, counselling also focused on other aspects of a woman's life. The effects of diet, exercise, stress, smoking and illicit drug use were all evaluated. Individual coping mechanisms were explored. Reproductive and childbirth education were provided to supple-ment that given by regular clinic staff. Family relationships, especially those with the baby's father, were discussed. Birth control options and their accept-ability were reviewed. Help with real-life situations was provided through practical suggestions and referral to appropriate hospital or community agencies. In some cases personal introductions to referral staff facilitated these transitions. Aftercare for the drinking problem as well as for parenting assistance were planned before delivery. In all cases, the woman's desire for a healthy baby was emphasized and reiterated.

Two-thirds of the women who participated in counselling were able to reduce consumption substantially or abstain before the third trimester. Newborn evaluations demonstrated that growth retardation occurred signif-icantly more frequently among children born to women who continued drinking heavily than among children born to rare and moderate drinkers. There were no differences observed between children born to rare and mod-erate drinkers. Newborns of women who drank heavily early in pregnancy and reduced consumption before the third trimester were comparable to those born to rare and moderate drinkers.

Long-term benefits

Improved neonatal outcome has been consistently associated with reduced levels of maternal drinking (Little *et al.*, 1984; Weiner & Larsson, 1987; Smith *et al.*, 1987; Autti-Rämö & Granström, 1991). In early childhood, children born to women who reduced heavy drinking demonstrated fewer morphological and developmental abnormalities than children born to women who drank throughout pregnancy (Aronson & Olegard, 1985; Larsson *et al.*, 1985). Psychological testing and language evaluation of 2-year-old children exposed to alcohol *in utero* showed no definite effect of alcohol exposure on mental or language development when mothers drank heavily only in the first trimester (Autti-Rämö *et al.*, 1992). Children born to women who drank heavily throughout pregnancy scored lower than all others on all measurements and more suffered from FAS and FAE. Children exposed for two trimesters showed some developmental delays but were not so severely affected as those exposed throughout gestation.

Animal models

Experimental findings underscore the efficacy of supportive therapy focused on reduction of heavy drinking as a preventive strategy (Weiner & Larsson, 1987). Maternal capacity to nurture improves when heavy drinking stops. In the absence of alcohol exposure, abnormalities and growth retardation that develop in later stages will be avoided. While structural malformations persist, experimental models suggest remediation and restitution of growth-related abnormalities when alcohol exposure ends. Abnormalities apparent on gestational day 9 following exposure on days 5–8, were no longer apparent on day 20 (Anders & Persaud, 1980). Similarly, alterations in neonatal brain size and structure were shown to recover (Volk *et al.*, 1981). Small nuclei were observed on day 7 among rat pups exposed to alcohol *in utero*; differences were gone by days 12 and 17. These studies suggest considerable capacity of the fetus to recover, yet it is important to remember that alcohol-exposed brains may not be similar to non-exposed brains on all neurological, physiological, or behavioral measures. The earlier in pregnancy – or even prior to conception – that treatment is provided, the greater is the potential for healthy babies. But it is never to late to improve outcome.

Designing successful prevention

Understanding addictive behavior

Prevention of alcohol-related birth defects requires cessation of drinking by the women who drink abusively. Successful programs will address the unique needs of addicted women, who require strategies relevant to their drinking behavior (Weiner *et al.*, 1989). Given the nature of their sustained drinking behavior, one may safely assume that problem drinking or incipient alcoholism is present. It is 'the nature of alcoholism and of all chemical dependence that its victims are rendered by the disease itself less and less capable of spontaneous recognition of the severity of their symptoms' (Johnson, 1986). Recognition of this demands carefully planned, individual intervention strategies with this population. The primary prevention paradigm of education must be replaced with more appropriate strategies which will redirect or rehabilitate the pregnant woman on an individual basis.

The disease concept of alcoholism offers invaluable heuristic utility in clinical situations. The effectiveness of this model stems from its ability, in part, to remove the moral stigma of alcoholism and its attendant guilt (Wallace, 1977). This, coupled with focusing intervention on the present with the hope of reconstructing the past and improving the future, takes on added significance with the population of at-risk pregnant women.

Viewing the drinking behavior as a moral or volitional issue has given rise to simplistic solutions manifesting as the slogan therapy of 'just say no' and to injunctions that a drinker stop lest she 'harm her baby.' The collective experience of alcoholism treatment specialists suggests that these approaches may not only be ineffective, but also quite destructive (Weinberg, 1974). Guilt is likely to create a vicious circle of self-recrimination and continuing alcohol abuse. An atmosphere of nonjudgmental acceptance makes the process of change possible. A supportive therapeutic climate facilitates intervention and sets the stage for referral to an appropriate alcoholism treatment specialist. An understanding of the dynamics of addiction in general, and alcoholism in particular, is the first step in the process of developing policies for prompt identification, intervention, and referral by health care providers.

Heavily drinking women report that physicians and/or other health providers are the best source of information leading to behavioral change (DHSS, 1986; Minor & Van Dort, 1982). At-risk women respond positively to supportive counselling offered in the prenatal setting (Larsson, 1983; Rosett *et al.*, 1983*a*; Little *et al.*, 1984; Smith *et al.*, 1987). In these four studies, between 35% and 80% of the women who reported heavy drinking were able to reduce their consumption before the third trimester. These high success rates may reflect the unique motivation of pregnancy and the desire of women to ensure as healthy a baby as possible.

Developing supportive therapy programs

The pregnant woman is inclined to respond favorably to therapeutic assistance focused on potential benefits to herself and her baby. Pregnancy is a normal crisis in every woman's life. Changes in physiology, body image and social role, particularly the sense of responsibility for another life, increase receptivity toward assistance from health professionals. The feelings that are engendered by bodily changes and new social roles should be recognized and utilized as a positive motivating factor. At Boston City Hospital, treatment capitalized on the woman's motivation to have a healthy baby. A positive hopeful message of the benefits of reduction and an attempt to build self-esteem in the women were emphasized in counselling.

Reports from smoking cessation programs have confirmed the value of positive supportive messages. Counselling which emphasized the benefits of quitting smoking and reflected a mood of realism, happiness, and accomplishment contributed to a higher 6 month abstinence rate as compared with participants who were not exposed to the positive message (Mogielnicki *et al.*, 1986). A review of health promotion campaigns also emphasized the need for positive rather than negative messages. Lack of success has been linked to fear or implied punishment in the message and to the lack of information on how to change undesirable behavior (Job, 1988). Successful campaigns are those in which the fear level is low, short- rather than long-term effects or benefits are emphasized, and specific behavioral techniques are provided. Target audiences may become immune to messages which pair undesirable behaviors with words of warning about what the public perceives to be an unlikely event. Lack of direct experience with the hazards of a product or behavior reduces the likelihood that the message will be effective (Richardson *et al.*, 1987). The audience is able to dismiss the warning by arguing to themselves that they know people who engage in particular behaviors and suffered no ill effects – for example, women who consumed alcohol during pregnancy and bore healthy children.

Conducting outreach

In spite of evidence that positive, supportive intervention is effective in preventing FAS, this information is not widely disseminated or incorporated in clinical settings or public health policy. Approaches are needed which will motivate the pregnant woman to seek care. Public health campaigns must convey the message that treatment is available, that it is successful, and that there are benefits to both mother and baby. Women who do not regularly receive health care can be reached through campaigns in non-medical settings. In addition to public service announcements on radio and television, messages can be disseminated through posters at diverse locations within the community, ranging from churches to laundromats. In Massachusetts, we distributed brochures at point-of-purchase in a drug store chain. Anecdotal reports revealed that many women responded to the information and requested help and/or information.

Training health care providers

At the same time that we are encouraging women to seek care, we must also prepare the health care community to respond to their needs. Health care providers must feel competent to intervene with pregnant, problem-drinking women. They must also be aware of the important role they can play. For prenatal providers, it is clear that intervention with the heavily drinking woman can have direct and positive effects. The role for pediatric providers is suggested by findings of an association between adverse outcome and high parity. Veghelyi *et al.* (1978) noted that the child with FAS was rarely the first born. Other studies have also found that the degree of retardation and fetal damage was increasingly severe with increasing parity (Palmer *et al.*, 1974; Bierich *et al.*, 1976; Fitze *et al.*, 1978; Iosub *et al.*, 1981). Similar observations have been made in experimental models (Dexter *et al.*, 1983). These data demonstrate that pediatricians can reduce the risk of additional cases in families which present with one child with FAS. In addition, identification of all parents who drink heavily provides an opportunity for referral and treatment. While it is never too late to improve pregnancy outcome, the optimal time for cessation of heavy drinking is pre-conception or peri-conception when there is contact with pediatric providers.

Addressing knowledge and attitudinal issues

Before intervention can be successful, there needs to be a change in the negative stereotypes about addiction, which influence multiple aspects of treatment from the ability and willingness routinely to take alcohol histories to the accurate diagnosis of FAS in a child. Alcoholism and illicit drug use are not regularly identified within medical settings. Among hospitalized alcoholic patients, less than half are correctly diagnosed as such, and even when diagnosed, only 29% are offered any treatment (Moore *et al.*, 1989). Patients in outpatient settings are no more likely to be identified. Studies have found that only 50% of patients are screened for alcohol problems and between 8% and 50% of alcoholics are diagnosed (Creek *et al.*, 1982; Leckman *et al.*, 1984; Mulry *et al.*, 1987; Woodhall, 1988). Only 54% of pediatricians reported that they routinely take maternal alcohol histories (Morse *et al.*, 1992). Negative attitudes towards addiction are cited as one of the most critical factors underlying the failure to identify at-risk patients across medical specialties (Coryell, 1982; Geller *et al.*, 1989; Coleman & Veach, 1990; Veach & Chappel, 1990). A recent editorial in *Obstetrics and Gynecology* noted how easy it is for physicians to assume addiction problems occur primarily in other people's practices (Schwarz, 1993).

Many health care providers receive their most powerful education about alcohol abuse in the emergency room, where they learn about the results of alcoholism but not about alcoholism itself. In this setting, only the most severe end of the spectrum of addiction is seen. The alcoholics who present have reached the end-stage of the disease syndrome. The disruption of their lives and their health overwhelm staff and medical students. The message that alcoholism is an important, albeit complex, disease which physicians have the knowledge and skills to treat is lost. Therapeutic pessimism persists. In contrast, experience with individuals recovering from alcohol problems increases a provider's willingness to engage patients in a positive manner. When treatment is successful, professional optimism increases and there is a greater willingness to treat additional patients. Educational strategies which force medical staff to encounter alcoholics break down stereotypes of 'skid-row' addicts (Weiner *et al.*, 1982).

Experience of the Fetal Alcohol Education Program

Intervention is most effective when a provider is comfortable discussing alcohol use with all patients, understands the dynamics of addiction, can provide accurate information about the risks of alcohol and the benefits of treatment, and is knowledgeable about referrals. The Fetal Alcohol Education program of Boston University School of Medicine has established and documented an effective curriculum for reaching health care providers with information regarding pregnancy and alcohol (Weiner *et al.*, 1988). Training sessions focus on three areas of importance to practitioners: knowledge about alcohol's mechanisms during pregnancy, attitudes towards alcohol use, and specific techniques for identification and treatment. Evaluations of training programs using the curriculum demonstrated improved clinical sensitivity to alcohol consumption among pregnant women. Respondents cited increased knowledge, more positive and hopeful attitudes, and greater willingness to discuss alcohol use with their patients. Clinical techniques were reported to be the most valuable aspect of the training. Six to 17 months after participation in training sessions, there was greater willingness and comfort in discussing alcohol issues with patients (88%). There was a significant increase (from 61% to 82%) in the number of clinicians who always took an alcohol history. Most clients at risk for FAS were identified and referred for treatment.

The ability of our training program to achieve success comes from several factors in its design. Presentations were made in the health care setting, enabling practitioners with full clinical schedules to participate. Experience has shown that while conferences are well attended by researchers, few

Table 14.1. *Ten question drinking history*

Beer:	How many times per week?
	How many cans each time?
	Ever drink more?
Wine:	How many times per week?
	How many glasses each time?
	Ever drink more?
Liquor:	How many times per week?
	How many drinks each time?
	Ever drink more?
Has your drinking changed during the past year?	

clinicians find the time to participate. More than 60% reported that they attended because it was part of in-service education at their institutions or agencies. Presenting to a cross-section of providers – physicians, nurses, nutritionists, social workers – helps to ensure that all those who deliver care will have the same information, and will present it similarly to their patients.

Information is presented in a scientific format, with quantification and documentation – a style to which health care providers respond favorably. The positive responses to the subject matter, its organization, and its capacity to stimulate thinking underscore the relevance of this format.

Training is directly relevant to patient populations. Strategies to identify drinking patterns are described. The Ten Question Drinking History (Table 14.1) which provides a brief, systematic format for evaluating alcohol use is reviewed. Positive and supportive approaches for counselling women at risk are provided. The technique of using positive statements as therapeutic tools is stressed. Statements such as, 'You have a better chance of having a healthy baby when you stop drinking,' are recommended. Sample drinking histories, trigger films, role-playing and suggestions for referral enable those who participate in the training to become comfortable asking patients about alcohol use and abuse.

Women's drinking patterns are often ignored by primary providers, who are reluctant to initiate discussion of alcohol use for fear that patients will become annoyed and not return for care (Russell *et al.*, 1983). When questions are asked in a direct, non-judgmental fashion, pregnant patients respond honestly to the doctor's concern. Professionals' negative attitudes may affect the accuracy of the drinking histories they obtain. Embarrassment or defensiveness on the part of the physician may be communicated to the patient and can contribute to underreporting. When patients sense the professional's discomfort and desire to avoid alcohol/drug problems they become reluctant to speak candidly. As the clinician's awareness of psychodynamic issues increases, negative stereotypes diminish. Their ability to obtain an accurate history and offer counselling and support improves.

Another explanation physicians give for failing to inquire about alcohol use is, 'I wouldn't know what to do if I found problems.' They feel that they lack both the knowledge and the time for problem drinkers, whom they perceive as difficult. This attitude may be overcome when clinicians learn, through experience, that patients appreciate professional concern and often respond rapidly when brief supportive therapy is integrated with prenatal care.

Primary providers are often unaware of existing referral resources and how to access them. Lack of knowledge of appropriate support programs decreases willingness to intervene with alcohol problems (Weiner *et al.*, 1982). In conjunction with a training program for house staff at Boston City Hospital on identifying drinking patterns among pregnant women, the Ten Question Drinking History described in Table 14.1 was printed in the clinic chart. The goal was to assess alcohol consumption routinely as part of the prenatal intake protocol. The number of charts containing histories was tabulated for several time periods. When the office of the training staff was in the clinic and their presence was a continual reminder, 92% of the charts included alcohol histories. This number decreased markedly (to 33%) when the trainers moved to an off-site office, even though they remained available for consultation. Utilization increased to 59% when the chairman of Obstetrics and Gynecology reinforced the need to ask and provided information about the availability of training staff for consultation and referral.

Effective alcohol treatment

To ensure that women receive appropriate and effective treatment, a network must be established between prenatal providers and addiction treatment specialists. Experience indicates that linkages between the two delivery systems helps provide comprehensive care. Addiction specialists need to reach out to primary providers and describe the availability and efficacy of treatment.

In addition, the treatment field needs to address the needs of pregnant women. Currently, there are too few treatment slots specifically geared to women and fewer for pregnant women. Adaptations from the male-oriented model are needed as women's alcoholism cannot be treated in isolation.

Women need to be viewed within their network of relationships. Programs must be family centred, offering comprehensive treatment in which the women's relationships to others are explored and services to the family are coordinated. Emotional, social, and economic issues need to be addressed through increased coordination of service agencies. Aftercare components for mother and child must be included in the treatment plan.

The alcohol problems which result in FAS are not confined to the pregnancy. While pregnancy offers a window of opportunity for treatment and prevention, alcohol abuse must be considered as a life-long problem. The prenatal provider has a unique opportunity to identify the woman at risk; however, it is the addiction specialist who will maintain a long-time interest in her alcohol use – before, during and after the pregnancy.

Treatment centers have been reluctant to accept pregnant women who are perceived as having complex medical problems. In-service education can increase the comfort level of the addiction specialist when information is provided on pregnancy in general and on benefits of addiction treatment during pregnancy. Presentations should provide accurate scientific information about the risks of abuse. It is also important to discuss the spectrum of maternal emotions such as guilt and fear of parenting. Unwarranted concerns about liability should be addressed.

Conclusion

From this review, it is clear that effective prevention of FAS will result from a multifaceted approach which utilizes existing resources and methodologies. Proper formulation of the problem constitutes the first step in developing policy. Public health strategies must match our understanding of alcohol's actions to the specific needs of the targeted population. While the precise level of maternal drinking which is dangerous or safe has not been determined, we do know that the greatest risk occurs for babies born to women who have high blood alcohol concentrations throughout pregnancy. There is a need for programs which motivate the at-risk woman to reduce alcohol consumption and to seek prenatal care. Campaigns which stress the potential benefits of reduction will improve participation. When there are expressions of alarm and concern about the ravages of maternal drinking, the woman's despair increases over her inability to stop drinking. She feels remorse for damage she may have done to the fetus and unable to master the problem. Information about the potential for success improves her ability to overcome her addiction.

Professionals who incorporate information about alcohol and pregnancy into their clinical practices are primary agents for the prevention of FAS and alcohol-related birth defects. Their role is critical in reducing abusive alcohol consumption and its associated risks. Among the various specialties involved in treating pregnant addicted women, there is ample expertise to provide effective care. Coordination of resources will ensure that the complex medical and social issues the families face will be addressed.

In the current arena of limited resources, it is crucial to define clearly the population at risk and to achieve an appropriate fit between the target population and intervention strategies. As direct interventions have been successful in reducing alcohol abuse among pregnant women, this represents the best approach. Until we develop appropriate policies, we will continue to see an overall reduction in drinking by pregnant women, but tragically there will be no lessening in the incidence of alcohol-related birth defects.

References

Abel, E.L. & Greizerstein, H.B. (1979). Ethanol-induced prenatal growth deficiency; changes in fetal body composition. *Journal of Pharmacology and Experimental Therapy*, **211**, 668–71.

Anders, K. & Persaud, T.V.N. (1980). Compensatory embryonic development in the rat following maternal treatment wth ethanol. *Anatomischer Anzeiger*, **148**, 375–83.

Aronson, M. & Olegard, R. (1985). Fetal alcohol effects in pediatrics and child psychology. In *Alcohol and the Developing Brain: Third International Berzelius Symposium*, ed. U. Ryberg *et al.*, pp. 135–45. New York: Raven Press.

Autti-Rämö, I. & Granström, M.L. (1991). The effect of intrauterine alcohol exposition in various durations on early cognitive development. *Neuropediatrics*, **22**, 203–10.

Autti-Rämö, I., Korman, M., Hilakivi-Clarke, L., Lehtonen, M., Halmesmäki, E. & Gramström, M.-L. (1992). Mental development of two-year-old children exposed to alcohol *in utero*. *Journal of Pediatrics*, **120**, 740–6.

Bierich, J., Majewski, F., Michaelis, R. & Tillner, I. (1976). Das embryofetale Alkoholsyndrom. (Embryofetal alcohol syndrome.) *European Journal of Pediatrics*, **121**, 155–77.

Bloss, G. (1994). The economic cost of FAS. *Alcohol Health and Research World*, **18**, 53–4.

Bonthius, D.J. & West, J.R. (1990). Alcohol-induced neuronal loss in developing rats: increased brain damage with binge exposure. *Alcoholism: Clinical and Experimental Research*, **14**, 107–18.

Boyd, T.A., Ernhart, C.B., Greene, T.H., Sokol, R.J. & Martier, S. (1991). Prenatal alcohol exposure and sustained attention in the preschool years. *Neurotoxicology and Teratology*, **13**, 49–55.

Casiro, O.G., Stanwick, R.S., Pelech, A., Taylor, V. & the Child Health Committee, Manitoba Medical Association (1994). Public awareness of the risks of drinking alcohol during pregnancy: the effects of a television campaign. *Canadian Journal of Public Health*, **85**, 23–7.

Clarren, S.K. (1981). Recognition of fetal alcohol syndrome. *JAMA*, **245**, 2436–9.

Coleman, P.R. & Veach, T.L. (1990). Substance abuse and the family physician: a survey of attitudes. *Substance Abuse*, **11**, 84–93.

Coryell, W. (1982). The organic dynamic continuum in psychiatry: trends in attitudes towards alcoholics. *American Journal of Psychiatry*, **139**, 89–91.

Creek, L.V., Zachrich, R.L. & Scherger, W.E. (1982). The use of standardized alcoholism screening tests in family practice. *Family Practice Research Journal*, **2**, 11–17.

Day, N.L., Richardson, G., Geva, D. & Robles, N. (1994). The effects of prenatal exposure on offspring growth and morphology at age six. *Alcoholism: Clinical and Experimental Research*, **18**, 786–94.

Dexter, J.D., Tumbleson, M.E., Decker, J.D. & Middleton, C.C. (1983). Comparison of the offspring of three serial pregnancies during voluntary alcohol consumption in Sinclair (S-1) miniature swine. *Neurobehavioral Toxicology and Teratology*, **5**, 229–31.

DHSS (1986). *Healthy Mothers, Healthy Babies: A Compendium of Program Ideas for Serving Low-Income Women*. DHSS Publication no. (PHS) 86-50209. Washington, DC: US Government Printing Office.

Dufour, M.C., Williams, G.D., Campbell, K.E. & Aitken, S.S. (1994). Knowledge of FAS and the risks of heavy drinking during pregnancy, 1985 and 1990. *Alcohol Health and Research World*, **18**, 86–92.

Du Ve Florey, C. (1988). Weak associations in epidemiological research: some examples and their interpretation. *International Journal of Epidemiology*, **17**, 950–4.

Fitze, F., Spahr, A. & Pescia, G. (1978). Familienstudie zum Problem des embryofötalen Alkoholsyndroms. (Embryofetal alcohol syndrome: follow-up of a family.) *Schweizerische Rundschau für Medizin*, **67**, 1338–54.

Freid, P. & Watkinson, B. (1990). 36- and 48-month neurobehavioral follow-up of children prenatally exposed to marijuana, cigarettes, and alcohol. *Journal of Developmental and Behavioral Pediatrics*, **11**, 49–58.

Geller, G., Levine, D.M., Mamon, J.A., Moore, R.D., Bone, L.R. & Stokes, E.J. (1989). Knowledge, attitudes and reported practices of medical students and house staff regarding the diagnosis and treatment of alcoholism. *JAMA*, **26**, 3115–20.

Gibson, G.T., Baghurst, P.A. & Colley, D.P. (1983). Maternal alcohol, tobacco and cannabis consumption and the outcome of pregnancy. *Australia and New Zealand Journal of Obstetrics and Gynecology*, **23**, 15–19.

Hankin, J.R., Sloan, J.J., Firestone, I.J., Ager, J.W., Sokol, R.J. & Martier S.S. (1993). A time series analysis of the impact of the alcohol warning label on antenatal drinking. *Alcoholism: Clinical and Experimental Research*, **17**, 284–9.

Hingson, R., Alpert, J.J., Day, N., Dooling, E., Kayne, H., Morelock, S., Oppenheimer, E. & Zuckerman, B. (1982). Effects of maternal drinking and marijuana use on fetal growth and development. *Pediatrics*, **70**, 539–46.

Iosub, S., Fuchs, M., Bingol, N. & Gromisch, D.S. (1981). Fetal alcohol syndrome revisited. *Pediatrics*, **68**, 475–9.

Jacobson, J.L., Jacobson, S.W., Sokol, R.J., Martier, S.S., Ager, J.W. & Kaplan-Estrin, M.G. (1993). Teratogenic effects of alcohol on infant development. *Alcoholism: Clinical and Experimental Research*, **17**, 174–83.

Job, R.F.S. (1988). Effective and ineffective use of fear in health promotion campaigns. *American Journal of Public Health*, **78**, 163–7.

Johnson, V. (1986). Intervention: missing link in nation's war against drugs. *Observer*, **9**, 1.

Kleinfeld, J. & Westcott, S. (eds.) (1993). *Fantastic Antone Succeeds!* Anchorage: University of Alaska Press.

LaPierre, R.T. (1967). Attitudes versus actions. In *Readings in Attitude Theory and Measurement*, ed. M. Fishbein, pp. 26–31. New York: Wiley.

Larsson, G. (1983). Prevention of fetal alcohol effects: an antenatal program for early detection of pregnancies at risk. *Acta Obstetricia Gynecologica Scandinavica*, **62**, 171–8.

Larsson, G., Bohlin, A.B. & Tunell, R. (1985). Prospective study of children exposed to variable amounts of alcohol *in utero*. *Archives of Disease in Childhood*, **60**, 316–21.

Leckman, A.L., Umland, B.E. & Blay, M. (1984). Prevalence of alcoholism in a family practice center. *Journal of Family Practice*, **18**, 867–70.

Little, R.E. (1977). Moderate alcohol use during pregnancy and decreased infant birth weight. *American Journal of Public Health*, **67**, 1154–6.

Little, R.E., Young, A., Streissguth, A.P. & Uhl, C.N. (1984). Preventing fetal alcohol effects: effectiveness of a demonstration project. In *Mechanisms of Alcohol Damage in Utero*, pp. 254–74. CIBA Foundation Symposium 105. London: Pitman.

Marbury, M.C., Linn, S., Monson, R.R., Schoenbaum, S., Stubblefield, P.G. & Ryan, K.J. (1983). The association of alcohol consumption with outcome of pregnancy. *American Journal of Public Health*, **73**, 1165–8.

Mills, J.L., Graubard, B.I., Harley, E.E., Rhoads, G.G. & Berendes, H.W. (1984). Maternal alcohol consumption and birthweight. *JAMA*, **252**, 1875–9.

Minor, M. & Van Dort, B. (1982). Prevention research on the teratogenic effects of alcohol. *Preventive Medicine*, **11**, 346–59.

Mogielnicki, R.P., Neslin, S., Dulac, J., Balestra, D., Gillie, E. & Corson, J. (1986). Tailored media can enhance the success of smoking cessation clinics. *Journal of Behavioral Medicine*, **9**, 141–61.

Moore, R.D., Bone, L.R., Geller, G., Mamon, J.A., Stokes, E.J. & Levine, D.M. (1989). Prevalence, detection and treatment of alcoholism in hospitalized patients. *JAMA*, **261**, 403–7.

Morse, B.A., Idelson, R.K., Sachs, W.H., Weiner, L. & Kaplan, L.C. (1992). Pediatrician's perspectives on fetal alcohol syndrome. *Journal of Substance Abuse*, **4**, 87–95.

Mulry, J.T., Brewer, M.L. & Spencer, D.L. (1987). The effect of an inpatient chemical dependency rotation on residents' clinical behavior. *Family Medicine*, **19**, 276–80.

Palmer, H.P., Ouellette, E.M., Warner, L. & Leichtman, S.R. (1974). Congenital malformations in offspring of a chronic alcoholic mother. *Pediatrics*, **53**, 490–4.

Pierce, D.R. & West, J.R. (1986). Blood alcohol concentration: a critical factor for producing fetal alcohol effects. *Alcohol*, **3**, 269–72.

Plant, M. (1985). *Women, Drinking, and Pregnancy*. London: Tavistock Publications.

Public Health Service (1981). Surgeon General's advisory on alcohol and pregnancy. *FDA Drug Bulletin*, **11**, 9–10.

Randall, C. (1982). Alcohol as a teratogen in animals. In *Biomedical Processes and Consequences of Alcohol Use*. Alcohol and Health Monograph 2. DHSS, 291-307. Washington, DC: US Government Printing Office.

Richardson, P., Reinhard, G., Rosenthal, A., Hayes, C. & Silver, R. (1987). Review of the research literature on the effects of health warning labels: a report to the United States Congress. Macro Systems, Inc. for NIAAA/ADAMHA.

Rosett, H.L. & Weiner, L. (1984). *Alcohol and the Fetus: A Clinical Perspective*. New York: Oxford University Press.

Rosett, H.L., Weiner, L. & Edelin, K.C. (1981). Strategies for prevention of fetal alcohol effects. *Obstetrics and Gynecology*, **57**, 1–7.

Rossett, H.L., Weiner, L. & Edelin, K.C. (1983a). Treatment experience with pregnant problem drinkers. *JAMA*, **249**, 2092–3033.

Rosett, H.L., Weiner, L., Lee, A., Zuckerman, B., Dooling, E. & Oppenheimer, E. (1983b). Patterns of alcohol consumption and fetal development. *Obstetrics and Gynecology*, **61**, 539–46.

Russell, M., Kang, G.E. & Uhteg, L. (1983). Evaluation of an educational program on the fetal alcohol syndrome for health professionals. *Journal of Alcohol and Drug Education*, **29**, 48–61.

Schwarz, R.J. (1993). Not in my practice (editorial). *Obstetrics and Gynecology*, **82**, 603–4.

Seidenberg, J. & Majewski, F. (1978). Zur Häufigkeit der Alkoholembryopathie in den verschiedenen Phasen der muetterlichen Alkoholkrankheit. (Frequency of alcohol embryopathy in the different phases of maternal alcoholism.) *Hamberg Suchtgrefahren*, **24**, 63–75.

Serdula, M., Williamson, D.F., Kendrick, J.S., Anda, R.F. & Byers, T. (1991). Trends in alcohol consumption by pregnant women: 1985 through 1988. *JAMA*, **265**, 876–9.

Silva, V.A., Laranjeira, R.R., Kolnikoff, M., Grinfeld, H. & Masur, J. (1981). Alcohol consumption during pregnancy and newborn outcome: a study in Brazil. *Neurobehavioral Toxicology and Teratology*, **3**, 169–72.

Smith, I.E., Lancaster, J.S., Moss-Wells, S., Coles, C.D. & Falek, A. (1987). Identifying high-risk pregnant drinkers: biological and behavioral correlates of continuous heavy drinking during pregnancy. *Journal of Studies of Alcohol*, **48**, 304–9.

Sokol, R.J., Miller, S.I. & Reed, G. (1980). Alcohol abuse during pregnancy: an epidemiologic model. *Alcoholism: Clinical and Experimental Research*, **4**, 1135–45.

Streissguth, A.P., Barr, H.M. & Martin, D.C. (1984a). Alcohol exposure *in utero* and functional deficits in children during the first four years of life. In *Mechanisms of Alcohol Damage in Utero*, pp. 176–96. Ciba Foundation Symposium 105. London: Pitman.

Streissguth, A.P., Bookstein, F.L., Sampson, P.D. & Barr, H.M. (1989). Neurobehavioral effects of prenatal alcohol. III. PLS analyses of neuropsychologic tests. *Neurotoxicology and Teratology*, **11**, 493–507.

Streissguth, A.P., Martin, D.C., Barr, H. & Sandam, B.M. (1984b). Intrauterine alcohol and nicotine exposure: attention and reaction time in 4 year old children. *Developmental Psychology*, **20**, 533–41.

Streissguth, A.P., Sampson, P.D., Carmichael Olsen, H., Bookstein, F.L., Barr, H.M., Scott, M., Feldman, J. & Mirsky, A.F. (1994). Maternal drinking during pregnancy: attention and short-term memory in 14-year-old offspring: a longitudinal prospective study. *Alcoholism: Clinical and Experimental Research*, **18**, 202–18.

Tennes, K. & Blackard, C. (1980). Maternal alcohol consumption, birth weight, and minor physical anomalies. *American Journal of Obstetrics and Gynecology*, **138**, 744–80.

Veach, T.L. & Chappel, J.N. (1990). Physician attitudes in chemical dependency: the effects of personal experience and recovery. *Substance Abuse*, **11**, 97–101.

Veghelyi, P.V., Osztovics, M., Kardos, G., Leisztner, L., Szaszovszky, E., Igali, S. & Imrei, J. (1978). The fetal alcohol syndrome: symptoms and pathogenesis. *Acta Paediatrica Academiae Scientiarum Hungaricae*, **19**, 171–89.

Volk, B., Maletz, J., Tiedemann, M., Mall, G., Klein, C. & Berlet, H.H. (1981). Impaired maturation of Purkinje cells in the fetal alcohol syndrome of the rat. *Acta Neuropathologica*, **54**, 19–29.

Wallace, J. (1977). Between Scylla and Charybdis: issues in alcoholism therapy. *Alcohol Health Research World*.

Weinberg, J.R. (1974). Interview techniques for diagnosing alcoholism. *American Family Physician*, **9**, 107–15.

Weiner, L. & Larsson, G. (1987). Clinical prevention of fetal alcohol effects: a reality. *Alcohol Health and Research World*, **11**, 60–3.

Weiner, L., McCarty, D. & Potter, D. (1988). A successful fetal alcohol training program for health care professionals. *Substance Abuse*, **9**, 20–8.

Weiner, L., Morse, B.A. & Garrido, P. (1989). FAS/FAE: focusing prevention on women at risk. *International Journal of the Addictions*, **24**, 385–95.

Weiner, L., Rosett, H.L. & Edelin, K.C. (1982). Behavioral evaluation of fetal alcohol education for physicians. *Alcoholism: Clinical and Experimental Research*, **6**, 230–3.

West, J.R., Goodlett, C.R. & Brandt, J.P. (1990). New approaches to research on the long-term consequences of prenatal exposure to alcohol. *Alcoholism: Clinical and Experimental Research*, **14**, 684–9.

Woodhall, H.E. (1988). Alcoholics remaining anonymous: residents' diagnosis of alcoholism in a family practice center. *Journal of Family Practice*, **26**, 293–6.

15

Social and public health aspects of alcohol abuse in pregnancy

ANNE-MARIE NYBO ANDERSEN AND JØRN OLSEN

Introduction

In most societies fetal alcohol syndrome (FAS) is rare, but being preventable makes it an important health issue. Should alcohol consumption during pregnancy below levels that cause FAS carry an increased risk of functional defects, it would, however, have even more important health implications, because such exposure is common in many countries whereas alcohol abuse is rare in young women.

Women whose intake of alcohol during pregnancy is high comprise a high-risk group that should be targeted for help and support for the sake of their own health and the health of their unborn child. Not only should we try to prevent FAS or other alcohol-related birth defects, but long-term side effects should also be taken into consideration. If the alcohol consumption remains at a high level, it interferes with breast feeding and the ability to take proper care of the child. Children growing up in homes where parents have an alcohol problem often become part of a broken family, they may be neglected or subject to sexual abuse, and sometimes they have to take over some of the parents' daily social responsibilities (National Board of Health, 1992; Bijur *et al.*, 1992). Therefore, preventing prenatal alcohol abuse is not only a social responsibility but is also imperative in families with small children. The damage caused by growing up in an alcohol-abusing family is probably not of lesser consequence than the damage that occurs during fetal development, and it is a far more widespread problem.

When setting up a prevention program, it will be useful to monitor the pattern of alcohol use in pregnancy to identify predictors of a high-level intake and to have empirical data on how different preventive strategies work. Unfortunately, most such data will vary over different cultures and subcultures and over different time periods. Specific information will be needed for specific populations and for different time periods. The lesson to be learnt from published results in the international literature is primarily how to approach the problem and how to identify the most promising methods of evaluation at the local level.

One positive aspect of preventing alcohol abuse in pregnancy is that resources are available in antenatal and perinatal care, because most countries currently invest a great proportion of their preventive medicine budgets in this field. To put more emphasis on the prevention of alcohol damage would, however, require more money or an adjustment of the priorities in the present policy setting. Most countries could make such changes in priorities without negative health effects, considering that several expensive and time-consuming procedures are performed to an extent that has no empirical justification (Huntington & Connell, 1994).

Any preventive program should have long-term goals and specific milestones to achieve at a fixed time schedule. Without such goals, we have no way of knowing if we are on the right track. Setting up realistic goals requires empirical data, not only on the present situation, i.e., baseline measures, but also on the outcome without any preventive interventions.

Alcohol use during pregnancy

A number of surveys on alcohol use during pregnancy have been conducted. In general, these do not provide reliable information on alcohol abuse, as women with a high level of alcohol consumption may be more likely to refuse to take part in the study or to underestimate their alcohol consumption when data are self-reported. Data on alcohol abuse require special and targeted questioning, and this questioning should be conducted in a clinical setting that provides substantial pressure on the woman to take part in the study.

Indirect methods of estimating alcohol use and abuse during pregnancy, based upon total sales data or the distribution of alcohol consumption in general or in the population of women of reproductive age, have not been developed for obvious reasons. Such estimates would most likely be merely particularistic and misleading over longer time periods.

The EUROMAC study (an EU-funded, concerted action on the impact of moderate alcohol consumption during pregnancy) showed that most pregnant women in Europe report some alcohol consumption during pregnancy (EUROMAC, 1992). Less than 10% of the participating women were reportedly abstinent, and in most countries less than 5% of the participating women reported abstinence during early pregnancy. The European countries taking part in this study included The Netherlands, France, Spain, Italy,

Scotland, Denmark, Germany, and Portugal. At the same time, less than 5% reported a consumption of more than 90 g alcohol per week during early pregnancy (slightly more than 1 drink per day), except in France (Roubaix region, 21%) and Portugal (Porto, 11%). This study was, however, not designed to provide data on high intake, and women were consecutively recruited to the study from different antenatal care centers in order to form a representative sample of 'normal' pregnant women.

According to the EUROMAC study, most women report a reduced alcohol consumption in pregnancy. This may be due to an effect on health behavior related to pregnancy, to reporting bias, or to metabolic changes in pregnancy. Most likely, the reduction in alcohol consumption for most women is real, and it is supported by the data from most other studies. However, an Italian study showed that pregnant women were more inclined to stop smoking than to stop drinking during pregnancy; nevertheless 26% of the heavy drinkers (defined as women drinking between meals) stopped drinking during pregnancy (Bonati & Fellin, 1991). A study from the United States also indicated a reduction in alcohol consumption in late pregnancy for all drinking levels compared with consumption prior to pregnancy (Bruce *et al.*, 1993). According to a Norwegian study, even a low consumption of alcohol during pregnancy was reduced by 50% over a 5 year time period. This probably reflects the strength of public opinion against alcohol consumption during pregnancy (Ihlen *et al.*, 1993). Telephone interviews with almost 27 000 women between 18 and 44 years conducted in the United States in 1991 showed that 50% of the subjects reported themselves to be non-drinkers, and 12% reported an alcohol consumption of 2 drinks or more per day. Only 1.3% reported alcohol consumption on one occasion of 5 drinks or more. Alcohol consumption was higher in the northern States (MMWR, 1994), and these results show a lower alcohol consumption in women than is usually found in European studies.

Little is known about trends in heavy drinking during pregnancy. Data from the United States shows that the proportion of women aged 21–34 years who consume 60 drinks or more per month increased from 4% in 1964 to 7% in 1984, and the proportion of binge drinkers (5 drinks or more on at least one occasion per week) in the same age range increased from 3% to 8% over the same time period. At the same time, alcohol use in pregnancy has been reported to have decreased dramatically and, furthermore, alcohol use during pregnancy continues to decrease from the time of conception to the time of confinement (Day *et al.*, 1993).

Few data are available to illustrate whether heavy drinking in pregnancy is an increasing or decreasing problem. In some countries, such as Sweden, alcohol consumption during pregnancy has probably declined, but little is known about the frequency of alcohol abuse.

Previously mentioned studies indicate a rather large variation of alcohol consumption during pregnancy in different countries or regions, and reports indicate secular changes. It is reasonable to believe that these results also reflect changes in a high alcohol consumption during pregnancy. High alcohol consumption in women of childbearing age would also pose a risk of high intake during the early phases of pregnancy, especially in populations using unreliable contraceptive methods, thus leaving little room for pregnancy planning and modification of risk behavior.

Indicators of high-risk behavior

Some pregnant women show clear signs of alcohol abuse, and occasionally they are even intoxicated on arrival at the antenatal care centers. Often women with alcohol problems are concerned about the risk to their babies and some of these ask for help. In most cases, however, the problem is hidden and women in high-risk groups attend the normal antenatal care service late or not at all.

For moderate drinkers who are pregnant, the situation is quite different in many countries. At least in some countries it has been shown that better-educated multipara, and older pregnant women, tend to drink more than younger and less-educated pregnant women (Heller *et al.*, 1988; Olsen, 1989). In the study by Heller *et al.* (1988) an association was found between anxiety, as measured by the GHQ subscale, smoking and coffee drinking, and the amount of alcohol consumed during pregnancy.

Heavy drinking was found to be more common in less privileged groups, among those who were not married, and those who had a history of psychiatric problems. Pregnant women who lived with a partner with a heavy alcohol or drug use were, themselves, also more likely to be heavy users of drugs or alcohol (Bresnahan *et al.*, 1992).

Alcohol use in pregnancy is much more likely to be underreported than alcohol consumption prior to pregnancy. Because alcohol use in pregnancy is closely correlated with alcohol use prior to pregnancy, pre-pregnancy use may be a better way of identifying high-risk groups. Indicators of problem drinking could also be used in screening. Questions about blackouts, friends who worried about the subject's drinking, inability of the subject to stop drinking when they wanted to, experiences of alcohol-related problems in the family, occasional morning drinking, perceived need to reduce consumption, or whether the subject had sought help to solve alcohol problems have all been shown to predict potential alcohol-dependent adverse outcomes of pregnancy, regardless of the actual reported use of alcohol during pregnancy (Russell & Skinner, 1988). Length of the drinking history and alcohol tolerance are strong predictors of alcohol use during pregnancy (Smith *et al.*, 1987).

In many countries, alcohol abuse during pregnancy remains undetected, mainly because no systematic screening is applied (Donovan, 1991). Asking questions about alcohol consumption during pregnancy is difficult for the doctor as well as for the midwife, who tend to see themselves more as the advocate of the woman rather than of the anonymous unborn child. Asking questions about alcohol use in the household or in the pre-pregnancy time period is not quite as sensitive an issue, and this information may provide valuable predictive data. A quick screening test could also be incorporated into either a structured, self-administered questionnaire or interview. The following (so-called CAGE) questions have been proposed: (1) 'Have you ever felt you ought to cut down on your drinking?' (2) 'Have people ever annoyed you by criticizing your drinking?' (3) 'Have you ever felt guilty about your drinking?' (4) 'Have you ever had a drink, an eye opener, in the morning to steady your nerves or to get rid of a hangover?' (Klein *et al.*, 1993; US Preventive Services Task Force, 1989). These four questions may be of use in some situations, but not all. They were found to be unsuitable for use in a busy antenatal clinic in London (Waterson & Murray-Lyon, 1988).

It would be much better to use a valid biomarker, and the development of bio-markers of alcohol use, such as carbohydrate-deficient transferrin, is improving and may in future surveys be applied when appropriate and with informed consent (Jeppson *et al.*, 1993; Kanitz *et al.*, 1994).

Pregnant women do not want to expose their unborn child to any hazards, and this also applies to women with alcohol problems. For many pregnant women with an alcohol problem it will be a relief to discuss the issue and to receive help in reducing the risk for the fetus. If no one asks the pertinent questions, these women are left in a difficult position of having to open the discussion on a topic that is difficult to talk about and is subject to self-denial.

There is, however, no need to screen unless acceptable and effective help can be provided, and there is still a great need for developing forms of social intervention that are appropriate to these demands.

Sociomedical contributions in the prevention of alcohol-related fetal damage

Several strategies are available in preventing alcohol-related reprotoxic effects, including legislation, creating (or trying to influence) social norms concerning drinking in pregnancy, special intervention programs for heavy users, and education for care providers that prepare them to recognise and cope with alcohol-abusing pregnant women.

A program would need a basic philosophy about who should be given the benefit of the doubt. We still have limited information on the potential consequences of low to moderate alcohol consumption during pregnancy (such as 1 drink or less per day). In fact, the empirical data point towards no effect of such use. Still, many clinicians would advocate no alcohol use during pregnancy due to moral considerations or as a safety factor for a substance that is a known teratogen when consumed in large doses. On the other hand, it should be taken into consideration that many researchers have looked for all kinds of effects of a low to moderate alcohol consumption in pregnancy without reporting any significant findings. Women who consume low to moderate levels of alcohol during pregnancy and subsequently give birth to a child who is born either prematurely or with malformations or growth retardation need not feel guilty about their alcohol consumption. No data point towards low or moderate alcohol consumption during pregnancy as a potential cause of birth or developmental defects.

A public preventive program could be based on legal procedures such as labelling alcohol products according to their reprotoxic effects, or it could aim at changing behavior concerning alcohol use during pregnancy. Behavior-modifying programs could focus on high-risk groups or on the population of pregnant women in general. It is interesting that informal, social norms for not drinking during pregnancy are present and effective in some countries that have a tradition of frequent alcohol use.

A program directed towards a reduction in alcohol consumption during pregnancy among all non-abstinent women has to be justified on moral rather than scientific grounds unless a shift in the general distribution of alcohol consumption is the only way of reducing high-level consumption.

It is possible that a high total consumption of alcohol during pregnancy is correlated with a high consumption of alcohol in doses that cause concern. It is also reasonable to assume that a general reduction in consumption also involves a reduction of the right-hand tail of the alcohol distribution in the population. Data from Sweden indicate the existence of such an effect

(Olegård, 1992; Larsson, 1992). The mechanism probably operates by strengthening the social norm of abstaining from alcohol during pregnancy, but as a side effect it is likely to become even more difficult to approach the problem drinker, because stigmatization is a likely outcome of such a mass strategy in prevention.

The labelling of alcohol products follows a procedure that is based on well-documented animal and human studies and serves to warn against reprotoxic substances in the consumer products sold in most European countries. Since 1989, all alcohol beverage containers for sale in the United States must have the following warning label: 'Government warning: (1) According to the Surgeon General, women should not drink alcohol beverages during pregnancy because of the risk of birth defects. (2) Consumption of alcohol beverages impairs your ability to drive a car or operate machinery, and may cause health problems.' Labelling of this type may be justified because it is an easy way of fulfilling the obligations of public authorities to warn against a hazardous substance. The United States labelling procedure, however, goes beyond the empirical evidence and takes a moral standpoint by warning against the use of any alcohol during pregnancy. It is, furthermore, questionable whether labelling has any preventive effect in high-risk situations, and it would be stigmatizing even to pregnant women with low levels of alcohol consumption during pregnancy. The advantage of labelling alcohol beverages is, however, that the message more often reaches heavy consumers than others, and a study from the United States *did* indicate this, albeit without showing any effect on risk behavior (Kaskutas & Greenfield, 1992).

Mass strategic alcohol reduction programs aimed at the general population of pregnant women have been tried in several countries, and most countries offer some information on the potential health hazard to the pregnant woman of drinking during pregnancy. In Denmark, a large group of pregnant women were subject to a general intervention program called 'Healthy Habits for Two' which had the philosophy of improving lifestyle in general during pregnancy. This involved reducing alcohol consumption, reducing or stopping smoking, and improving dietary habits. In spite of good public acceptance of the program and increased knowledge, no change in behavior was recorded over time in comparison with a control area and in comparison with the intervention time period (Olsen *et al.*, 1989). Contrary to this, an intervention in a much smaller group of pregnant women in Norway resulted in a substantial reduction in alcohol use during pregnancy in the intervention group, as well as in the control group (Meberg *et al.*, 1986).

Most comprehensive and focused prevention programs combine mass strategic means of public education and identification of high-risk women who need special care (Waterson & Murray-Lyon, 1989). Some pregnant women with heavy alcohol consumption will be capable of reducing alcohol intake when they are informed about the risk. The majority of heavy drinkers, however, are unlikely to reduce abuse unless extensive measures are taken to help the women achieve profound changes in their general social situation. Depending on local socioeconomic and cultural conditions, an optimum efficiency in controlling alcohol abuse may be reached through diverse measures such as housing programs and education. In most societies this presupposes an improvement of the present collaboration between the social and the health care systems.

The most vulnerable women with the highest risk are not likely to ask for help unless help is offered on their terms and when they feel they need it. Open facilities such as a 24 hour telephone service, activity centers, women's houses, self-help organizations, or open clinics may be useful and could be justified in areas with a high concentration of women at risk due to, for example, prenatal drug and alcohol abuse or substance abuse by their partners.

It has been said that the heaviest abusing women refuse the offers of help, but in a Swedish study it was found that half the women who consumed more than 125 g absolute alcohol per day during the month prior to the first visit to the maternal health clinics were deeply concerned about the harm they might have caused their fetus (Larsson, 1983).

Screening in antenatal care is often needed and alcohol consumption in pregnancy should always be discussed early in pregnancy as part of the normal visit. In countries with a high proportion of binge drinkers, such as in the population of the northern part of Europe, among Native American Indians and the Innuits, this problem should be discussed in order to avoid binge drinking throughout pregnancy. The most vulnerable time period for brain development is from gestational week 5 to 13, but the brain develops throughout pregnancy, and binge drinking should also be avoided during the period of breast feeding. Most of the suggested alcohol prenatal programs in pregnancy have mentioned some of these elements (Little *et al.*, 1980; Masis & May, 1991; Huntimer, 1987; Stephens, 1987; May & Hymbaugh, 1989; Weiner *et al.*, 1989; Smith & Coles, 1991; Ottenblad, 1992).

Evaluation

Most of the prenatal alcohol intervention studies have not been properly evaluated (Schorling, 1993). In spite of the fact that most people would agree to give prevention of alcohol-related birth defects high priority, we usually do not know if our activities actually work.

Unfortunately, we have very limited knowledge about the impact that the different intervention programs have in reducing alcohol-induced fetal defects, partly because very large studies are needed to demonstrate this. Nor do we have good process evaluation in well-controlled studies. One aim of the intervention program must be to make sure that pregnant women are aware of the potential health consequences of high alcohol consumption early enough in the pregnancy. In many countries, several visits to health professionals take place from early pregnancy to months or years after delivery. The facilities are thus available and the problem is well described, but better-controlled studies are needed before we will be able to formulate health prevention programs on scientific grounds.

Schorling (1993) has listed guidelines for such studies that include: (1) comparison of the intervention group with an adequate control group, (2) adequate description of the study cohort, (3) adequate determination of alcohol use, (4) adequate determinants of changes in behavior, (5) adequate follow-up of study participants, (6) adequate sample size, (7) adequate documentation on how the cohort was assembled, and (8) adequate description of the cohort. He was able to identify only five studies that to some extent met these criteria. All these studies showed some reduction in alcohol consumption during the intervention, even among heavy users.

This list should not be understood as the authors' 'gold standard' for the evaluation of such studies. Especially in social development projects, it is extremely difficult to select adequate and comparable control groups, apart from the fact that the procedure followed in such studies raises some ethical considerations.

Society has an obligation to protect its weakest members, and alcohol-related birth defects have serious consequences for the child, the parents, and for society. In the United States it has been estimated that the annual cost to society of problems related to alcohol consumption during pregnancy is about $250 million, and more than half of this is due to alcohol-induced mental retardation (Abel & Sokol, 1991).

Closing remarks

Warnings against drinking appear in the Bible, and most women are probably aware that heavy drinking should be avoided during pregnancy. FAS was, however, not described before 1968 in France nor before 1973 in the United States. Only a few pregnant women are familiar with the syndrome and not even health professionals in antenatal care have any detailed understanding of fetal-alcohol-related hazards. In most countries, only a few clinicians are able to diagnose an FAS child, not to mention less obvious alcohol related defects. Professional training should, therefore, be part of the program.

Health education often widens the social gap in the occurrence of disease, because the best-educated are the first to respond. The challenge lies in reaching high-risk women for whom an alcohol problem is only one of many problems that need to be addressed. If the alcohol problem is solved for these groups, benefits could be high, not only for the unborn child but also for the women themselves and for society. Prevention should be continued after pregnancy, because even a healthy newborn may be socially or psychologically handicapped by growing up in a family that abuses alcohol or other drugs.

Acknowledgment

Support was given by the Danish Medical Research Council j.nr.12-1663-1.

References

Abel, E.L. & Sokol, P.J. (1991). A revised estimate of the economic impact of fetal alcohol syndrome. *Recent Developments in Alcoholism*, **9**, 117–25.

Bijur, P.E., *et al.* (1992). Parental alcohol use, problem drinking, and children's injuries. *JAMA*, **267**, 3166–71.

Bonati, M. & Fellin, G. (1991). Changes in smoking and drinking behavior before and during pregnancy in Italian mothers: implications for public health intervention. *International Journal of Epidemiology*, **20**, 927–32.

Bresnahan, K., Zuckerman, B. & Cabral, H. (1992). Psychosocial correlates of drug and heavy alcohol use among pregnant women at risk for drug use. *Obstetrics and Gynecology*, **80**, 976–80.

Bruce, F.C., Adams, M.M. & Shulman, H.B. (1993). Alcohol use before and during pregnancy. *American Journal of Preventive Medicine*, **9**, 267–73.

Day, N.L., Cottreau, C.M. & Richardson, G.A. (1993). The epidemiology of alcohol, marijuana and cocaine use among women of childbearing age and pregnant women. *Clinical Obstetrics and Gynecology*, **36**, 232–45.

Donovan, C.L. (1991). Factors predisposing, enabling and reinforcing routine screening of patients for preventing fetal alcohol syndrome: a survey of New Jersey physicians. *Journal of Drug Education*, **21**, 35–42.

EUROMAC (1992). A European Concerted Action: maternal alcohol consumption and its relation to the outcome of pregnancy and child development at 18 months. *International Journal of Epidemiology*, **21**, Supplement 1.

Heller, J. *et al.* (1988). Alcohol in pregnancy: patterns and associations with socio-economic, psychological and behavioral factors. *British Journal of Addiction*, **83**, 541–51.

Huntimer, C.M. (1987). The utilization of antenatal care in the prevention and intervention of the consequences of parental alcohol use. *South Dakota Journal of Medicine*, **40**, 25–30.

Huntington, J. & Connell, F.A. (1994). For every dollar spent: the cost-savings argument for prenatal care. *New England Journal of Medicine*, **331**, 1303–7.

Ihlen, B.M., Amundsen, A. & Trønnes, L. (1993). Reduced alcohol use in pregnancy and changed attitudes in the population. *Addiction*, **88**, 389–94.

Jeppsson, J.O., Kristensson, H. & Fimiani, C. (1993). Carbohydrate deficient transferrin quantified by HPLC to determine heavy consumption of alcohol. *Clinical Chemistry*, **39**, 2115–20.

Kanitz, R.D., *et al.* (1994). New state markers for alcoholism: comparison of carbohydrate deficient transferrin and alcohol mediated (triantennary) transferrin. *Progress in Neuro-psycopharmacology and Biological Psychiatry*, **18**, 431–46.

Kaskutas, L. & Greenfield, T.K. (1992). First effects of warning labels on alcoholic beverage containers. *Drug and Alcohol Dependence*, **31**, 1–14.

Klein, R.F., Friedmann-Campbell, M. & Tocco, R.V. (1993). History taking and substance abuse counselling with the pregnant patient. *Clinical Obstetrics and Gynecology*, **36**, 338–46.

Larsson, G. (1983). Prevention of fetal alcohol effects: an antenatal program for early detection of pregnancies at risk. *Acta Obstetricia et Gynecologica Scandinavica*, **62**, 171–8.

Larsson, G. (1992). Diagnostic and preventive possibilities of excessive drinking in antenatal care. *International Journal of Technologic Assessment in Health Care*, **8**, 106–11.

Little, R.E., Streissguth, A.P. & Guzinski, G.M. (1980). Prevention of fetal alcohol syndrome: a model program. *Alcoholism: Clinical and Experimental Research*, **4**, 185–9.

Masis, K.B. & May, P.A. (1991). A comprehensive local program for the prevention of fetal alcohol syndrome. *Public Health Reports*, **106**, 484–9.

May, P.A. & Hymbaugh, K.J. (1989). A macro-level fetal alcohol syndrome prevention program for native Americans and Alaska natives: description and evaluation. *Journal of Studies of Alcohol*, **50**, 508–18.

Meberg, A. *et al.* (1986). Moderate alcohol consumption: need for intervention programs in pregnancy? *Acta Obstetricia et Gynecologica Scandinavica*, **65**, 861–4.

MMWR (1994). Frequent alcohol consumption among women of the childbearing age. *Morbidity and Mortality Weekly Report*, **43**, 328–9.

National Board of Health (1992). *Children in Families with Alcohol and Drug Problems*. (In Danish.) Copenhagen.

Olegård, R. (1992). Alcohol and narcotics: epidemiology and pregnancy risks. *International Journal of Technological Assessment in Health Care*, **8**, 101–5.

Olsen, J. *et al.* (1989). Changing smoking, drinking and eating behavior among pregnant women in Denmark. *Scandinavian Journal of Social Medicine*, **17**, 277–80.

Ottenblad, C. (1992). Support to pregnant women with drug abuse. (In Swedish.) *Nordisk Medicin*, **107**, 181–94.

Russell, M. & Skinner, J.B. (1988). Early measures of maternal alcohol misuse as predictors of adverse pregnancy outcomes. *Alcoholism: Clinical and Experimental Research*, **12**, 824–30.

Schorling, J.B. (1993). The prevention of prenatal alcohol use: a critical analysis of intervention studies. *Journal of Studies of Alcohol*, **54**, 261–7.

Smith, I.E. & Coles, C.D. (1991). Multilevel intervention for prevention of fetal alcohol syndrome and effects of prenatal alcohol exposure. *Recent Developments in Alcoholism*, **9**, 165–80.

Smith, I.E., *et al.* (1987). Identifying high-risk pregnant drinkers: biological and behavioral correlates of continuous heavy drinking during pregnancy. *Journal of Studies on Alcohol*, **48**, 304–9.

Stephens, C.J. (1987). The effect of social support on alcohol consumption during pregnancy: situational and ethnic/cultural considerations. *International Journal of Addiction*, **22**, 609–19.

US Preventive Services Task Force (1989). Screening for alcohol and other drug abuse. *American Family Physician*, **40**, 137–46.

Waterson, E.J. & Murray-Lyon, I.M. (1988). Asking about alcohol: a comparison of three methods used in an antenatal clinic. *Journal of Obstetrics and Gynecology*, **8**, 303–6.

Waterson, E.J. & Murray-Lyon, I.M. (1989). Screening for alcohol related problems in the antenatal clinic: an assessment of different methods. *Alcohol and Alcoholism*, **24**, 21–30.

Weiner, L., Morse, B.A. & Garrido, P. (1989). FAS/FAE: focusing prevention on women at risk. *International Journal of Addiction*, **24**, 385–95.

Index

Index